Textbook of Veterinary Sur

For Elsevier:

Commissioning Editor: Mary Seager
Development Editor: Rebecca Nelemans
Project Manager: Frances Affleck
Designer: Andy Chapman
Illustrator: Debbie Maizels
Illustration Manager: Bruce Hogarth

Textbook of Veterinary Surgical Nursing

Edited by

Carole Martin DipAVN(Surg) VN
Head Nurse, Clifton Villa Veterinary Surgery, Cornwall, UK.
Royal College of Veterinary Surgeons Veterinary Nursing Examiner.
Past President, British Veterinary Nursing Association.

Jo Masters Cert Ed VN
Practice Supervisor, Langport Veterinary Centre, Somerset, UK.
Royal College of Veterinary Surgeons Veterinary Nursing Examiner.
Past Honorary Secretary, British Veterinary Nursing Association.
Animal Nursing Assistant Head Examiner.

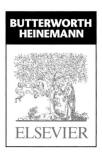

BUTTERWORTH
HEINEMANN

ELSEVIER

EDINBURGH LONDON NEW YORK OXFORD PHILADELPHIA ST LOUIS SYDNEY TORONTO 2007

BUTTERWORTH
HEINEMANN
ELSEVIER

First published 2007

ISBN 10: 0 7506 8813 0
ISBN 13: 978 0 7506 8813 0

British Library Cataloguing in Publication Data
A catalogue record for this book is available from the British Library

Library of Congress Cataloging in Publication Data
A catalog record for this book is available from the Library of Congress

Notice
Knowledge and best practice in this field are constantly changing. As new research and experience broaden our knowledge, changes in practice, treatment and drug therapy may become necessary or appropriate. Readers are advised to check the most current information provided (i) on procedures featured or (ii) by the manufacturer of each product to be administered, to verify the recommended dose or formula, the method and duration of administration, and contraindications. It is the responsibility of the practitioner, relying on their own experience and knowledge of the patient, to make diagnoses, to determine dosages and the best treatment for each individual patient, and to take all appropriate safety precautions.

To the fullest extent of the law, neither the publisher nor the author assumes any liability for any injury and/or damage.

The Publisher

Printed in China

Contents

Contributors

Nicholas J Bacon MA VetMB CertVR CertSAS DipECVS MRCVS
Surgical Oncology Fellow, Animal Cancer Center, Colorado State University, Fort Collins, Colorado, USA.

Stephen J Baines MA VetMB PhD CertVR CertSAS DipECVS MRCVS
RCVS Specialist in Small Animal Surgery European Specialist in Small Animal Surgery Lecturer in Small Animal Surgery Queen Mother Hospital, Royal Veterinary College, Hawkshead Lane, North Mimms, Hertfordshire, UK.

Alison Beck BVSc (Hons) CertSAS DipECVS MRCVS
Lecturer in Small Animal Surgery, Royal Veterinary College, Hertfordshire, UK. Queen Mother Hospital, Royal Vetinary College, Hawkshead Lane, North Mimms, Hertfordshire, UK.

Joanne Ewart DipAVN (Surg) VN
Veterinary Nurse, Davies Veterinary Specialists, Hertfordshire, UK.

Arthur House BVMS BVSc CertSAS DipECVS MRCVS
Veterinary Surgeon, Royal Veterinary College, Hertfordshire, UK. Queen Mother Hospital, Royal Vetinary College, Hawkshead Lane, North Mimms, Hertfordshire, UK.

Lucy Goddard DipAVN(Surg) VN
Veterinary Nurse, Davies Veterinary Specialists, Hertfordshire, UK.

Carole Martin DipAVN(Surg) VN
Head Nurse, Clifton Villa Veterinary Surgery, Cornwall, UK. Royal College of Veterinary Surgeons Veterinary Nursing Examiner. Past President, British Veterinary Nursing Association.

Jo Masters Cert Ed VN
Practice Supervisor, Langport Veterinary Centre, Somerset, UK. Royal College of Veterinary Surgeons Veterinary Nursing Examiner. Past Honorary Secretary British Veterinary Nursing Association. Animal Nursing Assistant Head Examiner.

Sue Mothersdale Dip AVN(Surg) VN
Veterinary Nurse, private practice, Buckinghamshire, UK.

Amanda Rock BVSc MRCVS
Lecturer in Veterinary Nursing, Rosewarne College, Cornwall, UK. Veterinary Surgeon, The Veterinary Hospital, Plymouth, UK.

Deborah Smeeton DipAVN (Surg) VN
Veterinary Nurse, Davies Veterinary Specialists, Hertfordshire, UK.

Anne Ward BSc DipAVN(Surg) VN
Lecturer in Veterinary Nursing, College of Animal Welfare, Edinburgh, UK.

Sandra Whiting BSc(Hons) Dip AVN (Surg) VN
Lecturer in Veterinary Nursing, College of Animal Welfare, Hertfordshire, UK.

Foreword

The surgical nurse plays a primary role in patient care, both directly and indirectly. This care is influenced by the individual's knowledge, skill and experience and affects not only the outcome of the surgery when fulfilling the role as a theatre nurse, surgical assistant or when monitoring and maintaining anaesthesia, but importantly during the pre-operative and recovery stages.

Owners often rely on the practice's VNs to provide them with accurate information and advice, to prepare for the procedure ahead and enable informed consent. This crucial communication roll continues throughout the patient's hospitalisation and importantly during discharge. The provision of a high standard of care to the owner, patient and the veterinary team following a surgical procedure cannot be overemphasised. Surgical nurses are well equipped to provide this.

Behind the scenes Veterinary Surgeons will often rely on their VNs to take charge of the patients' care. Their knowledge and skill come into play when, for example, the daily surgical list is organised and the patients are prepared for theatre. Theatre practice remains a primary role for the surgical nurse where the organisation of the equipment, materials and instrumentation required influences the smooth running of each procedure and can avert unnecessary delays for the patient and the surgeon.

Newly qualified VNs want to study surgical nursing, anaesthesia and radiography more than any other subjects, according to a recent CPD survey, (undertaken in 2005 by the RCVS VN Council and the BVNA in 2005). A high proportion of VNs also felt that reading professional journals and textbooks should be an accepted format of recordable CPD when considering a CPD framework as part of the approaching non-statutory regulation for VNs. Both points reflect the relevance of this textbook and at a time when there are further advances in veterinary medicine, necessitating the need for highly skilled veterinary nurses in this field. Many more practices, hospitals and referral centres are increasing the standard of patient care and expanding their provision; veterinary nursing will form part of this progression.

Looking into the future VNs are likely to take on more responsibilities in light of this and, following the changes made to the traditional and highly respected Diplomas in Advanced Veterinary Nursing, it is hoped that this will assist with the progression of our profession by making advanced nurse training accessible to all and a wider range of modules to develop in all disciplines. Surgical nursing will continue to be a largely studied area and will always be a role for most VNs throughout their career. For these reasons and many more this textbook is clearly extremely valuable for VNs.

Carole Martin and Jo Masters are both highly experienced and respected veterinary nurses and as such have produced a concise textbook enabling students, VNs and those holding or studying for the Diploma in Advance Veterinary Nursing (surgical) to experience and revise all aspects of surgical nursing, from asepsis to advanced surgical procedures. As the main veterinary nursing textbook in this area it amiably fulfils the title of the *Textbook of Veterinary Surgical Nursing.*

Dot Creighton VN DipAVN(surgical) MBVNA
BVNA Past President and Honorary Member
RCVS VN Council Vice Chairman

Preface

Surgical nursing is a discipline carried out by all veterinary nursing staff; whether in referral or general practice; and the development of good quality surgical care is often the remit of the VN in practice.

The popularity of the Diploma in Advanced Veterinary Nursing (Surgical) Dip AVN (Surg); shows that veterinary nursing staff have a genuine desire to increase their surgical nursing skills and knowledge; all practices can benefit from this motivation which undoubtedly improves patient care and practice success.

The aim of this book is to be a complete reference to veterinary surgical nursing care. Whilst it covers all surgical areas of the Royal College of Veterinary Surgeons (RCVS) Veterinary Nursing Syllabus and gives full coverage of the syllabus for the Dip AVN (Surg) it is also aimed at nurses and technicians who have a vested interest in improving the surgical care of their patients.

The contributors have been chosen for their expertise in the surgical field and we would like to thank them for their time and knowledge in supporting the veterinary nursing profession and its development.

This book has taken some time to get to publication due to our aim of getting the best people to contribute to the project. We hope that any reader will agree that it was worth the wait!

Carole Martin
Jo Masters
Truro & Langport 2006

Chapter **1**

Surgical conditions and intraoperative management

Amanda Rock

ANATOMY

Cutaneous system

Skin structure

The integument is a large body organ composed of an outer stratified epithelium (epidermis) and an underlying fibrous dermis (corium). The thickness of the epidermis varies, being thicker in the hairless areas such as the nose and digital pads. The dermis is composed of elastic fibres and collagen suspended in a mix of hyaluronic acid and chondroitin sulphuric acid. It contains the cutaneous circulation, nerves, hair follicles and glands and several cells can be found scattered through it including macrophages, mast cells and plasma cells.

Elasticity

Wound closure depends on the elasticity of skin, which is determined by the tightness of the collagen bundles and the numbers of elastic fibres present. Pliable skin, such as that in the axilla, flank and dorsum of the neck, has many elastic fibres and loosely packed collagen and so is often used in skin grafts. Conversely the skin in the tail, ear and digital pads does not stretch so well.

Thickness

This is related to the species, sex and body area with the thickest skin being found in the head, dorsum of the neck, back and sacrum. The ventral surface has much thinner skin, as do the underside of the pinnae and the medial surface of the limbs.

Hair follicles

These are found in the dermis and extend into the subcutaneous tissues. In dogs and cats an apocrine sweat gland is associated with each follicle. Some cats such as the Siamese have temperature dependent coat colour. This is due to an enzyme that converts melanin precursors to melanin at low temperatures. This has the implication that the coat grows back a darker colour in scar tissue and clipped areas and should be considered when planning surgery. The average coat takes over four months to grow back after clipping with growth being fastest during the winter months (0.4mm/day).

Sweat glands

There are sweat glands in the hairy skin of the dog and cat but they do not play a major role in thermoregulation, unlike the footpads – which contain most of the glands. A few apocrine glands have specialised functions such as the ceruminous glands of the ear, the anal sacs and the mammary glands.

Hypodermis

This is the layer known as the subcutis and is found beneath the dermis. It is composed of fat, collagen and elastic fibres and needs to be considered when elevating the skin for grafts. The panniculus muscle is included in this layer. The cutaneous trunci is the large muscle extending from the gluteals to the pectorals (but not over the limbs) that is responsible for making the skin shiver in response to stimuli and the cold. It is in this layer that the blood supply to the skin terminates. In dogs and cats direct cutaneous arteries supply the skin and run parallel to the skin surface. This is unlike humans where the blood vessels run through muscles first and then run perpendicular to the skin. Figure 1.1 shows the superficial arteries of the canine trunk that may be of use during skin grafting.

Healing

If only the epidermis and part of the dermis is damaged, the wound heals by adnexal re-epithelialisation. This means the hair follicles and sweat glands can utilise their epithelial components and serve as a source of epithelial cells for the damaged skin above. This is

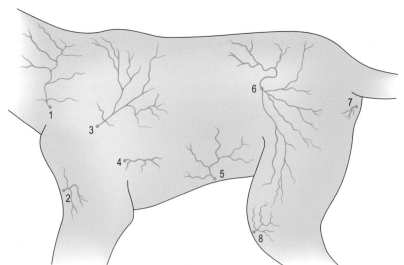

1 Superficial cervical branch of omocervical

2 Proximal collateral radial

3 Cutaneous branch of thoracodorsal

4 Lateral thoracic

5 Cranial superficial epigastric

6 Deep circumflex iliac

7 Perineal

8 Medial genicular

Figure 1.1   Superficial arteries of the canine trunk.

possible because of a shared ectodermal origin. Full-thickness wounds heal by wound contracture and epithelialisation from the boundaries of the wound.

Respiratory system

Nose
The thick keratinised epithelium that makes up the nasal planum is moistened by the remote nasolacrimal duct that opens up on the floor of the nasal vestibule just inside the nostril. Non-pigmented noses are prone to photosensitivity and melanomas. The nostrils (nares) can be stenotic in some breeds and are part of the brachycephalic airway obstruction syndrome (BAOS), a condition common in dyspnoeic British Bulldogs. The groove in the midline of the nose is called the philtrum and is continuous with the upper lip. Cat and dog nasal cavities differ, the dog having a membranous section to its nasal septum allowing it to push the tip of its nose upwards. The rest of the septum is cartilage with a bony outside which can be seen on dorsoventral radiographs of the nose. The nasal chambers are filled with scrolls of bone or cartilage called conchae or ethmoturbinates. These are lined with vascular and glandular mucous membrane.

Upper respiratory tract
The soft palate separates the nasopharynx from the oropharynx and is overlong in BAOS. Care must be taken when resecting it to prevent nasal aspiration of food. The two laryngeal valves, the glottis and epiglottis, deflect the air flow to aid olfaction and vocalisation. Figure 1.2 shows the intraoral view of the laryngeal cartilages. Surgery of the larynx is made more difficult due to the growth of fibrous strands postop. These can seriously compromise the airflow – plastic stents are sometimes inserted into the airway temporarily to prevent this occurrence. The dorsal cricoarytenoid is the only muscle that abducts the arytenoids and when the recurrent laryngeal degenerates, stridor results from a failure of the larynx to open up during inhalation. The blood supply to the area is via the external carotid through the cranial laryngeal artery. The external maxillary vein drains the blood and the lymph passes through the medial retropharyngeal lymph node. The larynx is supplied by two pairs of vagal nerves. The recurrent laryngeal nerves are given off inside the chest and run up the dorsolateral trachea until they reach the larynx where they change their names to the caudal laryngeal nerves.

Lower respiratory tract
The flexibility of the trachea comes from the alternating rings of cartilage and elastic annular ligaments. The cartilages are C-shaped with the ventral part thickest and the dorsal part bridged by smooth muscle which can contract to narrow the airway to reduce dead space and aid in the expulsion of mucus during coughing. Brachycephalics have narrow tracheas whereas Dachshunds and Basset hounds have relatively wide ones. The oesophagus passes dorsal to the trachea and the sternothyroid, sternohyoid and sternocephalic muscles lie ventral to it. The blood supply comes from the cranial and caudal thyroid

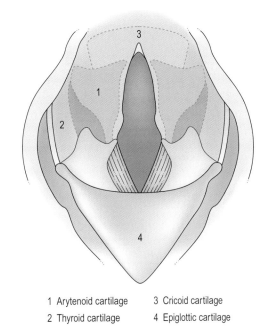

| 1 Arytenoid cartilage | 3 Cricoid cartilage |
| 2 Thyroid cartilage | 4 Epiglottic cartilage |

Figure 1.2 Intra oral view of the laryngeal cartilages.

arteries until the carina is reached where the broncho-oesophageal arteries take over. Surgical intervention to the bronchi often interrupts this blood supply leading to poor perfusion to the bronchi distal to the incision and subsequent poor healing.

Lungs and associated structures

The fissures that divide the lungs into lobes allow for movement when the spine flexes and the diaphragm moves. Both lungs have cranial and caudal lobes and the slightly larger right lung has a middle and an accessory lobe. The air within them gives great radiographic contrast so that the surrounding vessels and any tumours in the uppermost air-filled lung can be seen. The pulmonary vessels are under low pressure and due to the lack of arterio-venous anastomoses, all the blood flows through the lung capillaries. This means that any tumour cells, microthrombi and bacteria are filtered out in the lungs making them a common place for thromboemboli, infections and metastase. The pleura surrounding the lungs is thin and the mediastinal pleura, which separates the two sides of the thorax, often ruptures, meaning fluid and air from one side can enter the other pleural sac.

Alimentary system

Oral cavity

The muscles of the lips and cheeks are difficult to distinguish from one another. The trigeminal nerve supplies the sensory input and the motor output is via the facial nerve. The two sublingual veins are useful sites of venous access in anaesthetised patients and the whole tongue is highly vascular, aiding thermoregulation. The palate is especially important in neonates where the partition between the respiratory and digestive tract allows suckling to take place successfully. The caudal part of the soft palate is a free curved edge which has the epiglottis resting above it. The palate is often overlong in brachiocephalics and is also often thickened due to the permanent contracture of the muscle in the soft palate to try and keep the airway open.

Most of the lymphatic tissue is diffuse but there are some discrete encapsulated tonsils, as shown in Figure 1.3. Tonsils do not have afferent lymphatics but there are efferent lymphatics which drain to the retropharyngeal lymph nodes. The pharynx can dilate easily as it is surrounded by loose elastic tissue, but there are several important structures running through the area including the vagal nerve (which is important to the swallowing mechanism), the glossopharyngeal and hypoglossal nerves and some sympathetic nerves. In addition care must be taken during surgery to avoid the common carotid arteries and the mandibular and parotid salivary glands. The major salivary glands of the dog and cat are shown in Figure 1.4. The larger glands that are further away from the mouth produce the saliva needed to lubricate food where the smaller, nearer glands keep the local mucous membranes moist. During surgery of the parotid duct care must be taken to identify the maxillary artery and the facial nerve, which can be distinguished from the parotid duct by cannulation of the duct with stiff suture material. Salivary mucoceles occasionally form when there is damage to the duct of the

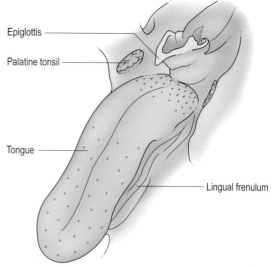

Figure 1.3   Palatine tonsils of the dog.

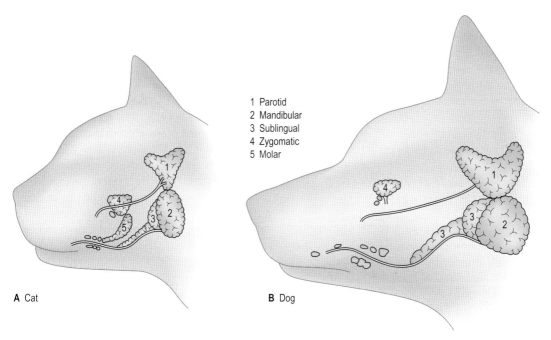

1 Parotid
2 Mandibular
3 Sublingual
4 Zygomatic
5 Molar

A Cat

B Dog

Figure 1.4   The salivary glands of the cat and dog.

sublingual gland due to leakage of saliva into the tissues.

Oesophagus
Due to difficult access and a segmental blood supply, the oesophagus is often feared surgically. The cranial portion receives blood from the thyroid arteries and can be accessed via a ventral midline approach. The thoracic section has poorer blood supply, coming from the broncho-oesophageal arteries and requires a right sided, fourth intercostal space thoracotomy for access. The terminal part receives blood from the gastric arteries and can be approached by a left sided tenth interspace thoracotomy. Hypomotility and poor wound healing result from damage to the blood supply so care must be taken during dissection in the area.

When closing incisions a two-layer approach is required and tension must be avoided to prevent dehiscence and stricture formation. The first layer comprises the mucosa and submucosa and the outer layer is placed through the muscle and the loose adventitia.

Stomach and small intestine
A cross-section of the stomach or intestines will reveal four layers – the serosa, the muscularis externa, the submucosa and the mucosa. Healing is relatively fast due to the good blood supply and capacity of the epithelium to regenerate despite the constant exposure to food, enzymes and bacteria. Initial healing involves a fibrin clot that helps to minimise leakage. By day three the epithelial cells have migrated across and by day 14 the collagen deposition means the wound nearly has full strength. The first 72–96 hours are when wound breakdown is most likely and so there is little logic in withholding food immediately after gut surgery as initially there is superior wound strength.

The submucosa carries the blood vessels and must be aligned when repairing the intestines so direct apposition of wound edges is preferred rather than inverting suture patterns. A two-layer closure is required in the stomach whereas in the intestines a one-layer closure is adequate. The suture holding layer with all the strength is the submucosa due to its collagen content and so sutures must pass through this layer. The fundus (Latin for bottom) of the stomach presses against the left part of the diaphragm.

Colon

Surgery of the large intestine has a higher potential risk due to a poorer blood supply and the fact that in initial healing stages collagen lysis exceeds collagen production.

The pancreas

The pancreatic blood supply is shown in Figure 1.5. The organ is found medial to the descending duodenum and has ducts that empty into the duodenum a few centimetres from the pylorus along with the main bile duct.

The liver

Sandwiched between the diaphragm and the stomach is the loosely fixed liver. The caudal vena cava runs through the middle of the liver which is comprised of seven main lobes. The falciform ligament attaches the liver to the ventral body wall and the lesser omentum courses over the surface of the liver carrying the bile duct, hepatic artery, the portal vein and some lymphatics and nerves. Several hepatic ducts join with the duct from the gallbladder to form the common bile duct which runs

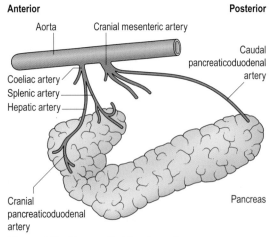

Figure 1.5   Pancreatic blood supply.

through the wall of the duodenum for a couple of centimetres before opening into its lumen.

The liver is highly vascular, about 15% of its volume being made up of blood filled spaces. The flow to the liver of about 35ml/min/kg comes from both the hepatic arterial and the portal venous supply. The portal vein runs from the gastrointestinal tract through the epiploic foramen into the liver, where it breaks up into seven major vessels supplying the principle lobes. Only in the foetus should the portal and systemic systems be in communication and the correction of portosystemic shunts of a congenital origin is an occasional reason for liver surgery.

Cardiovascular system

Approach

The anatomy of the thorax is best seen through either a lateral thoracotomy or a median sternotomy. A lateral approach through the fourth rib space allows access to the heart, the right ventricular outflow tract, main pulmonary artery and patent ductus arteriosus. It is important to incise through the centre of the intercostal space to avoid the vein, artery and nerve lying caudal to the rib. Muscles incised through include the latissimus dorsi under the skin, the scalenus and external abdominal oblique if performing a caudal thoracotomy and the serratus ventralis when performing a cranial procedure.

Vessels

The venous return to the heart is via the cranial and caudal vena cava, found to the right of the mediastinum, and the azygos vein which drains the dorsal intercostal veins and enters the cranial vena cava as it enters the right atrium.

The pulmonary trunk is in close contact with the aorta necessitating careful dissection to separate the two structures. The ligamentum arteriosum connects the two just before the bifurcation of the pulmonary artery and is usually patent in puppies for the first 6–8 days of life. The aortic arch normally arises embryologically from the left fourth arch but numerous anomalies of development have been reported. The brachiocephalic trunk leaves the aortic arch first, becoming the common carotids and the right subclavian artery. The left subclavian artery is the next branch to leave. The descending aorta gives off branches to the systemic organs before terminating in the iliac arteries.

Heart

The heart lies usually between the third and sixth rib, surrounded by the lungs except for the area at the cardiac notch on the right side, where access to the right ventricle can be gained. The outer fibrous pericardium continues over the vessels, unlike the inner serous part of the membrane. The space between the two is normally filled with a small amount of fluid but is a potential space for accumulation of blood or other fluids in pathological states.

The external grooves on the surface of the heart demarcate the atria and the ventricles, although there is often fat overlying the coronary vessels which supply blood to the myocardium. Figure 1.6 demonstrates the external anatomy of the heart. The fibrous tissue and cartilage in the heart separates the chambers

and restricts electrical communication to the bundle of His and Purkinje fibres shown in Figure 1.7. Note the Purkinje fibres cross the right ventricle in the trabecula septomarginalis (previously called the moderator band) to ensure the electrical activity is carried up the walls at the same rate.

There is a slit-like depression in the wall of the right atrium which marks the site of the foramen ovale, where blood flowed in the foetus between the atrium. In the left atrium, a membranous flap can be seen. There should be anatomical closure of this within the first few weeks of life due to the high pressure in the left side of the heart.

Defects in the interventricular septum most commonly occur in the dorsal membranous portion as the ventral part of the septum is much thicker and more muscular.

The tricuspid valve on the right side of the canine heart has only two cusps despite its name – the septal cusp and the parietal cusp. The mitral valve also has two similarly named leaflets but is a stronger valve due to the thicker papillary muscles and chordae tendinae. The semilunar valves have three leaflets. Surgery of the mitral or aortic valve demands careful dissection due to the close anatomical relationship between the two structures.

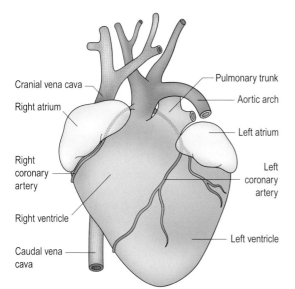

Figure 1.6   External anatomy of the heart.

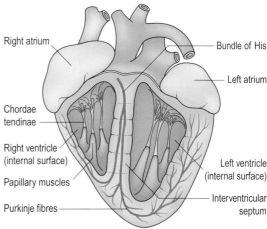

Figure 1.7   Purkinje fibres and the bundle of His.

Nervous system

The nervous system can be divided anatomically in several ways. The central nervous system consisting of the brain and spinal cord is often separated into those structures above the foramen magnum (to include the cerebrum, hypothalamus, midbrain, pons, medulla, vestibular system and cerebellum) and the regions of the spinal cord below the brain stem which are often split into the cervical, cervicothoracic, thoracolumbar, and lumbosacral areas. The peripheral nervous system involves the spinal, cranial and autonomic (involuntary) nervous trunks and their associated ganglia (collections of neurone cell bodies and their support cells).

Other divisions have more relevance to the physiology and describe the nervous system as either afferent (conducting impulses towards the brain and spinal cord) and efferent (those conveying impulses away from these structures). These are also referred to as sensory and motor pathways respectively.

The nature of the tissue innervated also permits further distinction of the peripheral nervous system into those involving voluntary muscle, termed somatic nerves, and those relating to the internal environment, called visceral nerves. These are concerned with the regulation of the heart rate, the control of digestion and other involuntary functions.

Peripheral nerves

The endoneurium that surrounds axons is made up of loose collagen fibres and fibroblasts. The next tough connective tissue sheath is the perineurium that encases bundles of nerve fibres. The entire nerve is encased in epineurium, which is collagen rich and whose fibroblasts provide strength to a repaired nerve. Severe or prolonged inflammatory responses cause excess collagen production with fibrosis and scarring of the nerve. When a nerve is traumatised, the disruption to the endoneurium results in disorganised regrowth of the axons down new Schwann cell tunnels – this leads to a nodular enlargement called a neuroma.

Meninges

The layers surrounding the brain and spinal cord are:

- the outer dura mater, which is fused with the periosteum of the skull
- the arachnoid, which has cerebrospinal fluid beneath it
- the pia mater, which adheres to the external surface of the nervous tissue.

Brain

The cerebrum is divided into two cerebral hemispheres by the longitudinal fissure and each has outward folds (convolutions) called gyri and inward folds called sulci. There is a band of fibres that course transversely from one hemisphere to the other in the depth of the fissure. This structure is called the corpus callosum and is sometimes sectioned in animals with epilepsy which are refractory to treatment without any undue effects on general function. The hemispheres are divided into lobes called the frontal, parietal, occipital and the temporal lobe relating to the portion of calvaria (skull) overlying them.

The cerebellum lies caudal to the cerebrum and dorsal to the fourth ventricle. The vessels in the pia around the ventricles form a dense network of capillaries called the choroid plexus which are involved in the secretion of cerebrospinal fluid into the ventricles.

Spinal cord

The cord is divided into segments corresponding to the vertebral bodies and a pair of spinal nerves leaves the cord at each intervertebral foramen. In the caudal cervical and midlumbar regions the cord thickens to innervate the limbs. These enlargements are called intumescence.

Between the dura of the spinal cord and the periosteum of the vertebrae is the epidural space, which contains loose connective tissue, fat and blood vessels. The blood supply to the cord comes from the longitudinal ventral spinal artery and the dorsal spinal arteries.

Locomotor

Structure of bones and joints
Cancellous bone consists of small spicules of trabeculae loosely arranged and is often referred to as spongy or woven bone – 2-mm pieces of this are used as bone grafts during fracture repair. Cortical or compact bone is denser and is found in the long bone cortices in concentric circles around a central canal.

Wolff's law states that 'bone adapts to the stresses put on it' and it is important to remember that bone remains active once growth is completed. Remodelling is a perpetual process with constant osteoclast (resorption) and osteoblast (deposition) activity. Table 1.1 illustrates the classification of joints.

Articular (hyaline) cartilage is smooth, glistening and whitish-yellow. It receives 90% of its nutrition from the synovial fluid with the remainder coming from the blood vessels in the subchondral bone. There is no innervation. The synovial membrane is continuous with the cartilage at the periphery of the joint and lines the joint capsule with its vascular connective tissue. The joint capsule and the ligaments of a joint each have a similar structure. They consist of dense fibrous tissue embedded in a matrix of proteoglycans. There is also a rich nerve supply, making them an important source of pain in clinical disease. Ligaments may be either a local thickening within the joint capsule, e.g. the collaterals, or a distinct entity, e.g. the cranial cruciate ligament.

Other intra-articular structures include the menisci and fat pads. The menisci are fibro-cartilaginous structures with a limited blood supply. They aid shock absorption, joint stability and weight distribution. The intra-articular fat pads fill the dead space and cushion bony prominences.

Axial skeleton
The atlanto-occipital membrane extends from the dorsal border of the foramen magnum to the dorsal arch of the atlas. This membrane is punctured during the collection of cerebrospinal fluid and in the administration of contrast media into the subarachnoid space during contrast myelography.

The atlantoaxial joint is enclosed in a single capsule. The two bones are held in apposition by a thin median ligament and paired alar ligaments. Surgical access to this region for correction of atlantoaxial instability is by a ventral approach through the paired sternomastoid and sternohyoid muscles and along the right side of the trachea, taking care to avoid the recurrent laryngeal nerve and the carotid sheath.

Access to the vertebral canal with a needle is difficult throughout the thoracic and lumbar regions as the interarcual spaces are narrow. The space at the lumbosacral junction is better

Table 1.1 Classification of joints

Types of joint		
Synarthoses	Immovable joints	Skull sutures
Amphiarthroses	Partially movable	Mandibular symphysis
Diarthroses	Freely movable	All synovial joints
Types of diarthrosis		
Enarthrosis	Ball and socket	Hip
Condylarthrosis	Condyloid	Carpus
Sellar	Saddle shaped	
Ginglymus	Hinge	Elbow
Trochoid	Pivot	Atlantoaxial
Arthrosis	Plain joint	Intercarpal

suited and can be located by palpation of the highest points of the wings of the ilia.

Most vertebrae are joined by the intervertebral discs, paired synovial joints and short and long ligaments. Discs degenerate with age. Fibrous tissue replaces the gelatinous material of the nucleus, consequently the lamellae forming the annulus separate and break up. The dorsal annular ligament is thinner than the ventral and this predisposes the disc to rupture upwards into the spinal cord if disease is present.

The nuchal ligament (absent in cats) must be spared during surgery as it plays an important role in support of the head. It runs from the spinous process of the axis to the tip of the first thoracic spinous process and is then continued as the supraspinous ligament following the tips of the remaining spinous processes.

The epaxial muscles running dorsal to the transverse processes must be separated and detached when access to the cord is needed. They are composed of a thin iliocostalis muscle, a thicker longissimus muscle and the complex transversospinalis muscle intimately associated with the vertebrae. The hypaxial muscles comprise the longus colli and longus capitis in the neck and cranial thoracic areas and the psoas muscle in the lumbar region.

Forelimb

The scapula and humerus form the shoulder and can be identified by the acromion on the distal end of the scapular spine and the greater tubercle of the humerus just distal to it. Deeper palpation also reveals the tendon of origin of the biceps and the deltoid tuberosity. The attachment of the pectorals to cranial parts of the bones prevents palpation of the medial surface of the joint. The scapula is covered laterally by the trapezius and the supra- and infraspinatus muscles. The capsule of the shoulder joint envelops the biceps tendon where it crosses the cranial aspect of the joint.

Surgical exposure of the scapular neck and glenoid requires an osteotomy of the acromion to allow distal retraction of the deltoid muscle. If proximal retraction of the supraspinatus is required the greater tubercle of the humerus is

osteotomised. Care must be taken to identify and protect the suprascapular nerve.

The proximal end of the humerus consists of the greater tubercle and the humeral head with the greater tubercle lying craniolaterally to it. The distal portions are termed the medial and lateral condyles, with the epicondyle an easily identifiable lateral prominence. The collateral ligaments arising from the epicondyles are also easily palpated. Luxation by lateral displacement of the radius and ulna is usual, due to the medial epicondyle being larger. As a result it is more difficult for the anconeal process (the proximal portion of the trochlear notch of the ulna) to snap over the medial epicondyle. Just cranial and slightly distal to the epicondyle is the extensor fossa, an important landmark in placing a screw for intercondylar fractures. The most prominent feature of the lateral surface is the musculospiral groove which houses the brachial muscle and the radial nerve. On the medial surface run the median, ulnar and musculocutaneous nerves and the brachial artery.

The olecranon is the proximal extremity of the ulna which serves as the attachment for the triceps. This results in proximal displacement of olecranon fractures. The medial surface of the radius is subcutaneous as is the distal cranial portion, which can be felt easily where there is only a thin covering from the extensor carpi obliquus and the tendons of other extensors. The ulnar is more deeply placed except at its distal end, where the styloid process connects with the carpal bones. There is a depression behind this process where the tendon of the flexor carpi ulnaris runs and the accessory carpal bone is found.

Paws

Elastic dorsal ligaments extend from the proximal end of the middle phalanx to the ungular crest of the distal phalanx to keep the claws elevated. The deep digital flexor opposes this action and protrudes the claws for digging or scratching. Cats have elastic dorsal ligaments of unequal length and oblique articular surfaces so that their claws can be fully retracted (Fig 1.8). Cats use their claws for climbing trees and initial prey contact unlike dogs, which make prey contact with their jaws. The characteristic clawing at furniture that cats perform that is thought to be a method of sharpening claws is actually related to territorial marking by the sweat glands on the digital pads.

Hind limb

The hip joints possess greater range and flexibility in the dog and cat than in any other species and the articular surface reflects this. The femoral head is almost a perfect hemisphere with a central fovea where the intracapsular ligament sits. There are no peripheral ligaments to restrict movement. Access to the joint from a craniolateral approach goes between the tensor and biceps muscles, exposing the vastus lateralis and the gluteals. The sciatic and caudal gluteal vessels should be caudodorsal and not at risk of damage.

Many of the features of the skeleton can be palpated in the stifle joint including the sesamoid bones within the origin of the gastrocnemius. The single patella ligament and

the medial and lateral collateral ligaments may also be distinguished – but not the femeropatellar ligaments which are overlain by the aponeuroses of the sartorius and semimembranosus on the medial side and the biceps laterally. The cruciate ligaments are set well back within the joint and assist the collaterals in opposing rotation and medial or lateral deviation of the leg. The synovial compartments are in free communication within the stifle joint and there is a thick fat pad between the patellar ligament and the synovial membrane.

The superficial flexor and gastrocnemius components of the common calcaneal tendon may be identified separately distal to the belly of the muscle of the caudal tibia. The lateral saphenous vein runs along the caudal border of the gastrocnemius before entering the popliteal fossa to join the femoral vein. The blood supply to the limb comes from the cranial tibial and saphenous arteries.

The prominent surface features of the lower limb include the calcaneus and its medial process the sustentaculum tali and the projections of the tibial and fibular malleoli at the lower limit of the leg.

Urogenital system

Kidney

The kidneys are relatively mobile, paired retroperitoneal organs, 2.5–3 times the length of the second lumbar vertebrae. The right is normally more cranial than the left and in the dog they are bean-shaped whereas in the cat they are more spherical. The tough inelastic fibrous capsule is perforated at the hilus by the renal artery and vein, lymphatics, autonomic nerve supply and the ureter. The renal arteries are direct branches of the aorta and supply the kidneys with 25% of the total cardiac output. There are also vessels supplying the kidney that anastomose with other abdominal vessels, meaning the kidney has an alternative source if disease obstructs a renal artery. The right renal vein drains directly into the vena cava whilst the left receives the ovarian/spermatic vein first. The lymphatic drainage is to the lumbar nodes.

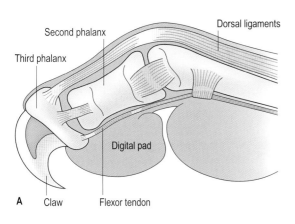
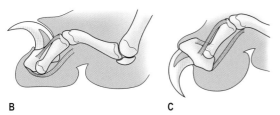

Figure 1.8 The cat's distal phalanx and claw (A), the claw fully retracted (B) and protruded (C).

Ureters

These paired fibromuscular tubes in the retroperitoneum transport urine from the renal pelvis to the bladder. They enter the lateral ligaments of the bladder in the region of the trigone and due to their oblique entrance into the bladder, progressive expansion with urine tends to occlude this opening and prevent urinary reflux. The ureteric arteries and veins run alongside the ureters.

Bladder

The bladder wall comprises three anatomically distinct layers:

1. an inner mucosal layer of transitional cell epithelium
2. layers of smooth muscle, the detrusor muscle, whose fibres run in all directions but converge to form the circular internal sphincter beyond the trigone at the urethral orifice
3. an outer serosal layer.

It is supported by two lateral umbilical ligaments which are continuous with the broad ligament of the uterus in the female. Ventrally the bladder is attached by the ventral umbilical ligament to the umbilicus. The arterial supply is from two sources: the cranial vesical artery from the umbilical artery and the caudal vesical artery from the urogenital artery. Venous drainage is to the internal pudendal vein and the lymphatic drainage is to the internal iliac and lumbar nodes. There is a somatic innervation from the pudendal nerve and an autonomic supply providing sympathetic innervation from the hypogastric nerve and parasympathetic fibres from the pelvic nerve.

Urethra

Extending from the trigone of the bladder to the urethral meatus, the urethra is divided into several segments in the male as shown in Figure 1.9.

- The prostatic segment is a short straight section within the gland itself and receives the prostatic secretions and sperm via the vas deferens.

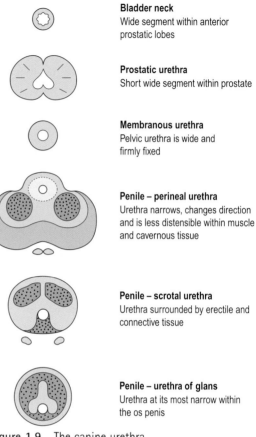

Bladder neck
Wide segment within anterior prostatic lobes

Prostatic urethra
Short wide segment within prostate

Membranous urethra
Pelvic urethra is wide and firmly fixed

Penile – perineal urethra
Urethra narrows, changes direction and is less distensible within muscle and cavernous tissue

Penile – scrotal urethra
Urethra surrounded by erectile and connective tissue

Penile – urethra of glans
Urethra at its most narrow within the os penis

Figure 1.9   The canine urethra.

- The membranous part has a large diameter and is firmly attached to the pelvic floor.
- The cavernous section has a reduced diameter and distensibility due to the surrounding muscle, cavernous tissue and the penile crura. The urethra turns ventrally and then cranially around the ischium.
- The penile urethra is the distal segment. It is surrounded by the corpus cavernosum and spongiosum and then the os penis.
- In the cat there are several differences including an elongated bladder neck and a reduced diameter of the terminal segment, especially at the glans.

Uterus

The organ comprises a uterine body, two horns and a cervix. It is supported by the mesometrium, part of the broad ligament which attaches the uterus to the dorsolateral abdominal wall. The round ligament, a continuation of the suspensory ligament, attaches the tip of the uterine horn to the deep inguinal ring. The ovarian artery anastomoses with the uterine vessels and supplies the cranial uterine horns. The uterine artery, a branch of the urogenital artery which runs in the broad ligament from the cervical level, gives off branches to the cervix, vagina, body and caudal horns of the uterus before anastomosing with the ovarian vessel.

Ovary

The ovaries are located caudal to the kidney, enclosed in a double peritoneal reflection, the ovarian bursa. They are supported by the mesovarium, an extension of the broad ligament, the suspensory ligament, which attaches the ventral ovary to the last ribs, and the proper ligament, an extension of the suspensory ligament which in turn attaches to the round ligament. The vascular supply is via the ovarian artery, a direct branch of the aorta, and the venous drainage is to the vena cava from the right ovarian vein and to the renal vein from the left.

Testicle

The testes are positioned obliquely within the scrotum and are covered along with the epididymes and spermatic cords with peritoneum originating from within the abdomen. The parietal vaginal tunic is the outer layer, whereas the visceral vaginal tunic is continuous with the parietal peritoneum of the abdominal cavity. Deep to the vaginal tunic is the tunica albuginea, a dense white fibrous capsule containing superficial branches of the testicular artery and vein. The testes and epididymes are connected to the parietal vaginal tunic by the caudal ligaments of the epididymes.

The testicular arteries are direct branches of the aorta and arise at the level of the fourth lumbar vertebra. The lymphatics drain into the iliac lymph nodes.

Penis

The penis is divided into three sections: the root, body and distal portion. The root is attached to the tuber ischii by the left and right crura. Each crus is composed of the proximal part of the corpus cavernosum and the ischiocavernous muscle covering it. The distal portion, the glans, is subdivided into a smaller proximal portion, the bulbus glandis, and a larger distal portion, the pars longa glandis. The right and left cavernous bodies are separated by a fibrous median septum.

Dogs have four paired extrinsic penile muscles: retractor penis, ischiocavernous, bulbocavernous and ischiourethral muscles. The blood supply branches from the internal pudendal artery and the venous drainage is via the internal and external pudendal veins. Nervous innervation comes from the pelvic and sacral plexuses.

Prostate

The prostate gland continues to increase in size throughout life by hyperplasia. It also moves cranially from the pelvic canal where it is found until 4 years of age, to become completely abdominal by 10 years in most dogs. The mature gland is ovoid and has a dorsal and ventral sulcus within a fibromuscular capsule. The dorsal portion encircles the urethra close to the neck of the bladder and the vasa deferentia enter each side of the craniodorsal prostate. From here they pass caudoventrally through the gland and empty into the urethra. The rectum is located dorsally and a fascial band connects the caudal third of the prostate to the ventral rectum.

Blood supply is from the prostatic artery, which penetrates on the dorsolateral surface, whilst the venous blood drains to the internal iliac vein. The innervation is from the hypogastric and pelvis nerves.

PHYSIOLOGY

Anaesthetic considerations in surgery

Anaesthesia involves the loss of consciousness in addition to the provision of analgesia and muscle relaxation. No one agent is sufficient to provide all of these components in every patient due to the range of surgical procedures and health states of the patients. Polypharmacy is employed, resulting in a wide range of effects on the cardiovascular, respiratory and nervous systems.

Central nervous system

The autonomic nervous system controls the involuntary muscles, glands and organs and is divided into sympathetic and parasympathetic pathways. The autonomic areas of the hindbrain include cardiovascular, respiratory and alimentary centres, but these are really no more than ill-defined pools of neurones in the medulla oblongata. There are two regions which control the heart and blood vessels, the vasomotor depressor centre and the vasomotor pressor centre. Collectively they are called the medullary cardiovascular centre. The two regions which influence breathing are the inspiratory centre and the expiratory centre. Together they are called the medullary respiratory centre. In the pons there is a pneumotaxic centre, which inhibits the inspiratory centre by negative feedback. Also in the pons is an apneustic centre which applies a steady excitatory drive on the inspiratory centre.

Frightened or injured patients can mask clinical problems due to activation of the sympathetic nervous system and the cardiac, renal and hepatic systems require evaluation in high-risk patients to determine the amount of agent required for chemical restraint or anaesthesia.

Tranquilisers and sedatives

Both are used to calm patients and are often used as preanaesthetic medications, sometimes in combination with opioids (known as neuroleptanalgesics). An advantage of this group is the potential for reversal or antagonism.

Acepromazine is a phenothiazine that depresses the reticular activating system (groups of small neurones concerned with consciousness and sleep) and brain stem, inhibiting the effects of the central neurotransmitters

dopamine and noradrenaline. This is responsible for the calmness and muscle relaxation seen with their use. The synapses are a logical site for pharmacological manipulation because transmission across them is chemical. The transmitter agents are synthesised, stored in the nerve endings and released near the neurones on which they act. They bind to receptors on these cells, thus initiating their characteristic actions and they are then removed from the area by reuptake or metabolism.

The reticular activating system (RAS) arouses the whole cerebral cortex, thereby enabling specific stimuli (touch, temperature, special senses etc) to be perceived by the sensory areas, visual areas etc. Pain sensations ranging from itching to agony are also transmitted by the RAS. General anaesthetics probably selectively depress the RAS by blocking transmission at its synapses, thereby providing narcosis and analgesia.

The hypotension is caused by the blocking of the alpha$_1$-adrenoceptor and has clinical implications when operating on shocked or hypovolaemic patients.

Benzodiazepines

Diazepam and midazolam are popular due to the lack of effect on the medulla oblongata, where the neurones in the vasomotor centre control blood pressure. This means therefore, they have little cardiopulmonary depressant effects. They are also used as appetite stimulants and for their ability to inhibit seizures and cause muscle relaxation.

Non-opioid analgesics

Xylazine and medetomidine produce analgesia, sedation and muscle relaxation by binding to alpha$_2$-adrenoceptors in the central nervous system, reducing sympathetic nervous outflow. Their binding to the peripheral receptors produces marked cardiopulmonary depression.

Opioid analgesics

Opioids can act as agonists, partial agonists or antagonists to produce their range of effects including analgesia. The receptor type also affects the amount of sedation and respiratory depression seen, for example fentanyl acts on the Mu receptor and produces far more respiratory depression than morphine which acts on the Kappa receptor.

Anticholinergics

Atropine and glycopyrrolate reduce salivary and tracheal secretions, dilate airways, prevent parasympathetically induced bradycardias and cause mydriasis. Impulses in the cholinergic vagal cardiac fibres decrease the heart rate but parasympatholytic drugs such as atropine raise the heart rate due to the unopposed sympathetic tone. They are useful in surgery where vagally induced bradycardia is likely e.g. correction of patent ductus arteriosus and excision of bladder neoplasms. They are not recommended in trauma patients because they often increase heart rate and oxygen consumption while predisposing to cardiac dysrhythmias.

Barbiturates

The anaesthetic duration is related to plasma concentration and redistribution into muscle and fat, not metabolism and excretion, so hypovolaemic patients will suffer prolonged unconsciousness after small doses due to centralisation of blood flow and poor muscle perfusion. Trauma patients are often acidotic and hypoproteinaemic. This will slow elimination and increase the amount of free drug in the plasma respectively, both augmenting the effects of the drug. Barbiturates depress myocardial function and baroreceptor reflexes. The baroreceptors are stretch receptors in the walls of the heart and blood vessels that are stimulated by distension of the structures in which they are located.

Dissociative anaesthetics

Ketamine provides excellent superficial analgesia due to depression of various areas of the brain. There is poor muscle relaxation and an increase in arterial blood pressure due to an increase in sympathetic activity,

making it unsuitable for patients with heart disease.

Neuromuscular blocking drugs

Muscle paralysis can greatly aid fracture repair and delicate eye surgery but their use is limited due to the close nursing required to ensure adequate return of ventilation. When an impulse arrives in the end of a motor neurone, it increases the permeability of the synaptic bouton to calcium which enters and triggers a marked increase in exocytosis of acetylcholine-containing vesicles. The acetylcholine diffuses across the synapse and is taken up by the motor end plate where there is an influx of sodium and potassium ions. This results in depolarisation of the membrane and the production of an action potential along the muscle fibre, which in turn causes contraction. Acetylcholine must be rapidly removed from the synapse if repolarisation is to occur. The removal occurs by way of hydrolysis of acetylcholine, a reaction catalysed by the enzyme acetylcholinesterase. Non-depolarising drugs are preferred due to their predictability and the potential for reversal with acetylcholinesterase inhibitors.

Inhalation agents

These agents are as hypotensive as barbiturates but are safer as they are more controllable and homeostatic mechanisms have longer to compensate for the depressant effects. Nitrous oxide stimulates cerebral metabolism. It causes increased cerebral blood flow and increased intracranial pressure and is therefore contraindicated in head injuries.

Physiology of the gastrointestinal tract

Digestive and absorptive functions of the gastrointestinal (GI) system depend on mechanisms that soften food, move it through the tract and mix it with pancreatic digestive enzymes and bile. The intestinal smooth muscle, neurones intrinsic to the gut, reflexes involving the CNS, paracrine effects of chemical messengers and the GI hormones all play a part.

Saliva

Salivary amylase secretion is minimal in dogs and cats as they spend little time chewing food. The optimal pH for this enzyme is 6.7 meaning that its action is inhibited by gastric acid as food enters the stomach. The flow of saliva is continuous but is increased by both sympathetic and parasympathetic stimulation. Secretory function can be evaluated by dropping ophthalmic atropine solution onto the dorsal surface of the tongue to stimulate secretion. Some of the functions of saliva are:

- lubricates food for swallowing
- dissolves food allowing chemoreceptors to detect taste
- contains lysozymes and other bactericidal agents to prevent oral infections
- continuous washing of teeth to reduce decay
- evaporation during panting helps temperature regulation.

Swallowing

The process is initiated voluntarily but completed reflexly. The muscle of the tunica muscularis of the oesophageal wall is responsible for the movements of peristalsis. It consists of various combinations of striated and smooth muscle. In the dog it is composed of striated muscle throughout the length of the oesophagus, but in the cat the transition to smooth muscle takes place between the caudal third and caudal fifth of the oesophagus. The vagus is responsible for part of the afferent innervation which initiates reflex swallowing and it is also responsible for a large part of the efferent pathways. The afferent side of the reflex consists of stimuli from the mucosa of the oesophagus and the efferent side is carried in the recurrent laryngeal nerve as well as the vagus. The stages of swallowing can be considered as follows (Fig 1.10):

- bolus of food is pressed against the hard palate and squeezed caudally
- soft palate is elevated to close the pharyngopalatine arch
- tongue is jerked caudally to push the bolus onwards

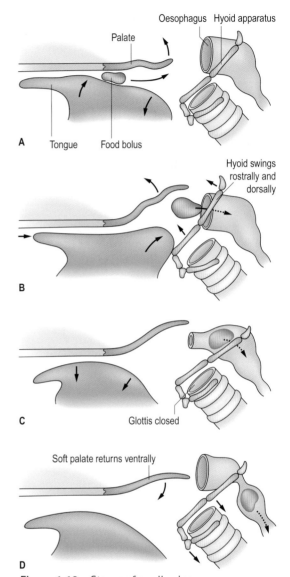

Figure 1.10   Stages of swallowing.

- hyoid is swung rostrodorsally bringing the pharynx to meet the bolus
- epiglottis bends back to contribute to closure of glottis
- the constrictors of the pharynx contract to propel the bolus caudally
- the tongue returns to resting position as the bolus enters the oesophagus

hyoid returns to resting position, the soft palate returns ventrally and the glottis reopens.

Stomach

Food is stored in the stomach, mixed with gastric secretions, broken down into small particles by contractions of the stomach wall and then released at a controlled rate into the duodenum. The major secretions are listed below and Figure 1.11 shows the locations in the stomach where they are produced (mucus is secreted in all parts of the stomach):

- hydrochloric acid to break down tissue and release nutrients, activate gastric pepsins, kill ingested bacteria and stimulate the flow of bile and pancreatic juices
- mucus forming a flexible gel coating the mucosa
- bicarbonate that forms an unstirred layer with the mucus to protect the mucosal surface from the gastric acid
- proteolytic enzymes (pepsinogens) secreted by chief cells in the inactive form to avoid self digestion
- intrinsic factor, a substance necessary for the absorption of cyanocobalamin (vitamin B_{12}) from the small intestine.

The rate of gastric emptying is related to the degree of gastric distension, the viscosity of contents and the presence of chyme in the duodenum. The peristaltic activity lasts for 15–20 minutes before the stomach resumes its fasting quiescence for about an hour.

Small intestine

The pancreas, liver and small intestinal mucosa all secrete substances that help digestion and absorption in the small intestine. The pancreatic juice is alkaline due to the high bicarbonate content – this neutralises the gastric acid, raising the duodenal pH to between 6.0 and 7.0. The powerful protein splitting enzymes of the pancreatic juice are secreted as inactive proenzymes, e.g. trypsinogen is converted by the brush border enzyme enteropeptidase.

Bile is secreted by the cells of the liver into the bile duct which drains into the duodenum. Between meals the gallbladder fills as the orifice of this duct is closed, but when food enters the mouth the sphincter relaxes and the gallbladder contracts as food enters the duodenum. Some of the components of bile are reabsorbed in the intestine and then excreted again by the liver (enterohepatic circulation). The principle functions of the liver are:

- formation of bile which reduces surface tension and emulsifies fat
- carbohydrate storage and release
- formation of urea
- cholesterol metabolism
- manufacture of plasma proteins
- many functions related to metabolism of fat
- inactivation of some polypeptide hormones
- conjugation of steroid hormones
- synthesis of 25-hydroxycholecalciferol
- detoxification of many drugs and toxins.

The small intestine is essential for life. Removal of short segments of the jejunum or ileum generally does not cause severe symptoms and there is hypertrophy of the remaining mucosa with return of the absorptive function towards normal.

Large intestine

Absorption of water from the faeces occurs in the proximal colon and caecum and the dry matter is stored in the distal segment. Absorption of water is a result of active absorption of

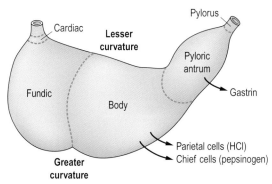

Figure 1.11   Secretions of the stomach of the dog and cat.

sodium which allows diffusion of water by osmosis. Potassium rich mucus is added to the faeces and bicarbonate is secreted to neutralise the acid produced by bacterial metabolism in the gut. The passage of faeces requires spinal reflexes to contract the colon, relax the anal sphincter, close the glottis and increase abdominal pressure. Defaecation can be overcome by voluntary contraction of the external anal sphincter.

The chyme in the jejunum contains few bacteria, the ileum has slightly more but it is only the colon that has large numbers. The relative sterility of the small intestine is due to the gastric acid and the quick transit time of the chyme. Antibiotic use improves growth rate as nutritionally important substances such as ascorbic acid, cyanocobalamin and choline are utilised by some intestinal bacteria.

Ammonia is produced in the colon and absorbed. When the liver is diseased, ammonia is not removed from the blood and hyperammonaemia occurs, causing neurological signs (hepatic encephalopathy). This is also seen with portosystemic shunts where the liver is bypassed by an abnormal blood vessel.

Physiology of the locomotor system

Motility has evolved from primitive neuroeffector cells that respond to stimuli by contracting. In animals, contraction has become the specialised function of muscle cells, whereas transmission of nerve impulses has become the function of neurones. The locomotor system also includes the connective tissues (tendons, ligaments, cartilage, bone) that provide support and organise its compartments.

Muscle

Muscle cells can be excited chemically, electrically and mechanically to produce an action potential that is transmitted along their cell membrane. The contractile proteins actin and myosin bring about contraction and there are several other proteins such as troponin that play an important role in linking excitation to contraction. The source of energy for muscle contraction is adenosine triphosphate. During muscular exercise the muscle blood flow is increased so that the oxygen supply is adequate for aerobic glycolysis – the breakdown of glucose to carbon dioxide and water. Lactate is produced when there is insufficient oxygen – this process is called anaerobic glycolysis. Box 1.1 shows the sequence of events in contraction and relaxation of skeletal muscle.

Most skeletal muscles begin and end in tendons. The muscle fibres are arranged in parallel between the tendinous ends so that the force of contraction of the units is additive. Muscular contraction involves shortening of the contractile elements, but because muscles have elastic and viscous elements in series with the contractile mechanism, it is possible for contraction to occur without a shortening of the muscle. This is called isometric con-

---

Box 1.1   Steps in contraction and relaxation

Contraction
1. Discharge of motor neuron
2. Release of transmitter (acetylcholine) at motor end plate
3. Binding of acetylcholine to nicotinic acetylcholine receptors
4. Increased sodium and potassium conductance in end-plate membrane
5. Generation of end-plate potential
6. Generation of action potential in muscle fibres
7. Inward spread of depolarisation
8. Release of calcium into the muscle fibres
9. Binding of calcium to troponin, uncovering the myosin binding sites on actin
10. Formation of cross-linkages between actin and myosin and sliding of the muscle filaments producing shortening

Relaxation
1. Calcium pumped back into the sheath surrounding the fibres
2. Release of calcium from troponin
3. Cessation of interaction between actin and myosin

traction. When the muscle shortens the action is called isotonic contraction.

Bone

Bone has many functions in structural support, protection of organs and as a reservoir for minerals. Articular cartilage covers the articulating surfaces and the synovial membranes line the joint capsules and tendon sheaths. The periosteum is a membranous structure surrounding the whole bone. The ends of the bone called the epiphysis contain the secondary centres of ossification and below that is the growth plate or physis. The next region, the metaphysic, contains woven lamellar cancellous bone and the compact cortical bone surrounds a marrow cavity in the diaphyseal region.

Bone mineralisation is in equilibrium with body fluids. Resorption of bone with a decrease in density and therefore strength occurs when intake of calcium, magnesium and phosphorous is inadequate. This occurs in vitamin D deficiency rickets, or when loss of mineral is excessive, as in secondary renal hyperparathyroidism.

The main function of the bone marrow in dogs and cats is haematopoiesis of non-lymphoid cells. It occurs within the medullary areas of the long and flat bones. As the animal ages, the diaphyseal region is replaced by adipose tissue, leaving active marrow confined to the epiphyseal and metaphyseal areas. Therefore in the young animal bone marrow is a red colour and in older animals the colour changes to yellow with white fat mottling. Access to the marrow for sampling is best achieved through the dorsal iliac crest and samples for transplantation are best taken from the femur, tibia and humerus.

Connective tissues

All connective tissues are composed of cells, extracellular fibres and ground substance. Fibroblasts are the main cell producing the matrix and collagen is the main component. Collagen is the most abundant mammalian protein and provides great tensile strength. It is a constituent of blood vessels and thus is found in all tissues but that found in bones, tendons and ligaments – type I collagen – is the most common form. The other fibrous component of the connective tissue matrix is elastin, a much more extensible material. Tendon collagen can only be stretched to five times its length before breaking whereas elastin can be extended to 100 times its length before it breaks.

The large proteoglycans and glycosaminoglycans provide resilience and flexibility to the matrix. Many form giant complexes by associating with hyaluronic acid, which gives the tissue the viscoelastic, semipermeable properties needed for cartilage, synovium and intervertebral discs. Also synthesised by connective cells are peptide growth factors which regulate the proliferation and differentiation of cells. Some of these growth factors have been implicated in cartilage and bone disease and some are being used therapeutically to aid wound management.

Physiology of the urogenital system

Urinary system

Blood is filtered through the glomerular capillaries into the renal tubules, where the volume is reduced and the composition is altered by tubular reabsorption (removal of water and solutes from the tubular fluid) and tubular secretion (secretion of solutes into the tubular fluid) to form the urine that enters the renal pelvis. From here it is passed to the bladder and expelled by the process of micturition. The kidneys are also endocrine organs, making kinins, secreting renin and erythropoietin and forming dihydroxycholecalciferol.

The dog has over twice as many nephrons as the cat, which has about 190 000 per kidney and this, along with the higher protein levels in their diet, may account for the increased prevalence of renal disease seen in this species. The kidneys receive 25% of the cardiac output – higher than that to the heart, brain or liver – and the blood flow is determined by the renal vascular resistance.

Renin is released from the juxtaglomerular cells in response to a fall in blood pressure.

A plasma protein made in the liver called angiotensinogen is activated by rennin. The product, angiotensin I, is converted in the blood vessels of the lungs to angiotensin II which is a potent systemic vasoconstrictor and stimulates proximal tubular resorption of sodium. It also stimulates the release of aldosterone from the adrenal cortex, resulting in an increase in blood pressure.

Renal function is assessed by analysis of urine and measurement of serum concentrations of creatinine and blood urea nitrogen. Urea is passively filtered through the renal glomeruli whereas creatinine is excreted through filtration and proximal tubular secretion in dogs. Abnormal values are only seen in animals with marked renal impairment as normal values can be seen when there is as little as 25% of kidney function.

During the storage of urine the bladder muscle (detrusor) relaxes to allow expansion of the organ which triggers the detrusor reflex by activation of stretch receptors in the bladder wall. Nervous impulse is carried to the sacral spinal cord and to the brain where parasympathetic fibres return to the bladder to stimulate urination. Both contraction of the bladder and relaxation of the urethra are required. Urethral resistance depends on both smooth muscle fibres (internal sphincter) innervated by sympathetic fibres and striated muscle fibres (external sphincter) innervated by the pudendal nerve.

Genital system

In both species the gonads have a dual function: the production of germ cells (gametogenesis) and the secretion of sex hormones. The androgens are the steroid sex hormones that are masculinising in their action and the oestrogens are feminising. Both are normally secreted in both sexes although the testes secrete mainly testosterone and the ovaries secrete oestrogen, progesterone, a steroid that has special functions in preparing the uterus for pregnancy, and, during pregnancy, relaxin, to loosen the ligaments of the pubic symphysis. The secretory and gametogenic functions of the gonads are both dependent upon the secretion of the anterior pituitary gonadotrophins – follicle stimulating hormone (FSH) and luteinising hormone (LH).

Pyometra is a disease of the dioestrous phase of the ovarian cycle, when the corpus luteum is actively secreting progesterone, which increases secretions of the uterine glands, inhibits myometrial contraction and maintains closure of the cervix. Long-acting progestational compounds administered to intact bitches cause endometrial hyperplasia with progression to pyometra in some individuals. Even though infection is not the primary cause of pyometra, it is usually present, as the progesterone primed uterus is more susceptible to infection.

Physiological response to trauma and sepsis

Trauma is derived from the Latin word for 'doing harm' and is used to describe injury from such events as road traffic accidents, falls and wounds from animal interactions and sharp objects. Tissue strength is related to the amount of elastin, collagen and water present. Tendons with little water and lots of collagen are stronger than liver for example. The orientation of fibres in tendons also gives them strength in tension but results in weakness if torn. The area of the body traumatised also has an effect on the pathology caused, e.g. what would be a severe contusion in a muscle may be a fatal contusion in the lungs or brain.

Wound healing

The first response to injury is vasoconstriction of the small vessels in the local area whilst a clot forms to control bleeding. Then vasodilation occurs and fluid leaks out of the venules into the damaged tissue. Histamine released from mast cells and platelets increase the permeability of the vessels and leucocytes migrate out through the endothelium. Initially the predominant cell is the neutrophil whose primary role is to destroy bacteria but because these cells are short-lived, they are soon superseded by monocytes, which predominate in older wounds. On entering a wound, monocytes become macrophages. A growth factor from the platelets attracts inflammatory cells to the site of injury, a process known as chemotaxis.

Macrophages help with the next phase of wound healing, the laying down of collagen, which starts when infection is under control. New capillaries (angiogenesis) grow behind the fibroblasts and then the fibrin network is destroyed. If haematomas, necrotic tissue or bacteria are present these processes are blocked.

Epithelialisation, proliferation and migration of cells occur in a wound even before any new connective tissue has formed. Epithelial cells migrate across a sutured wound within 2 days and are responsible for the strength of a wound for the first 5 days. When a full thickness portion of skin is lost, the wound edges initially retract, enlarging the wound, but soon after wound contraction occurs and continues until the wound edges meet. The collagen content of a wound stabilises after 3 weeks but the increase in wound strength may continue for years. Scar tissue is never as strong as the tissue it replaced.

Tissue regeneration

There is a relationship between the degree of tissue differentiation and its regenerative capacity. The more differentiated cells such as neurones do not regenerate whereas epithelial cells are capable of dividing and replacing themselves. With the exception of the liver, regeneration is limited to simple tissue such as epithelium; compound structures such as the skin, organs and the nervous system heal only by synthesis of scar tissue.

The liver has the capacity to restore its original size within 6 weeks of losing 80% of its mass. It does this by increasing cell division and hypertrophy of the remaining cells. Skeletal muscle can also regenerate but only if the cut ends of a muscle are apposed, preventing connective tissue from migrating in between the transected muscle.

When a nerve fibre is traumatised the severed ends retract and the axon starts to degenerate in both directions. Unmyelinated fibres degenerate more quickly. The Schwann cells (which are phagocytic) ingest clumps of myelin and debris. Sprouting of the damaged ends occurs within 48 hours and some may reinnervate the motor end plate or peripheral sensory receptors if connective tissue does not obstruct their path. The axon grows down a tube formed from the regenerating Schwann cells. This is why repair does not take place in the CNS because the oligodendrocytes that form myelin in the CNS do not regenerate in this way. Surgeons can aid the process of nerve regeneration by removing damaged tissue from the injury site, excising epineurium that could produce an obstructive scar and properly coapting the nerve ends to reduce loss of regenerating fibres.

Sepsis

When there is inadequate tissue oxygenation for normal cellular respiration, the body is defined as being in shock. In septic shock, this is due to hypovolaemic, distributive and cardiogenic forms of shock coupled with cellular dysfunction as the cells are unable to metabolise. Sepsis is the occurrence of systemic illness associated with infection and any illness or injury can depress the immune system and predispose the animal to sepsis. Causes include bacteraemia, burns, trauma, shock, peritonitis, mastitis, prostatic and other abscesses, metritis, intestinal ischaemia, enteritis, liver disease and gastric dilatation volvulus.

There is increased energy expenditure in sepsis due to the increased load on the heart, increased oxygen consumption by the wound, the utilisation of oxygen in the conversion of lactate to glucose in the liver and the effect of increased body temperature. A tissue insulin resistance also impedes glucose use. Initially there is an increased use of fat stores to provide energy but with time, there is an inability to use this energy source also. This means that nutritional support of the septic patient is critical and use of alternative fuels such as branched chain amino acids may be important. Disseminated intravascular coagulation is often seen and oedema is present due to an increase in capillary permeability.

PATHOPHYSIOLOGY

Inflammation and healing

The wound healing process is often divided into three overlapping phases:

- haemostasis and inflammation
- proliferation
- maturation and remodelling.

Haemostasis and inflammation

The first response to injury is vasoconstriction of the small vessels in the local area whilst a clot forms to control bleeding. Then vasodilation occurs and fluid leaks out of the venules into the damaged tissue. The classic signs of inflammation (redness, swelling, heat and pain) are the result of this vasodilation, fluid escape and obstruction of the local lymphatic channels. Pressure, chemical stimulation and stretching of nerve endings result in pain. Histamine released from mast cells and platelets increase the permeability of the vessels and leucocytes migrate out through the endothelium. Initially neutrophils (whose primary role is to destroy bacteria) predominate but they are soon superseded by monocytes, which on entering the wound become macrophages.

Growth factor produced by the platelets attracts inflammatory cells to the site of injury (chemotaxis). The activation of the macrophages also leads to the release of additional cytokines and nitric oxide (NO) which aid new capillary growth (angiogenesis). There is lots of interaction between the macrophages and released factors such as interferons, interleukins and tumour necrosis factor alpha. All of these help to modulate the healing process and are the subject of much study in the development of drugs to speed wound healing.

Proliferation

Macrophages help with the next phase of wound healing, the laying down of collagen, which starts when infection is under control. New capillaries grow behind the fibroblasts and then the fibrin network is destroyed. If haematomas, necrotic tissue or bacteria are present these processes are blocked. Severe tissue trauma results in the lowering of the wound pH owing to accumulation of lactic acid secondary to lymphatic and vascular compromise. This environment stimulates the release of potent proteolytic enzymes from the lysosomes of granulocytes. These enzymes break down local connective tissue and promote the formation of abscesses and infection.

Epithelialisation, proliferation and migration of cells then occur as described above. Lymphatic channels develop much more slowly than blood vessels so lymphatic drainage of wounds is poor in the early stages. The tissue that fills the wound space, called granulation tissue, is a mixture of branching capillary loops surrounded by mesenchymal cells and extracellular matrix. This tissue is highly resistant to infection because of the outer protection provided by the granulocytes and macrophages.

Maturation and remodelling

Collagen content of the wound stabilises after about 3 weeks but wound strength may increase for years, e.g. it is prolonged in tendon healing. The scar tissue is never as strong as the original tissue despite constant remodelling, dissolution and reformation of collagen fibres to produce a more efficient weave. After 1 week a wound only has 3% and after 2 weeks 20% of its final strength.

Pathophysiology of gastric dilatation volvulus

There are many local and systemic pathophysiological effects associated with gastric dilatation volvulus (GDV) (Table 1.2). The syndrome presents acutely and the effects are attributable to the accumulation of gas in the stomach, which becomes misplaced. Aerophagia, bacterial fermentation of carbohydrates and chemical diffusion from the bloodstream all contribute to the gas accumulation. There is also fluid found in the stomach which is a mixture of ingesta, gastric secretions and transudate from venous obstruction.

The displacement of the stomach is usually in a clockwise direction as viewed with the

Table 1.2   Pathophysiological effects associated with GDV

Intestinal ileus and gastric atony	Thoracic and diaphragmatic impingement	Decreased blood flow in caudal vena cava and portal vein	Gastric ischaemia
Fluid sequestration and electrolyte imbalance	Decreased tidal volume Ventilation perfusion mismatch	Decreased venous return Decreased cardiac output Decreased arterial blood pressure Decreased tissue perfusion Splanchnic hypoperfusion Reperfusion injury and myocardial injury	Gastritis and gastric mucosal necrosis Absorption of bacteria and endotoxins Septic-endotoxic shock Blood, fluid and protein loss Anaemia Perforation and peritonitis

dog in dorsal recumbency. The pyloric antrum passes from the right abdominal wall towards the ventral midline and passes over the gastric fundus and body to lie alongside the left abdominal wall (Fig 1.12).

The omentum, which is adhered to the greater curvature of the stomach, is seen lying over the ventral aspect of the displaced stomach. Because the gastrosplenic ligament holds the spleen close to the stomach, it too is often involved in the torsion, becoming quickly congested due to compromise of its blood supply.

The hypotension caused by the decreased cardiac output and the vascular stasis result in a cellular hypoxia and a shift to anaerobic metabolism. Other pathophysiological effects such as decreased hepatic endotoxin clearance due to the occlusion of the portal vein exacerbate the hypotension even further. The acidosis that results from the hypoxia predisposes to the development of disseminated intravascular coagulopathy.

Pathophysiology of intestinal obstruction

Small intestinal obstruction is a frequent occurrence and is the most common reason for surgery of the intestines. Figure 1.13 shows the

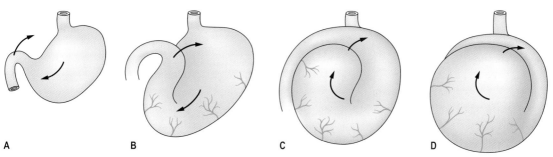

A   B   C   D

Figure 1.12   GDV–clockwise rotation as viewed with the dog in dorsal recumbency.

pathophysiological changes associated with a simple obstruction. High obstruction involving the pylorus, duodenum or proximal jejunum carries a poorer prognosis as there is hydrogen ion loss with a resulting metabolic alkalosis often associated with a hypokalaemia. Large amounts of fluid are lost with obstructions distal to the pancreatic and biliary ducts, which leads to a high loss of bicarbonate ions and a resultant metabolic acidosis.

Intramural pressure, i.e. the pressure in the intestinal wall, rises significantly and circulatory compromise in the segment can be so severely affected that blood is shunted away from intestinal capillaries directly into the venous system. The duodenum appears particularly susceptible. Large foreign bodies can cause pressure necrosis, which can lead to loss of viability and increased permeability to endotoxins.

The pathophysiology of a strangulated intestinal obstruction is slightly different (Fig 1.14). These obstructions occur when a loop of intestine becomes incarcerated into a hernia or rupture and the blood supply becomes quickly compromised. An intact arterial supply allows intramural sequestration of blood with resultant intramural oedema. Proximally the bowel will distend with gas and fluid which contains significant amounts of blood. The wall quickly becomes necrotic

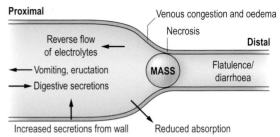

Figure 1.13 Pathophysiology of a simple obstruction of the small intestine.

and endotoxic shock results. Intussusception results in similar changes.

Pathophysiology of ileus

Ileus is a lack of motility of the gastrointestinal tract that produces signs similar to intestinal obstruction. Rough handling of the intestines during surgery can predispose to its development, as can peritoneal infection, dehydration of the intestines and some drugs such as opioids. When the intestines are traumatised, there is a decrease in intestinal motility caused by direct inhibition of smooth muscle. When the peritoneum is irritated, there is a reflex inhibition due to increased discharge of noradrenergic fibres in the splanchnic nerves. Because of the diffuse decrease in peristaltic

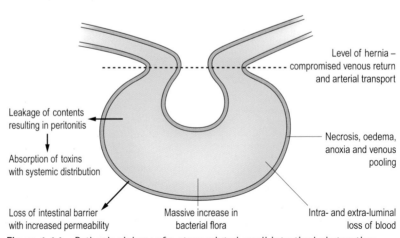

Figure 1.14 Pathophysiology of a strangulated small intestinal obstruction.

activity in the small intestine, its contents are not propelled into the colon and it becomes irregularly distended by pockets of gas and fluid. Intestinal peristalsis returns usually within 6–8 hours of surgery, quickly followed by gastric peristalsis. Colonic activity, however, takes 2–3 days to return to normal.

Electrolytes such as sodium, potassium and chloride are lost into the intestinal lumen and as potassium is essential for the synthesis of acetylcholine, a neurotransmitter, the loss contributes to the ileus.

Pathophysiology of urinary obstruction

The effects of urinary obstruction must be considered both during and after relief of obstruction as the kidneys can be significantly affected. Urine concentrating function is the first function to be affected as the glomerular filtration rate (GFR) is reduced to 20% of normal. The blood flow to the blocked kidney decreases by 50% in the first 24 hours and can be as little as 10% of normal in chronic cases of obstruction.

After relieving the blockage there is an increase in the amount of urine produced and the solute loss is much greater than normal. This diuresis can lead to a loss of sodium which persists for several days after correction of the problem. A similar change is seen in plasma potassium levels which increase initially during acute bilateral obstruction but then fall during the postobstruction diuresis.

Dehydration occurs after unblocking the kidneys as there is a decrease in reabsorption of the filtrate and an increased osmotic load per nephron due to azotaemia. There is a change in urine pH and plasma bicarbonate is reduced.

Prolonged ureteric obstruction leads to dilation of the proximal segment and hydronephrosis. If the obstruction is relieved within 7 days little permanent damage is done to the kidney. Obstruction of the normal flow of urine has several important effects on the kidney. The dilation of the calyces and collecting ducts causes reduced renal blood flow and GFR and as a result of this tubular function (secretion and resorption) is impaired,

causing azotaemia, hyperkalaemia and metabolic acidosis. Permanent damage to the kidney occurs through the increased pressure giving rise to ischaemia or superimposed infection. The severity of the renal damage will depend on the degree, duration and level of obstruction as well as the presence of infection.

Urethral obstruction can impair the function of the bladder wall muscle resulting in an inability to contract the bladder after resolution of the obstruction. This is due to a loss of tight junctions between the bladder cells and an overstretching of the detrusor muscle.

Pathophysiology of respiratory tract trauma

Compromised respiratory function results in dyspnoea caused by either a low partial pressure of oxygen (hypoxaemia) or a high partial pressure of carbon dioxide (hypercapnia) in arterial blood. Both increase the drive for respiration, resulting in signs of respiratory distress unless the hypoxia is severe, when there is depression of the brain stem ventilatory motor centres and there is a paradoxical reduction in ventilation.

Oxygen supplementation should be considered in patients with haemoglobin saturation of less than 93%. Blood gas analysis, if available, assists in determining whether positive pressure ventilation is indicated. General indicators are a partial pressure of oxygen of 50 mmHg or less on oxygen supplementation or a partial pressure of carbon dioxide greater than 50mmHg.

The arterial hypoxaemia, hypercapnia and acidosis seen with thoracic trauma are caused by:

- alveolar hypoventilation
- impairment of diffusion
- pulmonary shunting
- ventilation/perfusion imbalance
- decreased inspired partial pressure of oxygen
- altered blood gas transport.

Pneumothorax is the most common result of blunt trauma to the chest. It is caused by leakage of air from the lung tissue or airways into the pleural space, resulting in collapse of the lung lobes. Tension pneumothorax is a serious condition where a large pulmonary leak occurs, allowing air to continuously enter the pleural cavity but not allowing any to leave. This increases interpleural pressure, further compressing the lungs and causing a mediastinal shift away from the pneumothorax. The obstruction to the venous return to the heart leads to hypovolaemic shock.

Pulmonary contusions are also a common finding following thoracic trauma. The patient is usually in hypovolaemic shock but care must be taken when administering fluids so as not to worsen the pulmonary haemorrhage or exacerbate the condition by causing pulmonary oedema.

Diaphragmatic hernias can become obstructed and vascular compromise associated with strangulation may cause tissue necrosis. Dyspnoea is caused by the physical presence of these organs as well as the accumulation of pleural fluid due to inflammation and occlusion of venous return from the viscera.

Acute lung injury (ALI) and acute respiratory distress syndrome (ARDS) refer to inflammatory lung injury which may be secondary to pulmonary contusions. In ALI, pulmonary inflammation appears as vasculitis, interstitial and alveolar permeability oedema and infiltration of inflammatory cells such as neutrophils and macrophages. ARDS is a more severe form, manifest by inflammation, accompanied by proliferation of pneumocytes and interstitial fibrosis. Patients are dyspnoeic and hypoxic.

Complications of wound healing

Non-healing wounds and wound dehiscence
Conditions that impair circulation, physical agents, heat, radiation, prolonged inflammation, infection, tumours and improper nutritional support can impede steps in the three phases of wound healing. The surgeon can minimise complications by adhering to the basic surgical principles outlined by Halstead (Box 1.2) and Esmarch's principles of wound management (Box 1.3).

Box 1.2   Halstead's principles of surgery

- Minimal surgical trauma (gentle tissue handling)
- Accurate haemostasis
- Preservation of an adequate blood supply
- Aseptic technique
- No tension on tissues
- Careful tissue approximation
- Obliteration of dead space

Box 1.3   Esmarch's principles of wound management

- Do not introduce anything harmful
- Rest tissues
- Wound drainage
- Avoid venous stasis
- Asepsis

Some of the most common causes for dehiscence are:

- wound closure under tension, the sutures cut through the tissues due to ischaemic necrosis
- sutures placed too close to the wound edges – there is collagenase activity within 5mm of the skin incision
- incorrect suture material selection
- closure of compromised skin with resultant necrosis
- cutaneous circulation compromised
- moisture accumulation contributing to tissue overhydration and maceration
- underlying pocket of infection, necrosis, foreign body or neoplasia – healthy tissue is relatively resistant to infection but necrotic tissue can have devastating effects on the wound environment and should be excised whilst preserving the blood supply to the adjacent viable tissues.
- lack of postoperative protection from motion/trauma
- premature suture removal
- corticosteroid use delaying healing

- suture placement in scar tissue which has poor suture holding properties
- underlying systemic pathology, e.g. a healing disorder.

Wound contraction may fail to occur where there is undue tension in a wound or restrictive fibrosis, which mechanically impairs the skin from advancing across the deficit. Wound epithelialisation is independent from contracture but wounds that heal primarily by contracture are cosmetically better due to better hair growth. Epithelial cells require a viable vascular tissue bed for survival and repeated surface trauma from improperly applied bandages damage the delicate process. Tissue desiccation can have a similar effect so topical ointments and occlusive dressings are sometimes useful to provide a warm, moist protective environment.

Scarring

Scar tissue always forms as a normal response to healing and is only a problem when it restricts motion or function such as in flexion joints. Scarring is minimised by early wound closure and control of infection, as well as the use of Z-plasty techniques or free grafts, followed by physical therapy.

Necrosis and gangrene

The maintenance of perfusion and arterial oxygen tension are critical factors in resistance to infection. Although surgeons cannot alter systemic host defences they can promote infections and deter host defence mechanisms by adversely affecting local wound factors.

Abscess formation occurs when areas of cellulitis coalesce. Culture and sensitivity testing are not usually warranted unless the abscesses are deep, recurring or persistent, or form draining tracts. The most effective method of obtaining accurate culture from an infected pocket is to biopsy the wall. Cultures from the purulent exudates are likely to be contaminants rather than the primary infecting organism.

The kind of bacteria infecting a wound greatly affects the outcome of the infection. Skin infections in dogs are often caused by *Staphylococcus* spp. However, if the wound involves the gastrointestinal tract, the contaminants are often *E. coli* or *Clostridium* and this can lead to necrosis and gangrene with the build up of gas pockets, felt as crepitus under the skin. This is because the endotoxins that are produced cause direct cellular damage and stop the host from phagocytosing the bacteria and carrying out neutrophil chemotaxis. *Clostridium* is especially virulent as it produces exotoxins that cause a more rapid onset of infection with fewer bacteria numbers and it can protect other bacteria such as *E .coli* from host defences and thereby enhance the pathogenicity of mixed infections. *Clostridium* infection can be rapidly fatal, especially that caused by *C. perfringens*, which causes myonecrosis characterised by massive muscle necrosis and septic shock.

Sinuses and fistulae

Persistent or intermittent draining tracts have been seen with the presence of large pockets of necrotic tissue, bone infections, foreign bodies (including surgical implants) and neoplasms. It is useful to perform contrast radiography (fistulograms) to ascertain the extent of the tract and its relationship to the regional anatomy. Deep wound biopsy cultures should be taken to include fungal culture and the area should be excised around the tract to avoid spilling its contents into the tissues.

A fistula differs from a sinus in that it connects a mucosal surface of a viscus with the skin surface. Both are fibrous tracts lined by chronic, oedematous granulation tissue and are usually associated with purulent, serous or serosanguinous discharge. Fistulae may be lined with epithelium.

Seromas

The collection of serum in areas with dead space results from inflammation and lymphatic damage in the surgical field. Drains should be inserted into dead space to minimise their occurrence where possible. Other techniques for reducing dead space include tacking sutures and resection of extra skin, e.g. scrotal ablation following castration.

Exposed bone

A healthy bed of granulation tissue is required over the exposed bone before epithelialisation can commence. This arises from the viable periosteum, from the exposed viable medullary cavity or by creeping coverage from granulation tissue from soft tissue adjacent to the bone. Surgical promotion of this bed can be achieved by drilling small holes into the vascular medullary canal of the bones. Capillaries, fibroblasts and white cells extend from these holes to cover the cortical surfaces. Exposed bone that is sticking out of a wound needs debridement as granulation tissue will be unable to grow over this area.

Surgical sepsis

The use of routine perioperative antibiotics is common in veterinary practice and should be discouraged unless the procedure warrants the use. Such procedure masks breaks in surgical sepsis and encourages the development of resistance. Although it is impossible to sterilise skin surfaces there are many steps that can be taken to minimise the risks of infection such as:

- only perform clean procedures in operating rooms
- close off the surgical room from 'traffic'
- remove fur and clean the animal's skin for 5–7 minutes in a 'prep' area
- scrub the surgeon's hands following the guidelines in Box 1.4
- employ good surgical technique including minimising dead space, haemorrhage and removal of all devitalised tissues.

Complications of fracture healing

Malunion

This is where the fracture has healed but in poor axial alignment; the cause is inadequate or incorrect fixation. Treatment may require osteotomy and fixation.

Delayed union

This is when the fracture has not healed during the time period in which it should have

---

Box 1.4   Surgeon's scrub protocol

- Wash hands with soap to degrease
- Using chlorhexidine or povidone-iodine, wash hands and up to elbows for 1 minute
- Rinse hands only
- Scrub each hand and the ventral, axial and abaxial surfaces (not dorsal) for 1.5 minutes each hand
- Rinse to elbows and keep hand above them
- Wash hands and two-thirds of the way up to elbows for 1 minute
- Rinse hands only
- Wash hands for 30 seconds
- Rinse all the way to elbows keeping hands higher than elbows to prevent drips contaminating clean areas

---

repaired, although it will unite on its own eventually. The causes are as for non-union.

Non-union

This is when the fracture repair process has stopped and union will not occur without surgical intervention. There are no signs of osteogenesis and there is movement at the fracture site. The causes are:

- inadequate immobilisation
- gap between fracture fragments (soft tissue interposition, distraction of bones, inadequate reduction)
- loss of blood supply (damage to nutrient vessels, excessive stripping or injury to periosteum, comminution)
- infection and sequestra
- corrosion/reaction/failure of implants
- loss of bone due to underlying pathology.

The clinical and radiographic features of non-union are shown in Box 1.5. Treatment involves improving the fracture fixation, debriding old tissues (often necessitating opening of the marrow cavity), cancellous bone grafts and antibiotics. This complication is common in the radius of short-limbed dogs and occasionally is also seen in the femur.

Osteomyelitis

The term means inflammation of the bone, which may include the medullary cavity, cortex and the periosteum. The inflammation is usually associated with bacterial infection, although fungal and sterile inflammations occur. Usually the infection is introduced at the time of trauma, although haematogenous spread or from adjacent infected tissues can occur. The infection can cause thrombosis of blood vessels within the Haversian canals with resultant ischaemia of bone. Localised areas of cortex can become necrotic and separate off from the rest of the bone, forming sequestrum. Sinus formation is common.

Deep wound infections can progress to osteomyelitis and so should be treated aggressively. Once the symptoms of swelling, warmth, redness and pain are identifiable, swabs should be taken and antibiotic sensitivity testing performed. It is crucial to evacuate all haematoma, fluid and exudates and free pieces of bone. Gaps should be packed with cancellous bone graft and a drainage tube may be placed. Chronic osteomyelitis is when infection has been present for several weeks, months or years and may present after bony union has taken place.

Tumours

Nature and significance

A major study on the incidence rates of neoplasms in the dog and cat was conducted between 1963 and 1967 in California by Dorn et al. They showed an annual incidence rate of 1077 cases of cancer per 100 000 dogs and 188 cases per 100 000 cats. Of these, 67.6% of the canine cases were skin and connective tissue tumours and 44.8% were from these sites in the cat.

Benign tumours are given the suffix *-oma* whereas malignant neoplasms of ectodermal or neuroectodermal origin (epidermis and mucosa) are given the suffix *carcinoma*. A prefix such as *adeno-* (meaning glandular) can be added to describe the tissue type in the malignancy. Those tumours arising from mesoderm or endoderm are described using the suffix *sarcoma* and again a prefix determines the tissue type, e.g. *haemangio-*, meaning originating from blood vessels. Table 1.3 shows the full classification system.

There are several problems that can be associated with tumours, mainly haematological complications such as anaemia, leucopaenia, thrombocytopaenia and disseminated intravascular coagulation, and endocrine complications such as hypercalcaemia caused by lymphomas and other tumours. Tumours may metastasise in three ways:

- along tissue planes
- via lymphatics (carcinomas)
- haematogenously (sarcomas).

Some 21.5% of all canine tumours metastasise but less than 1% of the tumour cells released into the circulation manage to seed a second tumour due to mechanical destruction of the cell along the way. Tumour cells either lodge in the first capillary bed they encounter or else have tropisms for specific organs where they produce cytokines to allow the development of new capillary buds.

Clinical staging

The aim is to quantify the disease and to offer a more accurate treatment and prognosis.

Table 1.3 Classification of tumours

T – Primary tumour

Tis	Preinvasive carcinoma (in-situ)
T0	No evidence of primary tumour
T1	Tumour <2 cm diameter
	(a) without bone involvement
	(b) with bone involvement
T2	Tumour 2–4 cm diameter
	(a) without bone involvement
	(b) with bone involvement
T3	Tumour >4 cm diameter
	(a) without bone involvement
	(b) with bone involvement

N – Regional lymph nodes

N0	No evidence of RLN involvement
N1	Moveable ipsilateral nodes (those on the same side)
N1a	Nodes not considered to contain growth
N1b	Nodes considered to contain growth
N2	Moveable contralateral (on the opposite side) or bilateral nodes
N2a	Nodes not considered to contain growth
N2b	Nodes considered to contain growth
N3	Fixed nodes

M – Distant metastases

M0	No evidence of distant metastases
M1	Distant metastases

Clinical stage	TNM	Prognosis (% survival at 1 year)
I	T1a, N0, M0	100
II	T2a, N0, M0	75
III	T1b, T2b, T3a, N0, M0	35
IV	T, N2, M1	0

Box 1.6 Classification of tumours

Adenocarcinoma	Malignant tumour of glandular tissue
Adenoma	Benign tumour of glandular tissue
Carcinoma	Malignant tumour of epithelial tissue
Fibroma	Benign tumour of fibrous tissue
Fibrosarcoma	Malignant tumour of fibrous tissue
Lipoma	Benign tumour of adipose cells
Lymphosarcoma	Malignant tumour of lymphatic tissue
Malignant melanoma	Malignant tumour of Melanocytes
Melanoma	Benign skin tumour of melanocytes
Osteosarcoma	Malignant tumour of osteoblasts
Papilloma	Benign tumour of epithelial cells (wart like)
Sarcoma	Malignant tumour arising from connective tissue
Squamous cell carcinoma	Malignant tumour of squamous epithelium (often affecting skin, mouth and conjunctiva)

Staging should define the site, origin and extent of the primary tumour, the sites of metastases (local and distant) and the histological type. The system is called the WHO-TNM classification. Box 1.6 gives an example of an oropharyngeal malignancy TMN classification.

The role of surgery in oncology

Surgery has five main roles in oncology:

- biopsy
- prophylaxis
- definitive excision
- cytoreductive surgery
- palliation.

It is essential to remember that surgery only gives a local cure and must be considered as one arm of a multidisciplinary approach to the cancer patient.

Handling and transport of pathological specimens

Swabs, scrapings or brushings

Cells are harvested and either transferred to glass slides or else inserted into the correct transport media before sending to the laboratory. Cotton swabs can be used for collecting cells from vaginal and ear canals and mucosal surfaces. A scalpel is more appropriate to harvest a thin layer of cells from the surface of oral lesions or from surgical biopsy tissues.

Fluids

Fluids from body cavities can be retrieved by centesis. Once a fluid sample is obtained, aliquots should be placed in both EDTA and clotted tubes since effusions will occasionally clot.

Cytological examination of body cavity fluids usually involves determination of the protein concentration, nucleated cell count and a morphological description of the cells. When cellularity is low, concentrated smear preparations are required. The handling of a sample during slide preparation is crucial to preserving the pathology. For fine needle aspirations and fluids the needle tip should touch the slide as the plunger is advanced to push a small drop of material onto the glass surface. Each drop should be the size of a pin head otherwise the cells do not spread thinly over the slide. To spread the sample either the 'drawback and push away' technique is used as for blood or, if the sample has cell aggregates, a 'squash' technique is recommended, where a slide is placed on top of the sample and the two slides are separated by a horizontal sliding force. Air drying must be accomplished quickly to attain optimal cytoplasmic and nuclear detail.

Biopsy material

Biopsies should be well planned, the site should not compromise or modify further treatment, and it should be within the proposed surgical field. Furthermore it should minimise the potential spread of neoplastic cells. The techniques include:

- fine needle aspirate
- tru cut biopsy (using a needle with an outer sleeve that can be withdrawn once in the sample, allowing tissue to drop into an inner cavity)
- grab biopsy
- incisional biopsy
- excisional biopsy.

All of the above biopsy samples require fixing before transporting – 10% buffered neutral formalin is the agent of choice. Sample pots should not be filled with more than 50ml of fluid and each tissue sample must be sectioned less than 1cm thick to allow good penetration of the formalin into the whole sample. A ratio of one part tissue to ten parts formalin is ideal. Biopsy specimens should be handled carefully to avoid distorting the tissue architecture. Do not handle the samples with forceps or suction prior to fixation.

If an excisional biopsy has been performed, an essential element of the pathology report is the interpretation of tissue margins to ascertain completeness of resection. A good method is to tag the edges of a sample with suture material and indicate to the pathologist which colour suture is which margin. A preferable method is the use of Indian ink to mark deep and lateral margins so that after sectioning the pathologist can see if tumour cells reach the black line at the deep edge of the tissue.

Further reading

Pavletic M 1999 Atlas of small animal reconstructive surgery, 2nd edn. W B Saunders, New York

Luis Fuentes V, Swift S (eds) 1998 Manual of small animal cardiorespiratory medicine and surgery. British Small Animal Veterinary Association, Cheltenham

Slatter D 2003 Textbook of small animal surgery, 3rd edn. W B Saunders, New York

Hall E, Simpson J, Williams D (eds) 2005 Manual of canine and feline gastroenterology, 2nd edn. British Small Animal Veterinary Association, Cheltenham

King A S 1999 Physiological and clinical anatomy of the domestic mammals. Blackwell Science, Oxford

Ganong W F 2001 Review of medical physiology, 20th edn. McGraw-Hill, New York

Dyce K, Sack W, Wensing C J G 2002 Textbook of veterinary anatomy, 3rd edn. W B Saunders, Oxford

Williams J M, Birchard S J 2002 BSAVA Continuing Education Courses Advanced Soft Tissue Surgery.

King A S, Cox J E 1982 Notes on abdominal and pelvic anatomy of domestic mammals. University of Liverpool, Liverpool

Chapter **2**

Ophthalmological surgery

Sue Mothersdale

CHAPTER OBJECTIVES

- Preoperative considerations
  Suitability for surgery
  Housing a patient for ocular surgery
  Restraint of the patient
  Diagnostic aids
  Skin and eye preparations
  Preoperative ocular medication
  Topical preparation prior to
    intraocular surgery

- Anaesthetic considerations
  Local anaesthesia
  General anaesthesia in ocular surgery
  The anaesthetic plan
  Monitoring anaesthesia
  Recovery
  Anaesthesia for the diabetic patient

- Surgical preparation
  Corneal and intraocular procedures
  Extraocular procedures
  Positioning

- The operating theatre
  The nurse's role in theatre

- Postoperative nursing care and
  medication
  Postoperative care
  Postoperative medication
  Postoperative complications
  Discharge

- Surgical equipment and techniques
  Ophthalmic surgical instruments
  Drapes
  Illumination
  Magnification
  Haemostasis
  Scalpel blades
  Suture materials and needles
  Irrigating solutions
  Viscoelastic substances
  Intraocular lenses
  Phacoemulsification
  Cryosurgery
  Electrolysis
  Electrocautery
  Laser therapy
  Care and sterilisation of ophthalmic
    instruments
  Glossary

Eye disease requiring surgery is common in companion animals and veterinary surgeons often perform various procedures that can range from eyelid surgery in healthy young animals to advanced intraocular procedures in older animals with concurrent disease. The outcome for the patient not only depends upon the skill of the surgeon but on the care provided by the nursing team where knowledge and understanding of ocular disease (Fig 2.1, Table 2.1) and surgical procedures is necessary. Meticulous attention to detail is essential to achieve a successful outcome and improve the patient's quality of life.

PREOPERATIVE CONSIDERATIONS

Suitability for surgery

When acquiring patient history it is important to assess the patient's temperament. Patients undergoing ocular surgery of any kind will require considerable handling of the head during examination, preceding and following surgery, along with pre- and postoperative medication.

Patients who have become nervous, head shy or snappy due to discomfort or disorientation as a result of their condition generally return to their friendly self once treated and may still be considered for surgery. However, aggressive unmanageable patients may not be considered suitable.

It is important that all considerations are explained to the owner before the procedure is booked in. They themselves must be able to manage the postoperative medication regime, which may last in excess of 6–8 weeks along with regular re-examinations to achieve successful results.

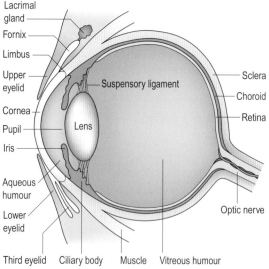

Figure 2.1   Transverse section of the eye.

Labels: Lacrimal gland, Fornix, Limbus, Upper eyelid, Cornea, Pupil, Iris, Aqueous humour, Lower eyelid, Third eyelid, Ciliary body, Muscle, Vitreous humour, Suspensory ligament, Lens, Sclera, Choroid, Retina, Optic nerve

Housing a patient for ocular surgery

Unless there is excessive rubbing of the head or eyes or obvious ocular discharge patients may have had ocular disease for some time before being brought to the practice for examination. Patients cope extremely well in their home environment with gradual loss of vision and the disease can go unnoticed for some time until the owner sees an obvious change in the colour of the globe or the pet begins to bump into objects or fails to return when called. Patients with ocular disease may therefore become distressed when removed from their familiar surroundings.

- The patient should be hospitalised in a quiet area of the kennels, they should be kept calm and must not be allowed to bark or jump up in their kennel – sedation may be required.
- All kennel surfaces should be flat; this includes the door, to prevent the patient pushing the nose through the bars and risking damage to the eye. A Perspex shield may be fitted to the door for this purpose.
- The kennel should ideally have immediate/close access to an outside run where the patient can be lead-walked to urinate and defecate. Cats will require a litter tray placed at a safe distance from the bedding area. For those cats which chose to sleep in the tray it is advisable to remove the tray and offer it periodically so that litter material does not contaminate the surgical site.
- Soft bedding should be provided (Vet bed). Avoid the use of solid plastic or wicker beds, even if they are familiar to the patient, to avoid stumbling and possibly knocking the eye on the bed or the side of the kennel.
- The patient should not be offered toys because of the risk of banging the head whilst playing.
- Food and water bowls should be shallow and always be kept in the same place (treat as though they are blind).
- It is important that you talk to patients when approaching them and maintain physical contact.

Table 2.1   Conditions of the eye

Eyelids and nictitating membrane

Coloboma	A congenital absence of tissue – eyelids or lens
Lagophthalmos	Condition where the eyelids do not close properly due to protrusion of the globe, common in brachycephalic breeds
Ophthalmia neonatum (neonatal conjunctivitis)	Infection within the conjunctiva before the eyelids are open
Ankyloblepharon	Continued fusion of the eyelids after 14 days following birth, requires surgical intervention
Macropalpebral fissure	Overlong palpebral fissure often seen in bloodhounds
Entropion	Inversion of the eyelid
Ectropion	Outward turning of the eyelid
Diamond eye	Combination of entropion and ectropion
Cherry eye	Prolapse of the nictitans gland
Neoplasia	Squamous cell carcinoma – commonest eyelid neoplasm
Trauma	Lacerations due to fighting

Disease of the orbit and globe

Retrobulbar swellings due to:

Abscess/cellulitis	Cellulitis – diffuse inflammation as a result of infection. Abscess due to bite, tooth root or zygomatic gland infection
Neoplasia	Nasal carcinoma, meningioma, lymphoma
Glaucoma	A group of diseases resulting in increased intraocular pressure, classified as congenital, primary or secondary
Extraocular polymyositis	Inflammation and swelling of the extraocular muscles producing bilateral exophthalmos without third eyelid protrusion
Zygomatic salivary gland mucocoele	Fluid filled mass of stagnant saliva in the ventral orbit causing exophthalmos
Arteriovenous shunt	Congenital vascular malformation in the orbit causing exophthalmos
Microphthalmos	Congenitally small eye
Strabismus	Where one eye cannot focus with the other due to imbalance in the eye muscles: cross eyed, squint
Prolapse of the globe	Acute anterior dislocation of the globe due to attack from larger dog, more common in brachycephalic breeds

Conditions of the cornea

Dermoid cyst	A choristoma – a mass of tissue skin, sebum and hair that develops not normally at that site. Dermoids develop on the corneoscleral limbus and may also be found on the conjunctiva and lids
Keratitis	Inflammation of the cornea: causes include trauma, infection, preocular tear dysfunction, immune mediated problems
Corneal ulcer	Superficial: loss of epithelium with or without stroma. Deep: loss of epithelium and stroma, may extend as far as the Descemet's membrane
Descemetocoele (keratocele)	A herniation of the Descemet's membrane as a result of a deep corneal ulcer
Corneal sequestrum	Black or dark brown discolouration of the cornea, which is unique to cats; common in Persians
Corneal lipidosis	Opacity within the cornea due to cholesterol deposits
Corneal trauma	Iris prolapse as a result of a cat scratch. Foreign body – thorn etc

table continues

Table 2.1   continued

Conditions of the lacrimal system	
Keratoconjunctivitis sicca (dry eye)	A deficiency in the production of the aqueous part of the tears.
Conditions of the conjunctiva	
Conjunctivitis	Inflammation of the conjunctiva
Symblepharon	Extensive conjunctival adhesions
Trauma	As a result of fighting, or foreign body – grass seed
Conditions of the uveal tract	
Uveitis	Anterior uveitis:
	Inflammation of the iris – iritis
	Inflammation of the ciliary body – cyclitis
	Posterior uveitis:
	Inflammation of the choroid – choroiditis
Iris bombe	A bulging forward iris
Iris cyst	Small-pigmented fluid filled body that becomes detached and floats freely in the anterior chamber
Conditions of the lens	
Cataract	Opacity of the lens and or its capsule. Can be the result of hereditary disease, diabetes mellitus, glaucoma, penetrating trauma, hypocalcaemia, retinal detachment or retinal atrophy
Lens subluxation	Partially displaced lens, still held by some intact zonular fibres
Lens luxation	Dislocation of the lens due to rupture of the zonular fibres
Papilloedema	Abnormal swelling of the optic disc
Optic neuritis	Inflammatory swelling of the optic nerve
Retinal atrophy	Degeneration of the retina affecting the photoreceptors and the pigment epithelium
Retinal detachment	Partial or total detachment of the retina as a result of inflammation, neoplasia, dysplasia, hypertension or hereditary – CEA
Retinal haemorrhage	Bleeding between the retina and the choroid

Restraint of the patient

When restraining a patient for ocular examination and medication *less is more*.

Manual restraint

To walk with a patient place a lead around the front of one shoulder and behind the other, alternatively use a harness. For examination or medication sit the patient and rest its chin on your hand, placing your other hand behind its head. Avoid scruffing patients as this alters the conformation of the face and lids. Heavy restraint around the neck should be avoided; holding too firmly around the neck may result in a false increase in intraocular pressure due to the occlusion of the jugular vein. Tension of the retrobulbar muscle may also lead to rupture of a deep corneal ulcer.

Chemical restraint

Light sedation may be used; however, this can cause enophthalmos and elevation of the third eyelid, thereby restricting examination of the globe.

Restraining aids

Any firm restraint, be it manual or by the use of restraining aids, is undesirable. They are best avoided if possible as they can excite the patient, causing a false increase in intraocular pressure. There is a risk that the patient may knock its head in the process of applying a muzzle and in particular tape muzzles alter the conformation of the face and lids.

Diagnostic aids

Before surgery commences a thorough assessment of the patient's condition is essential and a range of diagnostic tests may be performed:

- *Ophthalmoscopy* – assessment of pupillary light reflexes, fundus, lens and adnexal examination
- *Schirmer tear test* – to measure tear production
- *Fluorescein staining* – to assess damage to the corneal epithelium
- *Tonometry* – the means of measurement of intraocular pressure. Indentation tonometry assesses intraocular pressure by indenting the cornea using a Schiotz tonometer. Applantation tonometry assesses intraocular pressure by flattening the cornea using an electronic device called a Tono-Pen
- *Electroretinography* – assesses retinal function (Fig 2.2). A contact lens electrode is placed on the cornea; a light is flashed into the eye. A waveform of rod and cone activity is recorded. Primarily used for patients that are predisposed to progressive retinal atrophy by age, breed or retinal dysfunction
- *Ultrasonography* – to examine for retinal detachments.

Skin and eye preparations

Surgical ophthalmic procedures can be divided into corneal (ocular), intraocular or extraocular procedures. Patient condition and the surgical procedure to be performed will affect how the patient is prepared for surgery.

Preoperative ocular medication

To apply ocular drops (Figs 2.3, 2.4), elevate the patient's nose and place a finger across the medial canthus so as to occlude the ventral nasolacrimal punctum. One drop is sufficient, over-infusing the eye will cause lacrimation – diluting the medication, reducing its efficacy and washing it out of the eye. Keep the nose elevated for one minute. Allow at least 5 minutes between administering each medication to prevent one drop washing out the next.

Topical preparation prior to intraocular surgery

Before any intraocular procedure is performed adequate preoperative preparation is essential to reduce any existing inflammation and to minimise intraoperative and postoperative complications. The type and frequency of medication varies widely and is based on the surgeon's preference. Medication generally consists of a combination of topical anti-inflammatories, mydriatics and antibiotic drops.

Solutions (drops) are preferable to ointments to prevent oily bases entering the eye –

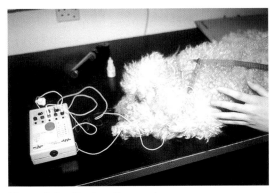

Figure 2.2   Electroretinography.

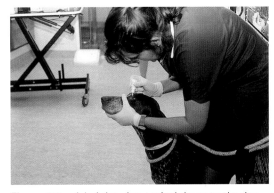

Figure 2.3   Administering topical drops to the dog.

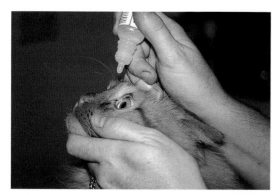

Figure 2.4　Administering topical drops to the cat.

preservatives found in them may irritate the wound. Ointments should not be used within 12 hours of intraocular surgery; if an ointment has been used it can be effectively removed by gentle ocular lavage. Preparations used include:

- anti-inflammatory agents to reduce intra-operative and postoperative inflammation; they also stabilise the blood aqueous barrier
- mydriatics to dilate the pupil; often a combination of mydriatics are used and they are essential to provide access to the operating field – during surgery a miotic pupil would increase the need for intraoperative manipulation, resulting in postoperative inflammation and possibly jeopardising the outcome of surgery
- topical prophylactic antibiotics to prevent would breakdown.

Patients undergoing cataract extraction are admitted the day before surgery. That evening topical ocular medication begins (Sheet 2.1) and continues on the morning of the surgery.

ANAESTHETIC CONSIDERATIONS

Local anaesthesia

Topical anaesthesia
Often used to assist ophthalmic examination and for minor procedures such as superficial foreign body removal, grid keratectomy for a non-healing superficial corneal ulcer or the

removal of sutures. It provides pain relief for the cornea but should not be used frequently as it inhibits corneal re-epithelialisation and impairs lacrimation.

Regional anaesthesia
This technique is used to achieve a central eye position for corneal and intraocular surgery. Regional anaesthesia of the eye/orbit is produced by blocking the ophthalmic branch of the trigeminal nerve. Paralysis of the globe results and so care must be taken to provide lubrication (false tears) to the cornea and surrounding tissues due to the loss of tear formation for several hours.

Retrobulbar block
This involves injecting local anaesthetic behind the globe (under general anaesthesia). There is a rapid onset (<10min) and long duration (2–3h) of action. This technique provides excellent intra- and postoperative analgesia and is effective in preventing oculocardio reflex. The risks include initiation of the oculocardio reflex during local infiltration, subarachnoid injection, retrobulbar haemorrhage and penetration of the globe; the procedure is generally retained for enucleation.

General anaesthesia in ocular surgery

General anaesthesia is used for all but the most minor of ophthalmic procedures and one anaesthetic protocol for all patients does not exist. A thorough examination should be performed, along with preoperative haematology, biochemistry and electrolyte analysis. Ideally patients over 6 years of age should have thoracic radiographs. Concurrent eye disease, systemic disease and concurrent medication must be considered when planning and performing anaesthesia.

Concurrent and intraoperative medication
Most ophthalmic drugs are applied topically either to prepare the eye for surgery or to treat the eye disease itself. These may include steroids, non-steroidal anti-inflammatories, antibiotics, carbonic anhydrase inhibitors,

Sheet 2.1 – Preocular medication sheet

PRE-OCULAR MEDICATION FOR CATARACT EXTRACTION

ANIMAL NAME .... OWNER ....

Eye(s) to prep .... DATE ....

Atropine drops (dilate pupil)
    Once evening before, twice in 2 hours prior to surgery
Phenylephrine drops (dilate pupil)
    Three times in 2 hours prior to surgery
Ocufen drops (stabilise blood–aqueous barrier)
    Once evening before, four times in 2 hours prior to surgery
Chloramphenicol drops (antibiotic)
    Once evening before, once in 2 hours prior to surgery

EVENING BEFORE SURGERY

Drop to apply	Time to give	Initial when given
Atropine	19.00	
Ocufen	19.30	
Chloramphenicol	20.00	

DAY OF SURGERY

Drop to apply	Time to give	Initial when given
Atropine	07.00	
Phenylephrine	07.10	
Ocufen	07.20	
Chloramphenicol	07.30	
Ocufen	07.40	
Atropine	08.00	
Phenylephrine	08.15	
Ocufen	08.30	
Ocufen	08.45	
Phenylephrine	09.00	

mydriatics and miotics. They have limited systemic effects; however, in susceptible patients some medication such as cholinergics (pilocarpine) for the treatment of glaucoma can cause bradycardia. Adrenergic agonists such as adrenaline and phenylephrine used topically may lead to hypertension and tachycardia, predisposing the patient to arrhythmias during surgery. An older dog may be currently receiving systemic non-steroidals for arthritis, ACE inhibitors/beta-blockers for cardiac disease or steroids for atopy. Systemic effects need to be considered as this medication may affect the choices made with respect to the anaesthetic plan.

Concurrent disease

Glaucoma is a group of eye diseases characterised by abnormally high intraocular pressure (IOP). The increase in pressure can lead to damage of the optic disc, with hardening of the eyeball that may result in partial or total blindness. The rise in IOP is almost always due to reduced outflow of aqueous humour, the inflow remaining constant.

It is classified as congenital, primary or secondary glaucoma. Congenital is present at birth, primary relates to anatomical abnormalities within the drainage angle (narrowing or malformation) and secondary as a result from another disease such as lens luxation or intraocular inflammation (uveitis). The commonest condition is primary glaucoma where the obstruction is in the trabecular meshwork

Intraocular pressure

In the normal eye the ciliary body continuously produces aqueous humor. The fluid flows through the pupillary opening into the anterior chamber and exits the anterior chamber into the uveal veins through the trabecular meshwork at the iridocorneal angle. Fluid production and drainage is constant – aqueous humor supplies nutrients to and removes waste from the eye. Anything that causes an obstruction to the drainage of fluid results in increased intraocular pressure. The normal intraocular pressure in dogs is 10–25mmHg.

It is vital that IOP is controlled if there is to be a successful surgical outcome. Too high a pressure may complicate the surgery and turn a standard conjunctival graft for a deep corneal ulcer into a more complex procedure to salvage a ruptured globe. Too low a pressure may cause distortion of the globe hindering surgery and the placement of sutures. Intraocular pressure is influenced by several factors, which include the following.

Venous pressure   Venous pressure increases blood volume in the eye. It may be caused by occlusion of the jugular veins for blood sampling, during restraint, a tight collar or lead around the neck, poor positioning of the neck for surgery or allowing equipment to lie upon the neck.

Ventilation   Airway obstruction due to poor positioning of the head and neck for surgery causes dramatic increases in venous pressure. Inadequate gaseous exchange in the lungs results in hypoxia and hypercapnia, causing vasodilatation and thus increasing IOP.

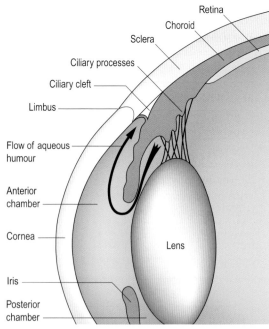

Figure 2.5   Aqueous flow. Reproduced from Seymour & Gleed 1999, with permission from BSAVA.

Blood pressure IOP remains stable over slight variations in blood pressure. Sudden changes in systemic blood pressure will cause changes in blood flow and thus changes in IOP.

Drugs Anaesthetic agents can increase or decrease IOP and so may help or hinder the surgery. Drugs such as medetomidine and opioid analgesics such as morphine, which may induce vomiting, should be avoided as retching and vomiting increase IOP. The use of ketamine or xylazine is not recommended for ocular procedures – they initially increase muscle tone, including the extraocular muscles, elevating IOP. Drugs which increase IOP should not be used for patients suffering perforated globe, iris prolapse, corneal foreign bodies or deep corneal ulcers – a raised IOP would result in rupture of the globe. Succinylcholine, a depolarising neuromuscular blocking agent, is contraindicated; it produces an initial increase in skeletal muscle tone along with extraocular muscles before producing muscle relaxation. Premedicants used for sedation such as acetylpromazine and benzodiazepines may lower IOP or at the least cause no change. Thiobarbiturates and propofol relax extraocular muscles and increase aqueous outflow, resulting in a lowering of IOP.

Hypertonic osmotic agents Traditionally osmotic diuretics are administered either orally (glycerol 2ml/kg) or by intravenous infusion (mannitol) to reduce IOP. They may be used preoperatively to reduce IOP, if there is a risk of vitreous prolapse, or at the end of intraocular surgery to reduce the risk of increased IOP in breeds predisposed to glaucoma. Mannitol is a sugar-based hypertonic osmotic diuretic; it is given by slow intravenous infusion 1–2 hours prior to surgery administered at a rate of 1–2g/kg for 20–30 minutes. It works by drawing fluid from an area of high osmolarity into an area of low osmolarity, in this case from the eye into the venous circulation; this produces a rapid, although short-lived (5–6h), reduction in IOP.

The benefits must be weighed against the potential problems that this therapy may induce. A thorough clinical examination including assessment of the patient's hydration, cardiac, renal and electrolyte status must be made before its administration. Due to the nature of a hypertonic solution the infusion results in rapid systemic diuresis, there is an increase in plasma osmolarity, circulating blood volume and central venous pressure, and hypokalaemia can occur – all of which are detrimental to those with pre-existing cardiac disease. Rapid diuresis may also result in dehydration and in some cases prerenal azotaemia and renal failure may also occur. Due to the undesirable effects of intravenous osmotic diuretics topical carbonic anhydrase inhibitors, which effectively reduce intraocular pressure, are becoming more favourable.

Oculocardio reflex

The oculocardio reflex is initiated by a stimulus to the eye such as direct pressure on the globe, manipulation of the eyelid muscles or traction of the extraocular muscles. The stimulus is transmitted via the ciliary nerves to the ophthalmic branch of the trigeminal nerve and continues to the trigeminal sensory nucleus. This continues through the visceral motor nucleus of the vagus to the vagus nerve, finally reaching the heart – initiating bradycardia and arrhythmias. Prevention of the reflex can be achieved by gentle handling of the eye. Should the reflex occur surgical manipulations are stopped. Administration of anticholinergic drugs (atropine and glycopyrrolate) act upon the vagal component of the reflex, blocking the stimulus.

The anaesthetic plan

Premedication

It is important not to premedicate before the surgeon has examined the patient on the morning of surgery. The surgeon will map out the procedure to be performed and agents that offer a sedative effect may cause enopthalmos, altering conformation of the eye and lids. This can, for example, affect the tissue removed in entropion, resulting in over- or under-correction.

Sedatives Premedicants used for sedation such as acetylpromazine and benzodiazepine provide good sedation, especially in combination with an appropriate analgesic, resulting in a relaxed patient suitable for induction.

Analgesics Ocular pain presents itself in different forms depending on the eye disease; a patient with sore irritated eyes (distichiasis or entropion) may paw or rub the head/eyes along surfaces. Foreign bodies and corneal ulcers present with acute sharp pain and again the patient may rub the head, potentially causing further damage or rupture to the globe. Glaucoma produces a dull deep pain and patients often present as stoic and withdrawn.

Pain requires prompt relief to reduce the risk of further damage; this relief may come in the form of systemic analgesia, protective dressings or collars. The partial opioid buprenorphine is a potent analgesic and is commonly used; it provides good analgesia pre- and postoperatively and has a relatively long duration of action.

Premedication with pure opioid analgesics can cause miosis and should be avoided, as should anticholinergics, which induce mydriasis. Topical control of the pupil provides the surgeon with more flexibility. Systemic NSAIDs (non-steroidal anti-inflammatory drugs) help control postoperative swelling whilst also providing analgesia.

Antibiotics Topical antibiotics are given as part of the ocular preparation to eliminate bacteria and microflora from the surgical site. Systemic prophylactic broad-spectrum antibiotics are given subcutaneously either 24 hours prior to surgery to provide optimum antibiotic blood levels during surgery or at the time of premedication. Alternatively, intravenous antibiotics are given at the time of induction.

Venous access

Hind limb venous access is preferable. Placement of a catheter into the saphenous vein requires practice; ideally the catheter is placed whilst the patient is in a standing position, as restraint in lateral recumbency often causes struggling, resulting in increased IOP. A 'T'-port extension is attached to the catheter to improve access whilst reducing the risk of dislodging the catheter. This site allows intra-operative venous access to the patient without disruption to the surgical site or surgeon. If catheter placement into the saphenous vein has not been possible in the conscious patient, cephalic catheter placement should be used for induction. Once induced it is advisable to place a catheter into the saphenous vein for access and intraoperative fluids during surgery.

Induction and maintenance of anaesthesia

Induction A smooth induction is vital. The patient must not be allowed to struggle, become excited or bark – all increase venous pressure and in turn increase intraocular pressure. Venous access via the saphenous vein comes into its own – the patient is stood calmly with its body resting against the handler, the induction agent is administered and the patient is calmly induced. The patient then relaxes into lateral recumbency.

Induction agents Induction by inhalation anaesthesia is not recommended as animals tend to struggle, thus increasing IOP and potentially cause further damage to the eye.

Anaesthesia is most commonly induced using a thiobarbiturate such as thiopentone sodium or propofol. Both provide a smooth induction, reduce IOP, and facilitate a smooth recovery. Propofol has the benefit of a smooth complete recovery with no hangover effect.

Ketamine, though infrequently used for ocular procedures, when used on its own produces nystagmus and the palpebral reflex remains strong throughout. Ketamine also produces a rough recovery from anaesthesia where the patient is disorientated and may stumble, inducing postoperative complications. When used in combination with acetylpromazine or benzodiazepines (diazepam or midazolam) these problems can be avoided. Ketamine should not be used for patients suffering perforated globe, iris prolapse, corneal foreign bodies or deep corneal ulcers – a rise in IOP would result in rupture of the globe.

Intubation Endotracheal intubation should only be attempted when the patient is in a deep enough plane of anaesthesia to allow the procedure. Attempting to intubate a lightly anaesthetised patient will result in laryngeal spasm and coughing, thus increasing intraocular pressure. Topical lignocaine can be sprayed onto the larynx before intubation. Tubes should be cut to fit the patient from mid-neck to level with the incisor teeth. Gauze bandage should be tied securely around the endotracheal tube connector, not the tube itself, to provide security. This should then be tied to either the mandible or behind the head to avoid distortion of the face and lids, which can occur if tied to the maxilla.

Airway obstructions can be difficult to detect due to the impaired access from draping and the position of the surgeon. This loss of access to the endotracheal tube and its connections with unnatural or extreme positioning of the head may result in undetected airway obstruction. Ideally armoured endotracheal tubes should be used – they are made from silicone, have a steel coiled wire embedded into the wall and do not kink when the head is flexed.

Maintenance Halothane, or more commonly isoflurane, vaporised through oxygen is used to maintain anaesthesia. Re-breathing circuits which minimise the amount of tubing and valves around the headspace of the patient are suitable e.g. Bain, Lack, Circle or modified Ayres 'T'-piece.

Central eye position

The production of a central immobile eye position is an essential requirement for corneal and intraocular surgery. Under light anaesthesia the eye is central but surgical stimulation will cause the eye to retract into the socket. A level of general anaesthesia suitable for surgical procedures produces a ventromedial rotation of the eye – limiting access to the cornea, anterior chamber and anterior segment. As the globe rotates the nictitating membrane prolapses to nearly cover the cornea and enophthalmia develops, further reducing exposure to the globe for surgery (this is exaggerated in the giant breeds). Deeper planes of anaesthesia that do produce a central

eye are associated with cardio and respiratory depression and possible arrest and cannot be recommended.

Several techniques have been developed to correct globe rotation and exposure difficulties but all carry their own risks.

Surgical techniques Surgical techniques employed to produce a central eye position involve the use of scleral clips or stay sutures, which are placed into the anterior sclera or rectus muscles and then anchored to the eyelid speculum or drapes. Sutures and mosquito forceps may be used to retract the nictitating membrane and rotate the globe dorsolaterally. These methods may cause trauma to the eye.

Local anaesthesia Local anaesthesia techniques employed are retrobulbar or regional anaesthesia – both carry their own risks as previously described.

Neuromuscular blocking agents The most reliable technique is the use of non-depolarising neuromuscular blocking agents. They produce a central immobile eye that does not vary its position with the depth of anaesthesia. On administration they produce relaxation of the extraocular muscles and the eye returns to its normal axis, facilitating surgical access. The disadvantage is that they cause paralysis of all skeletal muscle and therefore the patient must receive intermittent positive pressure ventilation either manually or mechanically. Mechanical ventilation is preferred as there is limited access to the patient's head and re-breathing bag due to the position of the patient, drapes, surgeon (seated), instrument trolley and operating microscope.

The most commonly used non-depolarising neuromuscular blocking agents (Table 2.2) are atracurium, pancuronium and vecuronium. Their onset of action is around 2 minutes and duration from 15 to 40 minutes.

A 'Train of 4' (Fig 2.6) nerve stimulator measures the depth of muscle relaxation. Due to limited access around the front of the patient the electrodes are placed over a hind-limb nerve. The nerve is stimulated four times over a period of 2 seconds and the muscle twitches; as the twitches fade this indicates the blockade is taking effect. When twitches are absent there

Table 2.2   Neuromuscular blocking agents*

Dose rate and duration of action with non-depolarising blocking agents

Agent	Dose IV mg/kg	Duration of action (mins)
Atacurium	0.5	15–80
Pancuronium	0.06–0.10	20–40
Vecuronium	0.06–0.10	15–20

*Reproduced from Seymour & Gleed 1999, with permission from BSAVA.

is complete blockade and once the twitches start to return the effects of the blockade are wearing off. If stimulation occurs during surgery further doses of neuromuscular blocking agent are required as movement of the eye would be hazardous to the surgery.

Non-depolarising blocking agents may be reversed with an acetyl cholinesterase blocking agent such as neostigmine or edrophonium and should be given at the end of surgery. These reversing agents can have undesirable side effects such as bradycardia, increased bronchial and salivary secretions and defecation, which can be blocked with the pre-administration of anticholinergic drugs such as atropine or glycopyrrolate.

Fluid therapy

The rate of fluid administration varies depending on the patient's physical status and concurrent disease; however, the following may be used as a guide. Hartmann's given at an infusion rate of 10ml/kg/h is the standard infusion rate during anaesthesia and surgery and is safe for almost all patients. Patients suffering from concurrent disease such as renal, respiratory or cardiovascular disease are at a risk of over-hydration and benefit from a slower rate of 5ml/kg/h.

Monitoring anaesthesia

Monitoring the patient's depth of anaesthesia and physiological status can be challenging due to limited access. At best only the patient's head may be draped, e.g. lid surgery. However, during corneal or intraocular surgery the front two-thirds of the patient is surrounded by drapes, the surgeon, instrument trolley, operating microscope and infusion stand with infusion pump. During cataract surgery the back third is obstructed by phacoemulsification equipment. This leaves very little access for anaesthetic monitoring equipment and the anaesthetist.

Monitoring equipment

ECG   An ECG may be useful to monitor the heart in the event of arrhythmias, catecholamines or oculocardio reflex. However, should the electrodes become disconnected during surgery they will have to remain so – attempting to reconnect them may disturb the position of the patient and therefore jeopardise the outcome of the surgery.

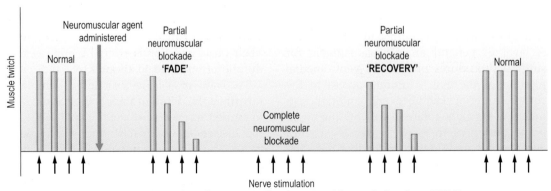

Figure 2.6   Train of 4. Reproduced from Seymour & Gleed 1999, with permission from BSAVA.

Doppler flow probe   Peripheral pulse and systemic blood pressure may be monitored using a Doppler flow probe. The Piezo crystal is placed over the coccygeal or digital pedal arteries; an audible pulse is heard and with the aid of a cuff systemic blood pressure may be monitored.

Pulse oximetry   Pulse oximeters are now commonplace in practice. They measure haemoglobin saturation and give an audible pulse. They are generally placed on the patient's tongue but are easily moved during ocular surgery; alternatively, the clip may be placed between the toes or ideally a rectal probe can be used

Train of 4 muscle stimulator   This is used to determine the degree of paralysis following administration of a non-depolarising neuromuscular blocking agent.

Temperature   Core temperature should be monitored regularly. Hypothermia is a common side effect caused by decreased muscle tone following administration of neuromuscular blocking agents along with ventilation with cold anaesthetic gases.

Regardless of the equipment and space available the following should be assessed and recorded:

- peripheral pulse should be frequently palpated
- pulse pressure – when the peripheral pulse is taken pulse pressure should be determined, giving an indication of peripheral perfusion
- capillary refill time – mucous membrane colour and capillary refill time can be taken using either the vulva or prepuce
- an oesophageal stethoscope with extension tubing can be used to auscultate the heart and monitor breathing sounds.

Recovery

Ensure that the patient has a calm and quiet environment for recovery where it can be readily observed. Avoid the patient crying, howling or barking (all of which increase intraocular pressure) and ensure that other patients recovering at the same time are also quiet. Provide a stable surface, preferably a solid non-slip floor with flat heat pad covered with a vet bed. Avoid the use of padded mattresses and hot water bottles that may increase the chance of the patient stumbling in the kennel. Do not allow the patient to recover in a disorientated manner as this will increase the risk of stumbling and banging the head or eye, resulting in postoperative complications. Sit with the patient if necessary until there is a complete recovery.

Observe for signs of patient discomfort – squinting or holding the eye closed, excessive wet discharge around the eye, pawing the eye or rubbing the head along the walls, floor or in the bedding. Give analgesics as prescribed.

Anaesthesia for the diabetic patient

A significant number of patients presented for cataract removal have diabetes mellitus that may or may not be well stabilised. Diabetic patients are controlled in a variety of ways and their regimes (Box 2.1) may be designed around their physiological status, i.e. obesity, age, concurrent illness and medication, along with the owner's lifestyle/work/family commitments.

Patients should be admitted at least one day prior to surgery to allow biochemistry and blood glucose assessment. This is particularly important when the veterinary surgeons are not those who normally care for the patient, e.g. as in a referral practice. Admitting the patient early also allows the nursing team to familiarise themselves with the patient's insulin and feeding regime – which should be adhered to as closely as possible along with any other concurrent medication.

Various anaesthetic regimes are used; the following is probably the most common.

Surgery is scheduled for first thing in the morning and short-acting agents are used where possible so that the patient returns to its normal routine whilst there are plenty of staff around to observe it. Water should not be withheld as patients are often polydypsic and can become dehydrated very quickly.

Blood glucose is measured on the early morning ward round when the surgeon examines the patient prior to surgery. The insulin dose is divided in two, the first of which is given at the time of premedication – when blood glucose is again checked.

An intravenous catheter should be placed into the cephalic vein for induction and administration of intravenous glucose saline and another into the saphenous vein to monitor blood glucose (better access during surgery). Blood glucose samples should not be taken from the catheter used to administer fluids. Blood glucose should be measured again at the time of induction and every 15 minutes until the patient recovers.

The patient is premedicated as for a normal patient. However, low-dose agents are given so that the patient is able to recover from anaesthesia and eat as soon as possible.

Short-acting intravenous anaesthetic agents should be used for induction – propofol or thiopentone sodium is suitable. However, propofol is preferred as it provides a rapid recovery with no hangover effect. Isoflurane is also preferred as a maintenance agent.

During anaesthesia the aim is to keep the blood glucose levels to the top end of or just above the normal range, around 8–16mmol/l. This can be achieved by administering an intravenous infusion of 5% glucose saline at a rate of 5–10ml/kg/h. Increasing the infusion rate of glucose saline above this in order to raise the blood glucose concentrations should be avoided as it may result in fluid overload, leading to pulmonary oedema. An infusion of hypertonic glucose should be administered to increase blood glucose concentrations.

Periods of hyperglycaemia are not detrimental to the patient – however, even a short period of hypoglycaemia could be fatal.

Once in recovery, when the patient appears able to eat it should be offered a small amount of food. Then 20–30min after it has eaten the test food, and if the patient has not vomited, it may be offered the remainder of its morning feed along with the second half of the insulin. Blood glucose should be monitored as neces-

sary and the evening feed should be given as normal. The patient's normal feeding and insulin regime should be returned to normal on the following day.

Box 2.1 Example of anaesthesia protocol for diabetic patient

Premedication
- Measure blood glucose on morning round
- Measure blood glucose on premedication
- Give half normal insulin dose

Induction
- Do as first surgery of the morning
- Measure blood glucose on induction
- If normal, use glucose saline infusion
- If low, use glucose infusion
- If high, use maintenance fluids without glucose

Maintenance
- Measure blood glucose every 15 minutes
- Adjust fluids as necessary

Postoperative
- Give small amount of food as soon as patient able to eat
- Give remainder of morning feed and second half of insulin 20–30 minutes after keeping test food down
- Give evening meal as normal
- Monitor blood glucose as necessary
- Return to normal feeding and insulin regime

SURGICAL PREPARATION

Corneal and intraocular procedures

Once the patient has been anaesthetised the eye can be prepared for surgery. The aim of surgical preparation is to eliminate microflora and potential pathogens from the surgical site to prevent postsurgical ocular infections. Corneal and intraocular surgical procedures, although most commonly unilateral, may be bilateral – as in some cataract removals or, less commonly, lens luxations.

- In a unilateral procedure the patient is placed into lateral recumbency with the surgical eye uppermost; the underside eye is protected with an ophthalmic sterile lubricant applied to the globe and eyelids and covered with a swab.
- Hair is not removed or clipped from around the eye – irritation caused by clipping may encourage the patient to rub the head postoperatively. During surgery hairs that are tiny to the naked eye appear large under magnification and obscure the surgeon's field of view.
- If the globe has been penetrated special care must be taken when handling the eye to avoid undue pressure that may rupture the globe and to prevent hair from entering into the eye and conjunctival sac.
- An absorbent pad/towel is placed under the head and a kidney dish is placed beside the head to collect the lavage fluids.
- Ocular lavage is begun using low-pressure irrigation. Sterile saline 0.9% (1–15ml) will flush out debris and reduce conjunctival bacteria. Sterile water should be avoided due to its hypotonicity; the resulting osmotic effect will draw fluid into the eye, increasing intraocular pressure.
- The cornea and conjunctival tissues are flushed twice with 1:50 povidone-iodine solution using gentle low-pressure lavage (1–15ml). Any debris within the eye should be removed using cellulose surgical spears or gauze swabs – care being taken to avoid abrading the cornea. Cotton wool should be avoided as it may shed fibres.
- 1:10 povidone-iodine solution is applied to the hair and extraocular tissues around the eye using a gauze swab.

If the procedure is to be bilateral both eyes are prepped and the underlying eye should be closed using non-stick tape (Micropore) to prevent drying out of the cornea. This is especially important in brachycephalic breeds. Once surgery has finished on the first eye, the eye should be covered with a sterile swab and the patient carefully turned. The uppermost eye is re-prepped as before, prior to head and eye being re-positioned for surgery.

Extraocular procedures

Clipping hair from around the eye is important when preparing the surgical site for extraocular surgery. The area of hair to be removed varies depending on the procedure to be performed but should exceed the area to be draped by 2cm.

- Sterile ophthalmic lubricant is placed into the conjunctival sac and across the globe to protect the eye, prevent hairs entering into the eye and assist in their removal.
- Curved scissors are coated with sterile water-soluble lubricant (e.g. KY jelly); coarse hairs, lashes, cilia or long facial hairs are removed to prevent them from entering the surgical site. The lubricant causes the hairs to stick to the scissor blades thus preventing them falling into the eye.
- To clip eyelid hair effectively and safely, the skin is gently stretched and the clippers are pushed slowly over the area against the direction of the hair growth; this allows close trimming of the hair and avoids damage to the adnexal tissues. Damage to the skin results in postoperative inflammation and oedema, which causes irritation and encourages the patient to rub the head. Small rechargeable cordless clippers are ideal for this purpose.
- After hair removal the area is flushed with sterile saline 0.9% to remove hair and debris – the ophthalmic lubricant is flushed out of the eye, taking along with it any small hairs that may have entered. The site is swabbed and gently cleansed with 1:10 povidone-iodine solution applied to gauze swabs, working in concentric circular motions starting at the eyelid margins working towards the periphery. After the eyelids have been prepped the conjunctival sac and corneal surfaces are gently irrigated with 1:50 povidone-iodine solution. Once the patient

is positioned for surgery the eyelids are finally swabbed with 1:10 povidone-iodine.

For unilateral procedures a sterile ophthalmic lubricant is applied into the conjunctival sac and across the globe to protect the eye that is not undergoing surgery.

For bilateral procedures both eyes are clipped and prepped before being positioned on the operating table, and as before the underlying eye should be closed using non-stick tape (Micropore) to prevent drying out of the cornea – especially in brachycephalic breeds. Once the first procedure is complete the patient is re-positioned and the eye re-prepped as before.

Povidone-iodine has a broad spectrum of activity and excellent tolerance of ocular tissues; however, it has a short residual activity and reduced efficacy in the presence of organic matter. Although chlorhexidine has a better residual activity and is effective in the presence of organic matter it has the potential for irritating the corneal and conjunctival tissues

Presurgical soap scrubs cannot be used in or around the eyes, as the detergent components can cause irritation, inducing corneal erosions, ulcers and chemosis – in turn stimulating the patient to rub the eye on recovery, causing self-trauma. Alcohol solutions should not be used in or around the eyes for the same reason.

Positioning

The patient's head is positioned (Fig 2.7) upon a vacuum pillow (e.g. Buster; Krusse UK). For intraocular procedures the surgeon will position the patient and operating microscope before going to scrub and gown up. While the surgeon prepares for surgery, the base brakes of the microscope must be applied and the microscope lamp switched off to prevent desiccation of the patient's corneal and adnexal surfaces.

Once the surgeon is seated, the instruments are in place (Fig 2.8) and the lamp is switched on, it is crucial that the table, patient, microscope and instrument trolley are not moved/knocked during surgery. Should this occur the

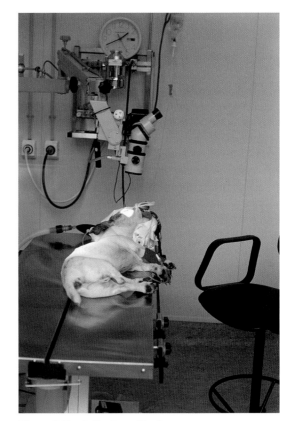

Figure 2.7   Patient positioning.

patient's eye may no longer be in the microscope's field of view and the surgeon will be required to re-position the patient and microscope then re-scrub.

THE OPERATING THEATRE

Ideally the surgical team is made up of the surgeon, scrub nurse, anaesthetist or anaesthetic nurse and circulating nurse. In practice, due to limited staff, the surgical team is usually made up of the surgeon, anaesthetist or anaesthetic nurse and circulating nurse. Each has a personal area of responsibility and they also work together as a team. However, the anaesthetist/anaesthetic nurse should not also perform the role of circulating nurse – this would seriously compromise the monitoring and thus welfare of the patient.

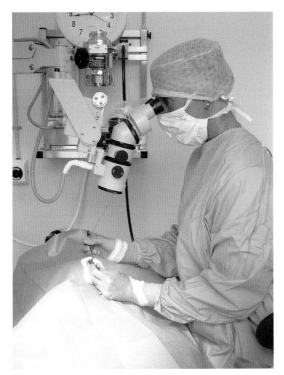

Figure 2.8 Intraoperative view: surgeon seated, using operating microscope.

The nurse's role in theatre

Circulating nurse

Surgical equipment set-up is time consuming and can even take more time than the surgery itself. It is important that the nurse has a good understanding of the ocular procedures and is familiar with the set-up of the theatre equipment and instruments required. The circulating nurse is responsible for the following:

- prepare the theatre ready for surgery
- position the table; all electrical equipment, bulbs, (operating microscope) etc require checking to ensure they are working prior to the patient being premedicated
- assist with the induction of the patient

- prepare the surgical site
- assist with the positioning of the patient and ensure that the patient's position is not moved/knocked by other theatre staff throughout the procedure
- assist the surgeon and scrub nurse with gowning
- assist during draping and connect any equipment – phacoemulsification, aspiration fluids etc
- unwrap instruments and fetch any further equipment as required
- apply foot dressings at the end of surgery
- clean and prepare theatre for subsequent surgery
- check, clean and sterilise equipment and surgical instruments.

Scrub nurse

Due to limited staffing a scrub nurse is usually not present but in some of the larger referral/teaching hospitals a scrub nurse may be used. The scrub nurse is responsible for the following:

- prepare and maintain the instrument trolley, keeping all instruments clean and tidy
- return instruments to the trolley, maintaining an unobstructed and aseptic operating field
- anticipate the needs of the surgeon (this skill comes with experience gained in assisting in ocular procedures and working with the same surgeon).

Veterinary anaesthetist/anaesthetic nurse

Patients with ocular disease that require corneal or intraocular surgery will be referred to a veterinary ophthalmologist at a referral practice/hospital. These practices generally employ a veterinary anaesthetist or an experienced veterinary nurse who holds a diploma to perform anaesthesia. Balanced anaesthesia is a key element to the successful outcome of ocular surgery and as such the anaesthetist should focus on anaesthesia alone and should not be required to assume the role of the circulating nurse. The anaesthetist or anaesthetic nurse (under direct supervision) is responsible for the following:

- ensure that all preoperative biochemistry is performed and interpreted prior to premedication
- set up and check the anaesthetic monitoring equipment, ventilator and supplies
- placement of intravenous catheters
- premedicate the patient
- induction – the patient must be induced by a veterinary surgeon so nurses will assist in this
- provide and maintain balanced anaesthesia
- provide and maintain fluid therapy
- monitor blood glucose levels in the diabetic patient
- administer non-depolarising neuromuscular blocking agents, provide intermittent positive pressure ventilation and monitor the blockade; it is usually for this purpose a veterinary anaesthetist provides anaesthesia care, as they are able to diagnose and act appropriately without disrupting the surgery
- recovery of the patient.

POSTOPERATIVE NURSING CARE AND MEDICATION

Postoperative care

Ophthalmic surgery is very delicate and prevention of self-trauma is important. Foot bandages (Fig 2.9) should always be applied prior to recovery to the corresponding forelimb and should include the toes and dew claws. This will prevent the patient from traumatising the lids and eye should any attempt be made to rub the area.

The use of Elizabethan collars is controversial and is generally dependent on the views of the surgeon and referral practice. Fitting a collar will often excite or upset the patient, who may try to remove it using the paws or by shaking the head, resulting in increased venous pressure and hence intraocular pressure. This upset increases the risk of the head or eye being knocked, causing postoperative complications, inflammation,

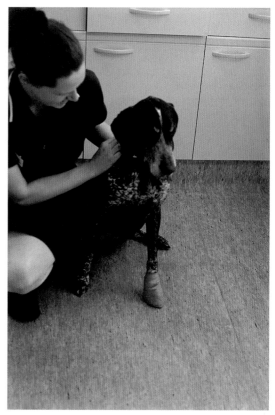

Figure 2.9   Foot bandage.

and potentially rupturing the sutures or even the globe if the collar is pulled off.

Regardless of whether the collar is fitted before or after recovery from anaesthesia the patient should always be sat with until you are confident that they have accepted the collar. Care must be taken to select an Elizabethan collar that fits appropriately – it must not be so tight around the neck that it restricts blood flow and increases intraocular pressure. The collar may need some modification – it should extend a couple of inches past the nose and should not flare out too much. A collar that is too wide will cause the patient to bump into furniture and doorways etc – especially important for a patient who has undergone surgery for cataract removal and will only have limited guidance vision for some weeks after the surgery.

The patient should be kennelled in a quiet area, kept calm and not allowed to bark or jump up; if this becomes a problem the patient may require sedation. All kennel surfaces including the door should be flat; a soft bed should be provided (no wicker or plastic beds) with no toys. Bowls should be shallow and kept in the same place.

It is inadvisable to take postoperative rectal temperature unless the patient is unwell – if this upsets the patient intraocular pressure may increase.

Avoid handling the patient's head except during the application of medication and observe for changes in shape or colour of the globe. Ocular discharge or wetness around the eye may be indicative of an aqueous leak.

Postoperative medication

Postoperative medication requires organisation and the medication record needs to be clear to all staff involved in the patient's aftercare. Medication comprises oral analgesics and antibiotics and a combination of topical mydriatics, steroids and antibiotics. Most patients tolerate their postoperative medication; in fact surgery generally provides enormous relief – especially for those with entropion or ectopic cilia. Do not struggle with a patient intolerant of medication but question why – often this is due to discomfort and further analgesia may be required. Postoperative analgesia should always be administered to ensure the patient is comfortable. The uncomfortable patient will not settle, may squint or hold the eye closed, rub or paw the head or become inappetent. An analgesic that offers a mild sedative effect such as buprenorphine often settles a fractious patient.

If antibiotics and analgesics are prescribed for oral administration ensure that they are swallowed – if not, inject under instruction. Some topical drops require refrigeration once opened and should be stored accordingly. Chilled drops may cause discomfort and others that are prescribed postoperatively (e.g. Ocufen) can cause mild irritation – it may be

necessary to sit with the patient for a couple of minutes following treatment. Atropine drops often leave a bitter taste and cause salivation that can become disconcerting to the patient, especially cats – the prescribing surgeon should be notified and atropine ointment may be prescribed as an alternative.

Postoperative complications

There are a number of conditions to be aware of that may cause postoperative complications after intraocular surgery.

- Uveitis. The uvea is made up of the iris and ciliary body (referred to as the anterior uvea) and choroid (the posterior uvea). Uveitis is inflammation of the uveal tract and can occur postoperatively due to over-manipulation of the chamber during surgery or as a result of inadequate preoperative medication. It can also be as a result of inadequate preparation of the surgical site or poor aseptic technique.
- Glaucoma. This is an increase in intraocular pressure, caused by excitement, crying, coughing or barking preoperatively, on induction or recovery from anaesthesia, or whilst being hospitalised.
- Secondary glaucoma. Occlusion of the drainage angle results in the restriction of aqueous flow and an increase in intraocular pressure. Occlusion can be due to a dilated iris, hyphaema (haemorrhage into the anterior chamber), or fibrin clots.
- Aqueous leak. An increase in intraocular pressure can cause pressure and tension on the sutures, resulting in leaking aqueous. If the leak does not seal there is a chance that the anterior chamber may collapse, causing permanent blindness.
- Dehiscence. Infection or wound breakdown due to inadequate surgical preparation of the eye, poor aseptic technique or aftercare.
- Corneal oedema. Usually due to over-manipulation of the chamber.
- Retinal detachment.

Discharge

On discharge the owner should be advised of oral and topical medication, including how to handle and store them. They should be shown how to medicate their pet effectively. Most topical medications are stored in opaque bottles, making it difficult to know when they are getting low. As a guide, 1ml yields approximately 20 drops, therefore a 5ml bottle contains 100 drops – a patient prescribed one drop into each eye every 12 hours will have sufficient medication to last approximately 25 days for bilateral and 50 days for unilateral.

Present the owner with a discharge sheet (Sheet 2.2). Explain how postoperative care differs from that of general surgery. Regardless of the type of ophthalmic surgery 'minimal lead exercise' should only be allowed until advised otherwise by the veterinary surgeon. Owners should guide the pet, always taking extra care when walking through doorways and climbing up or down steps. Patients who have undergone cataract extraction should still continue lead exercise even when guidance vision has returned. It may be several weeks before the surgical site has completely healed. Exercise in wet or windy weather should be avoided. If a mydriatic has been prescribed, owners should avoid taking the patient out immediately afterwards or in strong sunlight – the patient will be unable to constrict the pupil, which can be quite uncomfortable (photophobic). Advise the owner to avoid walking the pet in long grass, near trees or bushes and not to leave it unattended in the garden.

SURGICAL EQUIPMENT AND TECHNIQUES

Ophthalmic surgical instruments

Ophthalmic tissues are delicate and require the use of instruments specifically designed for ophthalmic surgery – instruments designed for general surgeries are not suitable and would cause tissue trauma. Ophthalmic instruments (Boxes 2.2, 2.3, 2,4; Figs 2.10, 2.11) should not be used for any other purpose and ideally should be divided into those suitable for adnexal tissue surgery (extraocular kit) or microfine instruments suitable for corneal and intraocular surgery (intraocular kit).

Instruments have a matt finish to prevent glare and have been designed for a specific purpose. Instruments should be used for that purpose alone – failure to do so will either result in damage to the delicate ocular tissues or damage to the instrument itself.

Drapes

Draping for adnexal surgery comprises the standard use of cloth field drapes that are positioned around the eye and held with towel clips. For corneal and intraocular procedures ophthalmic drapes are applied; they are purpose made disposable drapes that have a fluid resistant backing – an adhesive area where an appropriately sized fenestration can be cut then applied to the skin. Adhesive drapes prevent the drape from moving, stop penetration from moisture and bacteria and prevent fine loose hairs from falling into the operating field. Specifically designed adhesive drapes with fluid catch-bags are used for phacoemulsification procedures.

Illumination

Ophthalmic surgery is performed in a semi-darkened room with a focal light to reduce reflections. For extraocular procedures a standard operating light is suitable but for corneal or intraocular procedures a focal or head mounted light source that generates minimal heat is required to limit desiccation of delicate ocular tissue.

Magnification

Procedures that involve cilia or puncta require magnification – magnifying loupes (Figs 2.12, 2.13) with interchangeable lenses of different magnification are suitable for such surgery. For corneal or intraocular surgery an operating microscope is essential and the light intensity of the operating microscope should be adequate for the procedure. When the surgeon is not working on the eye the cornea should be

Sheet 2.2 – Discharge sheet

POSTOPERATIVE EYE CARE SHEET

AFTERCARE SHEET FOR .... DATE ....

Your pet has undergone surgery for an eye condition. These instructions are designed as a guide for caring for your pet in the postoperative period. It is important that you follow them closely since attention to detail can make the difference between success or failure of the operation undertaken.

    Make sure that a warm bed is provided away from disturbance from people or other pets. It is important that your pet is kept relatively quiet for several days or even weeks following the surgery. This means that dogs should have lead exercise and cats should be kept indoors with a litter tray provided. You will be given specific advice for your pet, but stick to these instructions unless informed otherwise.

OPERATION SITE
Handle the eye(s) as little as possible, gently clean away any discharge with damp cotton wool and apply treatment if dispensed. If the area is causing irritation, looks sore or is discharging excessively please seek veterinary advice immediately. If you have been supplied with an Elizabethan collar use it. Some patients have foot bandages instead to prevent self-trauma from rubbing – the nurse will give you instructions about keeping these dry and how often they need to be changed.

STITCHES
Most sutures in and around the eye are soluble so do not need removing – however on occasion they may need removing after 10–14 days.

MEDICATION
Dispensed ☐   Not dispensed ☐

Ointment / Drops – Apply to the LEFT / RIGHT / BOTH EYE(s) as follows

.... to be applied .... times daily for .... days/until re-exam

.... to be applied .... times daily for .... days/until re-exam

.... to be applied .... times daily for .... days/until re-exam

Always leave 5 minutes between different drops and apply before ointment if you have both

Tablets

.... to be given .... times daily for .... days

.... to be given .... times daily for .... days

.... to be given .... times daily for .... days

Comments

Re-examination

Box 2.2   Intraocular surgical kit

■ Beaver blade handle
■ St Martins rat toothed tying forceps
■ Adson fine plain tissue forceps
■ Colibri corneal forceps
■ Utrata capsularhexis forceps
■ Intraocular lens forceps
■ Vannus scissors
■ Iris scissors
■ Castroviejo corneal scissors
■ Castroviejo conjunctival scissors
■ Halstead curved mosquito haemostat
■ Halstead straight mosquito haemostat
■ Castroviejo needle holder
■ Castroviejo lid speculum
■ Barraquer eyelid speculum
■ Snellens vectis – lens loop
■ Iris repositor
■ Irrigating cannula
■ 5 × 5cm swabs
■ Cellulose sponges
■ Saline bowl

Box 2.4   Equipment required for cataract extraction by phacoemulsification

■ Operating microscope
■ Phacoemulsification machine
■ Phacoemulsification handpiece
■ Irrigation aspiration handpiece
■ Manifold set
■ Intraocular surgical kit
■ Sterile disposable drape for the patient
■ Ophthalmic drape with fluid catch bag
■ Insulin syringe
■ 8-0 Vicryl
■ Pointed Beaver blade No 65
■ Viscoelastic agent
■ Irrigation aspiration fluids
■ Intraocular lens

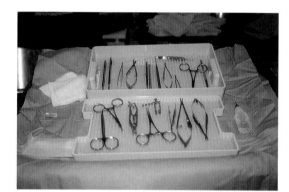

Figure 2.10   Examples of ophthalmic surgical kits.

Box 2.3   Extraocular surgical kit

■ Beaver blade handle
■ Paragon blade handle
■ St Martins rat-toothed forceps
■ Adson rat-toothed forceps
■ Adson fine plain tissue forceps
■ Von Graefes fixation forceps
■ Cilia forceps
■ Tenotomy scissors
■ Strabismus scissors
■ Halstead curved haemostat forceps
■ Halstead straight haemostat forceps
■ Castroviejo lid speculum
■ Desmarres chalazion clamp
■ Towel clips
■ Lacrimal cannula
■ 5cm × 5cm swabs
■ Cellulose sponges
■ Saline bowl

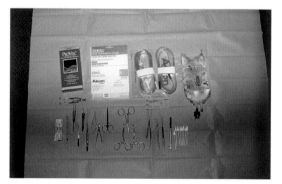

Figure 2.11   Examples of ophthalmic surgical kits.

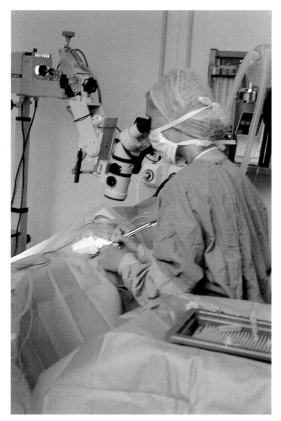

Figure 2.12   Operating microscope.

covered or the light source turned down or off to prevent desiccation of the delicate tissues and prevent retinal phototoxicity – a potentially serious complication, which can occur due to prolonged exposure to the bright microscope light source.

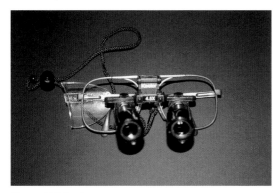

Figure 2.13   Loupes.

Haemostasis

Control of haemostasis in ophthalmic surgery includes mosquito haemostats, pressure with a gauze swab or cellulose sponges. The use of sterile cotton-tipped applicators (cotton buds) is not recommended because of the danger of cotton strands entering the eye.

Scalpel blades

- Paragon surgical handle with either a No 11 or No 15 blade – for lid surgery
- Beaver Blade Handle with either a No 64 or No 65 disposable blade – most commonly used in corneal and intraocular surgery to incise the cornea, limbus and sclera
- Keratome – used to incise the cornea and anterior capsule in cataract extraction
- Diamond Knives – extremely sharp reusable blades for corneal, limbal and scleral incisions.

Suture materials and needles

Suture material (Table 2.3) needs a minimum amount of tensile strength to hold the tissue securely and should last long enough in the tissue for the incision to heal by first intention. It needs to be well tolerated and the thickness of the suture material dictates the extent of tissue reaction. Braided sutures increase strength and knot security and the ends are softer than those of monofilament suture. Absorbable braided sutures are used for most procedures to eliminate the need for suture removal; nonabsorbable nylon or silk may be used in lid surgery. Suture needles need to be strong enough so as not to bend, yet be as atraumatic as possible for delicate ocular tissue. Suture material should be swaged on for this purpose.

Irrigating solutions

For preoperative preparation sterile saline may be used to flush the eye. During surgery, balanced salt solution is preferred to prevent drying of corneal and conjunctival surfaces as it causes less osmotic damage to the corneal epithelium. During phacoemulsification continuous intraocular irrigation is required and

Table 2.3   Ophthalmic suture material

Ocular tissue	Suture material	Suture size*	Suture type	Needle
Cornea	Polyglactin 910 (Vicryl)	6-0, 8-0, 10-0	Absorbable braided	Spatula tipped
Sclera	Polyglactin 910	6-0, 8-0	Absorbable braided	Spatula tipped or reverse cutting
Conjunctiva	Polyglactin 910	5-0, 6-0	Absorbable braided	Tapercut
Lids	Polyglactin 910	4-0, 6-0	Absorbable braided	Reverse cutting
	Nylon	4-0, 6-0	Non-absorbable Monofilament or pseudo monofilament	
	Silk	4-0, 6-0	Non absorbable	

*8-0 and 10-0 requires magnification

the following are added to a 500ml bag of Hartmann's solution:

- 500iu heparin – controls fibrin formation
- 1ml adrenaline 1:1000 – maintains pupil dilation and aids haemostasis
- 10ml sodium bicarbonate – protects corneal endothelium.

Viscoelastic substances

Viscoelastic substances are placed into the anterior chamber to:

- retain its shape during surgery
- prevent contact of intraocular tissues
- protect the corneal endothelium
- control small vessel haemorrhage
- facilitate intraocular lens insertion.

Intraocular lenses

Synthetic intraocular lenses (Fig 2.14) may be implanted in the remaining capsular bag after the cataract has been removed by extracapsular extraction or phacoemulsification. Lenses help to stabilise the internal structures by filling space left by the removal of the lens They are well tolerated in the canine eye and allow clear images to be seen on the retina.

Phacoemulsification

Phacoemulsification (Fig 2.15) is a technique whereby the cataract material is broken down

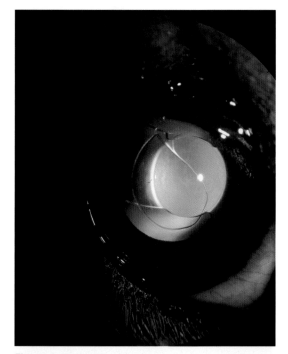

Figure 2.14   Intraocular lens.

and liquefied by ultrasonic energy, with simultaneous irrigation and aspiration. It can be used for most cataracts. The advantage of this method is the minute 3mm incision as opposed to the 15mm incision required for the extracapsular method of cataract removal. With phacoemulsification there is less manipulation of the chamber intraoperatively, thereby reduc-

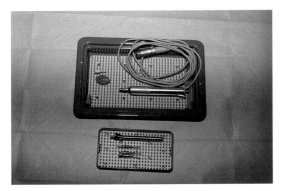

Figure 2.15   Phacoemulsification handpiece.

ing postoperative inflammation and further complications.

Cryosurgery

Cryotherapy (Fig 2.16) is used for the selective destruction of neoplasms, removal of luxated lenses, treatment of distichiasis, and destruction of ciliary bodies in the treatment of glaucoma. General cryosurgery units that use liquid nitrogen can be used for adnexal procedures to treat distichiasis and periocular tumours, but for intraocular procedures an ophthalmic cryosurgical unit cooled by nitrous oxide is preferred.

Electrolysis

Permanent destruction of distichia may be achieved by electrolysis. The procedure is performed using a commercial electroepilation unit – the needle electrode is placed into the eyelid alongside the shaft of the cilia and the current is turned on for 5–10 seconds so as to destroy the follicle; the cilia is then plucked. This method can be very time consuming and the owner should be warned that the cilia might grow back. Diathermy or electrocautery units should not be used for depilation as they may result in severe necrosis of the eyelids

Electrocautery

Electrocautery units have limited use in ophthalmic surgery. They are primarily used to coagulate blood vessels; they are not used for cutting ocular tissue as they may penetrate more deeply than expected. Small electrocautery units are adequate and safe for ophthalmic surgery. Hand-held battery-powered units that provide wet-field cautery are useful – they are effective in the presence of blood and do not require patient grounding. Batteries must be removed before sterilisation and replaced before surgery.

Laser therapy

Although there are many types of lasers used in human medicine there are fewer used in veterinary ophthalmology. The laser most commonly used is the semiconductor diode laser (Fig 2.17). It is a compact unit, emitting light in the near infrared range, which is absorbed by melanin-containing tissues

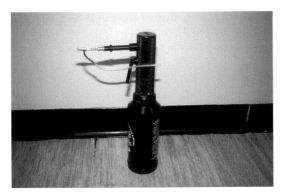

Figure 2.16   Liquid nitrogen cryosurgical unit.

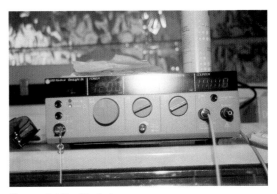

Figure 2.17   Diode laser.

resulting in coagulation necrosis. They are used for trans-scleral cyclophotocoagulation in the treatment of glaucoma, in the treatment of iris tumours and iris cysts, and in retinopexy (i.e. retinal reattachment).

Care and sterilisation of ophthalmic instruments

Ophthalmic instruments are delicate precision tools and require special care. They should be laid out flat and not grouped to be soaked in instrument cleaner as soon as they are finished with. They should be individually wiped to remove organic material – scrubbing can damage the delicate blades and tips so should be avoided. Ultrasonic cleaners may be used but instruments need to be laid out in the baskets so that they do not touch each other as this can also cause damage to the blades and tips. If an ultrasonic cleaner is used, instruments with moving parts will require lubrication. They should be rinsed then air-dried to minimise the risk of damage from towels. Instruments should be examined regularly for signs of blunting or damage and tubular silicone protective cuffs should be applied to all delicate ends. Ideally instruments should be placed into rubber matted ophthalmic instrument trays for sterilising and storage.

Methods of sterilisation commonly used are ethylene oxide and autoclaving. Ethylene oxide is least damaging to the instruments but toxic to tissues so instrument packs must be aired for 48 hours before use – this may make it impractical in a busy ophthalmic referral practice where there is a high turnover of instruments. Autoclaving is most commonly used and steam sterilisation will damage the fine tips and blades due to the high temperature and pressure of the process. To limit the damage it is advisable to autoclave at a lower temperature – 121°C porous load cycle.

Acknowledgements

The author would like to thank Sally Turner, MRCVS, for her assistance in writing the chapter, for the use of images and for the preoperative and postoperative medication sheets.

GLOSSARY

Adnexa – Lids, orbit, lacrimal system, conjunctiva, third eyelid
Anisocoria – Pupils of uneven size
Aphakia – Absence of the lens
Blepharitis – Inflammation of the eyelids
Blepharospasm – Spasm of the eyelids (squinting)
Buphthalmos – Enlargement of the globe
Chemosis – Oedema of the conjunctiva
Dehiscence – Breakdown of the sutures at the site of incision
Desiccation – Extreme drying of the tissues
Dyscoria – Abnormally shaped pupils
Enophthalmos – Sunken globe
Exophthalmos – Protrusion of the globe
Epiphora – Tear overflow
Aqueous flare – Increased protein of the aqueous
Hyperaemia – Increased redness e.g. in the conjunctiva
Hyphema – Blood in the anterior chamber
Hypopyon – White cells in the anterior chamber (resembles pus)
Intumescent – Becoming swollen
Miosis – Constriction of the pupil
Mydriasis – Dilation of the pupil
Microphakia – Abnormally small lens
Proptosis – Forward displacement of the globe

Further reading

Brearley J C 1999 Ophthalmic surgery. In: Seymour C, Gleed R (eds) Manual of small animal anaesthesia and analgesia. British Small Animal Veterinary Association, Cheltenham

Colitz C M H 2003 Eye and adnexa. In: Slatter D (ed) Textbook of small animal surgery. W B Saunders, New York
Gellatt K N, Gelalt J P 1994 Handbook of small

animal ophthalmic surgery. Volume 1:
extraocular procedures. Butterworth-
Heinemann, Oxford

Gellatt K N, Gelatt J P 1995 Handbook of small
animal ophthalmic surgery. Volume 2: corneal
and intraocular procedures. Butterworth-
Heinemann, Oxford

Johnson C 1999 Endocrine disease surgery. In:
Seymour C, Gleed R (eds) Manual of small
animal anaesthesia and analgesia. British Small
Animal Veterinary Association, Cheltenham

McKelvey D, Hollingshead W K 1994 Small animal
anaesthesia: canine and feline practice (Mosby's
fundamentals of veterinary technology). C V
Mosby, St Louis

Petersen-Jones S, Crispin S (eds) 2002 Manual of
small animal ophthalmology, 2nd edn. British
Small Animal Veterinary Association,
Cheltenham

Seymour C, Gleed R (eds) 1999 Manual of small
animal anaesthesia and analgesia. British Small
Animal Veterinary Association, Cheltenham

Tracy D L 1994 Small animal surgical nursing
(Mosby's fundamentals of veterinary
technology), 2nd edn. C V Mosby, St Louis

Wingfield W E 2000 Part IV: Ophthalmic
emergencies. In: Veterinary emergency medicine
secrets, 2nd edn. Hanley & Belfus, Philadelphia

Chapter 3

Surgery of the abdominal cavity

Arthur House

Surgery of the abdominal cavity is a common procedure and is performed for a number of reasons. A celiotomy is an incision into the abdominal cavity, though the term laparotomy is frequently used. Laparotomy technically refers to a flank incision as used in large animal abdominal surgery. Abdominal surgery may be indicated for diagnostic reasons, therapeutic reasons or for elective procedures such as ovariohysterectomy and elective gastropexy. In many circumstances abdominal surgery is performed on animals with chronic disease, though some patients require abdominal surgery for acute life-threatening disease. The success of abdominal surgery is dependent on an accurate diagnosis prior to performing a procedure, careful postoperative monitoring and patient care, sufficient knowledge of each disease process to anticipate potential complications and the ability to manage complications arising as a consequence of the disease or the surgical procedure.

The decision to perform abdominal surgery should be based on history, physical examination and ancillary diagnostic tests such as radiography, ultrasonography and laboratory analysis of bodily fluids. Patients with abdominal disease may present with non-specific clinical signs and history. Physical examination can be inaccurate in both predicting severity of disease and duration of disease, consequently ancillary diagnostic techniques are vital to aid surgical decision making.

ANATOMY

The abdomen extends from the diaphragm to the pelvis, the abdominal muscles and 8th to 13th ribs form the lateral and ventral walls and the vertebral column and musculature form the dorsal wall. The abdomen is continuous with the pelvic canal, with the transition from abdomen to pelvic canal occurring at the pelvic inlet. The abdominal cavity is lined by the peritoneal lining, termed the parietal peritoneum, which in dogs and cats is a thin transparent lining, unlike in humans in which it is a grossly identifiable structure. The peritoneal lining also covers abdominal organs, and here it is termed the visceral peritoneum.

The abdominal cavity may also be referred to as the peritoneal cavity, though these two terms are not strictly interchangeable. In the clinical setting the abdominal cavity is frequently divided into four quadrants by one transverse and one sagittal line – creating cranial right, cranial left, caudal right and caudal left quadrants. Another clinical description are the paravertebral gutters, which refers to the trough-like regions viewed from a ventral midline abdominal incision in the dorsal abdomen either side of the vertebral column. Fluid frequently accumulates during abdominal surgery in the paravertebral gutters, making them an ideal location from which to aspirate lavage or peritoneal fluid.

The retroperitoneal space refers to regions in the abdominal cavity outside the peritoneal cavity. Organs in the retroperitoneal space are covered on only one surface by parietal peritoneum. They include kidneys, ureter, aorta, adrenal glands, lumbar lymph nodes and vena cava.

The abdominal wall consists of the transverse, internal abdominal oblique, external abdominal oblique and the rectus abdominus muscles. The external oblique muscle is the most superficial and arises from the lateral surface of the ribs and from lumbar fascia; its fibres run caudoventrally. The internal abdominal oblique is immediately beneath the external abdominal oblique and arises mainly from the tuber coxae, the thoracolumbar fascia and the transverse processes of the lumbar vertebrae; its fibres run predominantly ventrocranially. The deepest muscle, the transverse abdominal, arises from the inner surfaces of the last ribs and the transverse processes of the lumbar spine; its fibres run transversely.

Fibres of the transverse abdominal, internal and external abdominal oblique muscles converge in the midline to form the fibrous linea alba. The linea alba is more obvious and developed in the cranial abdomen compared to the caudal abdomen. The rectus abdominus muscle forms a broad band to each side of the linea alba. It arises from the sternum and inserts on the pubic brim. The external abdominal oblique aponeurosis is always external to the rectus abdominus but the internal abdominal oblique is either internal or external depending on the location in a cranial-to-caudal plane.

On entering the abdominal cavity from a midline abdominal incision the first organ encountered is the omentum. The greater omentum consists of two layers of 'leafs' or sheets that extend from the greater curvature of the stomach, covering the duodenum, jejunum and ileum ventrally (Fig 3.1). Between the ventral and dorsal sheets of the greater

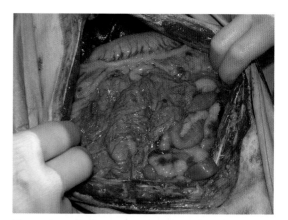

Figure 3.1 An intraoperative view of a ventral midline celiotomy in a dog. The omentum is extending from the greater curvature of the stomach, ventral and covering the small intestines. Notice that the liver occupies the cranial abdomen. This patient is suffering from peritonitis, which is causing the omentum to have increased vascularity. Photograph © Arthur House.

omentum is a cavity referred to as the omental bursa. The lesser omentum extends from the lesser curvature of the stomach, cranially to the hilus of the liver.

The liver is positioned cranially against the diaphragm, often covered by the last ribs. The liver consists of six lobes, left lateral and left medial on the left, quadrate lobe central with the gallbladder closely associated with it, right medial and lateral lobe on the right. The caudate lobe, which consists of the caudate and papillary processes, lies transversely and is the most caudally positioned. The right lateral liver lobe and the vena cava obscure the right kidney and adrenal gland; the left lateral liver lobe is dorsal to the left kidney and adrenal gland.

The stomach is immediately caudal to the liver with the ileum occupying the mid abdomen. The duodenum is positioned on the right and the descending colon on the left. The transverse colon is ventrally positioned and immediately caudal to the stomach. The pancreas is an L-shaped organ with the right or duodenal limb closely associated with the duodenum and the left or gastric limb in close association with the greater curvature of the stomach. The spleen is predominantly positioned on the left but can extend across the midline ventrally if engorged. The bladder is caudally located, extending into the pelvic canal in many animals.

INSTRUMENTATION FOR ABDOMINAL SURGERY

Appropriate instrumentation facilitates successful abdominal surgery. The basic surgical pack should include as a minimum multiple (6–8) straight or curved fine Halstead mosquito haemostatic forceps, large haemostatic forceps such as Rochester-Carmalt or Kelly haemostats, DeBakey or Brown-Adson tissue forceps, straight and curved Mayo dissecting scissors, curved Metzenbaum scissors, scalpel handle, Mayo-Hegar or Olsen-Hegar needle holders and four Backhaus towel clamps. In addition to the basic surgical kit, abdominal retractors are essential to achieve thorough

abdominal exploration. Abdominal retractors frequently used are Balfour and Gosset self-retaining retractors (Figs 3.2, 3.3). Suction to remove lavage and abdominal fluid is equally essential as it not only improves visibility but also facilitates reducing abdominal contamination. The Poole suction tip is the most suitable for abdominal surgery.

Large waterproof drapes that cover the entire patient are recommended as abdominal surgery frequently involves large volumes of fluid and exteriorisation of abdominal organs (Fig 3.4). Large radiopaque abdominal swabs (10 inch × 10 inch) as well as standard sized (4 inch × 4 inch) radiopaque swabs are frequently useful. All swab packs should be counted on opening the packs. Swab counts on the completion of surgery should be performed to ensure that no swabs are left in the abdomen. Radiopaque swabs allow identification of a retained swab if necessary. Large volumes of warm lavage solution are used during abdominal surgery. Isotonic saline is the lavage solution of choice. Lavage solution should be bought in bottles of isotonic saline for lavage instead of using intravenous fluid bags as the bottles allow easy and aseptic pouring (Fig 3.5).

Additional instrumentation that enhances surgery is extensive but includes Doyen bowel clamps, monopolar or bipolar diathermy, large bowls to hold lavage fluid, hand-held retrac-

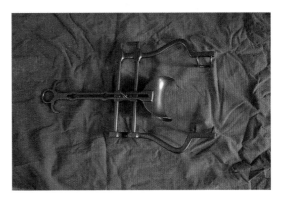

Figure 3.2   Balfour abdominal retractors. The large detachable 'blade' is positioned cranially under the xiphoid to help stabilise the retractors on the abdominal wall. Photograph © Arthur House.

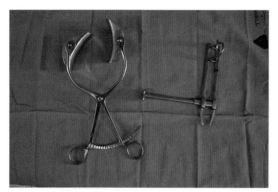

Figure 3.3   Posse abdominal retractors (left) and Gosset abdominal retractors (right). Both are useful in small dogs and cats but tend to not provide sufficient retraction in large dogs. Photograph © Arthur House.

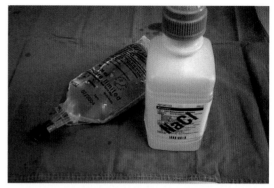

Figure 3.5   An intravenous fluid bag (left) and isotonic fluid in a bottle manufactured for use in theatre as lavage solution. The bottle allows easy pouring which reduces the risk of breaks in aseptic technique. Photograph © Arthur House.

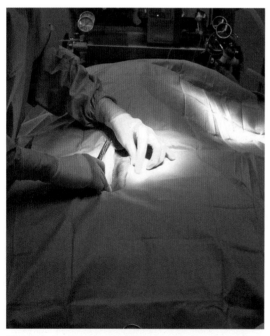

Figure 3.4   A waterproof drape covering the entire patient is recommended to maximise aseptic technique, particularly in abdominal surgery where abdominal organs are frequently exteriorised and copious amounts of lavage fluid are used. This is a male dog – the penis has been reflected laterally to remove it from the surgical field. Photograph © Arthur House.

tors such as Army-Navy retractors, Allis tissue forceps and endo surgical stapling devices.

ABDOMINAL SURGERY

The abdominal wall and celiotomy

A ventral midline celiotomy is the standard approach to the abdomen. The skin incision in many cases may have to extend from the xiphoid to the pubis. Consequently the surgical field that is prepared should begin cranial to the xiphoid, extend caudal to the pubis and lateral to the skin folds of both the fore and hind limbs. The patient is clipped and the skin aseptically prepared as discussed in Chapter 9. The patient is positioned in dorsal recumbency on the surgery table and stabilised with in a trough, with sandbags or ties from the limbs.

Circulating warm water blankets or BAIR huggers are essential to maintain the patient core body temperature, as heat is rapidly lost via the abdominal cavity. Electric blankets should be avoided due to the risk of accidental burns to the patient. Intravenous fluid bags heated in a microwave, used as warming devices, should be carefully monitored to avoid excessively hot bags been placed against the patient.

The celiotomy incision aims to incise through the linea alba, avoiding the muscles either side. In male dogs the penis does not prevent a ventral midline approach to the abdomen. A parapreputial skin incision is performed, the penis reflected and then the abdomen entered through a standard ventral midline incision. In dogs and cats a paramedian incision is rarely indicated and is performed by incising through the abdominal musculature parallel to the linea alba. Increased bleeding and potentially increased postoperative morbidity is observed wih paramedial incisions compared to the ventral midline incision.

Accurate closure of abdominal incisions is vital as the complication of incisional dehiscence is severe, with potential for abdominal organ herniation. The midline incision is closed in three layers – rectus abdominus and associated linea alba, subcutaneous tissue and lastly skin. Closure of the peritoneal lining is not required as serosal defects heal rapidly and it does not increase the tensile strength of the closure. Placement of sutures lateral to the transition between the linea alba and the rectus abdominus musculature is recommended. Sutures placed lateral to the transition between the rectus abdominus muscle and linea alba compared to the linea alba alone have approximately twice the pull-out strength. In the cranial abdomen both the internal and external sheath of the rectus abdominus should be included in the closure. In the caudal abdomen closure of the external rectus abdominus sheath is adequate.

Abdominal wall closure can be performed with either simple interrupted or simple continuous suture patterns. If simple continuous patterns are used then an adequate number of throws must be used on each knot for the suture material used. An absorbable suture with long to moderate duration of tensile strength is recommended. Commonly used suture materials are Polydioxanone and Polyglactin 910. Suture materials with rapid loss of tensile strength such as Poliglecaprone 25 and Polyglytone 6211 are not recommended for closure of the abdominal wall. Surgical catgut is unreliable, particularly as a continuous suture.

Both flank and paracostal approaches to the abdomen do not provide general access to the entire abdomen and have very specific indications. The flank approach is commonly used to access the uterus and ovaries in cats when performing ovariohysterectomy. The approach is made through the three muscles – external abdominal oblique, internal abdominal oblique and transverse abdominal. Each muscle is incised in the direction of their fibres, resulting in a grid incision that is shorter than the skin incision. The paracostal approach to the abdomen is virtually restricted to adrenalectomies in dogs (Fig 3.6). In rare circumstances a paracostal incision may be combined with a ventral midline incision to improve exposure of cranial abdominal organs. Closure of both flank and paracostal incisions is achieved by simple continuous sutures in each layer of muscle with an absorbable suture material.

Postoperative care for animals following celiotomy is largely dependent on the intra-abdominal procedures performed. Pre-emptive planning to facilitate invasive and non-invasive monitoring, enteral nutrition and pre-emptive analgesia combined with careful regular evaluation of both subjective and objective parameters optimises the care of the postoperative patient. Patients recovering from severe abdominal diseases such as peritonitis generally require intensive care.

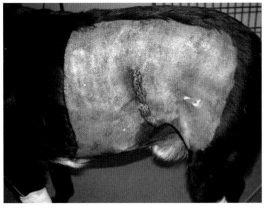

Figure 3.6 A typical incision following a paracostal approach to the abdomen. This dog has undergone a right-sided adrenalectomy. Photograph © Arthur House.

For all approaches to the abdomen the surgical wound is monitored for discharge and erythema. Complications following celiotomy include postoperative wound infection, seroma formation and incisional dehiscence. Midline celiotomies are considered to be at higher risk of developing seromas and abdominal wall dehiscence than a flank or paracostal celiotomies. If a seroma does develop postoperatively, careful evaluation of the swelling should be performed to differentiate a seroma from abdominal wall dehiscence with organ herniation. Management of a seroma should include exercise restriction and, in large seromas, drainage. Repeated drainage is avoided and if performed is done in an aseptic manner with a needle and syringe. Antibiotics are only indicated in the management of seromas if there is evidence of secondary infection.

All animals require a minimum of opiate analgesia postoperatively following a celiotomy. Provision of adequate analgesia is essential for both the welfare of the animal and to avoid the adverse physiological affects of persistent pain. Persistent pain is associated with immune suppression, delayed wound healing and increased tissue catabolism. Each patient should have an analgesia strategy that is pre-emptive and multimodal. Epidurals or regional anaesthesia, systemic opioids and non-steroidal anti-inflammatory drugs (NSAIDs) pre-emptively and systemic opioids and NSAIDs postoperatively is ideal. The duration of opiate analgesia is dependent on the individual's recovery. NSAIDs are used with caution in critically ill animals due to their multiple potential adverse side effects. Opiate choice and dose may be affected by cardiovascular function in the individual patient.

Abdominal exploration

There is no indication or justification for performing an exploratory celiotomy without some knowledge of what disease process may be occurring or without the intent to perform biopsies for the purpose of achieving a diagnosis. An exploratory celiotomy is not a substitute for a full diagnostic investigation and should only be performed when the initial investigation indicates a need for collection of biopsy samples of abdominal organs or surgical intervention to control a disease process occurring in the abdomen.

For thorough surgical abdominal exploration a ventral midline incision is made in the abdomen extending from the xiphoid to the pubis. Excision of the falciform fat may help visualisation of the cranial abdomen. In addition, a paracostal incision may rarely facilitate removal of large cranial abdominal masses. The use of suction to remove free fluid, and abdominal retractors such as Balfour or Gosset retractors are essential to achieve adequate exposure and visualisation of all organs.

Exploration of the abdomen must be performed in a systematic manner, utilising the consistent location of each organ between each individual. Thorough exploration of the abdomen is essential for identification of all abdominal pathology. The author's preference is to start the exploration in the cranial abdomen and progress caudally, systematically evaluating all organs. Reflection of the left lateral and medial liver lobes towards the right with caudal retraction of the fundus of the stomach and spleen reveals the gastric cardia and abdominal oesophagus, left aspect of the diaphragm, cranial pole of the left kidney and left adrenal. The quadrate, right medial, right lateral, and caudate and papillary processes of the caudate lobe are inspected visually and gently palpated. The gallbladder, cystic and common bile ducts should be carefully evaluated. The ability to express the gallbladder does not necessarily demonstrate patency of the common bile duct since reflux of bile into the hepatic ducts can also lead to gallbladder emptying.

The stomach is then traced to the pylorus and proximal duodenum. The gastric limb of the pancreas is closely associated with the dorsal leaf of the greater omentum. Visualisation is achieved by reflection of the greater omentum ventrally and cranially or by creating a window in the omental bursa. Elevation of the descending duodenum reveals the right kidney, right adrenal and portal vein. The right ovary and uterine horn are visualised in female dogs. The duodenal limb of the pancreas is inspected. The duodenum is traced to the duodenocolic ligament and beyond to the jejunum. The remainder of the intestinal tract is inspected in an oral to aboral direction. Elevation of the descending colon reveals the caudal pole of the left kidney and the left ovary and uterine horn in female dogs. Elevation of the bladder reveals the ureters entering the caudal and dorsal bladder trigone and both vas deferentia in male dogs.

Abdominal wall ruptures and hernias

A true hernia has an anatomically defined hernial ring with a complete sac of peritoneum surrounding the herniated abdominal organs. Defects in the abdominal wall caused by trauma are best referred to as abdominal wall ruptures rather than hernias. Hernias are either secondary to a congenital defect in the abdominal wall, such as umbilical hernias, or the result of abnormal displacement of organs into a potential space, such as inguinal hernias. Hernias are further classified by their location on the body wall – paracostal, dorsolateral, ventral, umbilical, inguinal, scrotal, femoral, and prepubic hernias have all been described.

To achieve closure of the hernias, the herniated contents are reduced back into the abdomen, the hernia sac excised and the defect closed with monofilament non-absorbable sutures or absorbable sutures that have prolonged tensile strength with a simple interrupted suture pattern. Debridement of hernia wound edges is not necessary. In circumstances where very large hernias are present it may not be possible to close the abdominal wall defect by primary apposition. In these cases the defect is closed with either synthetic materials such as polypropylene mesh or, if possible, by construction of local muscular flaps. If strangulation of the herniated organs has occurred then resection of any non-viable portions of these organs is performed. To facilitate exposure and resection of strangulated organs frequently a ventral midline celiotomy is performed in conjunction with an incision over the hernia.

Umbilical hernia

Umbilical hernias appear as soft swellings located at the umbilical scar. They may feel firm if entrapment of herniated contents occurs but are more frequently reducible. These hernias are frequently of little clinical significance. Spontaneous closure of small defects can occur up to 6 months of age; hence conservative management is advised initially. The decision to surgically close an umbilical hernia is subject to the size of the defect and the risk of potential complications. Hernias approximately the size of small intestine should be surgically closed as bowel herniation and strangulation are possible. Affected animals are neutered, as there is a genetic predisposition for these hernias. Umbilical hernias can be corrected during the closure of the abdominal wall following routine ovariohysterectomy.

Minimal postoperative care is required following uncomplicated hernia repair. Wound observation and limited exercise is advised for 14 days. If bowel strangulation has occurred then postoperative care may include the required care for intestinal surgery.

Inguinal hernias

Inguinal hernias occur due to a defect in the inguinal ring through which abdominal contents can herniate. The internal inguinal ring is bounded by the rectus abdominus muscle medially, caudal edge of the internal abdominal oblique cranially and the inguinal ligament laterally and caudally. The external inguinal ring is a slit in the aponeurosis of the external abdominal oblique muscle.

In females inguinal hernias may be either direct or indirect. In males inguinal hernias are direct, with indirect hernias termed scrotal hernias (Fig 3.7). Inguinal hernias are rarely congenital and are generally acquired. The most commonly affected animals are middle-aged intact bitches. Occasionally very large

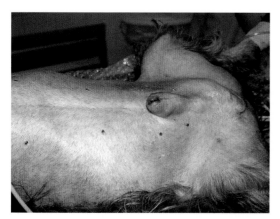

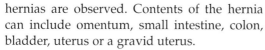

Figure 3.7 A direct inguinal hernia in a male dog. Indirect inguinal hernias occur when the herniated contents are within the sac formed by the tunica albicans. Normally the tunica albicans contains the spermatic chord, testicles and vas deferens in the male and hence these hernias are termed scrotal hernias in male dogs. Photograph © Arthur House.

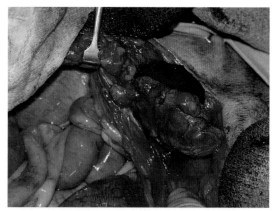

Figure 3.8 An intraoperative view of the same patient as Figure 3.7. This dog's hernia is complicated by strangulation of bowel within the hernia sac (dark red structure to the right). A midline ventral celiotomy has been performed to expose the abdomen (normal intestine light pink and to the left) to facilitate reduction of the herniated bowel and resection and repair of the strangulated bowel. Photograph © Arthur House.

hernias are observed. Contents of the hernia can include omentum, small intestine, colon, bladder, uterus or a gravid uterus.

Several risk factors have been identified for inguinal hernia formation. Bitches may be predisposed to inguinal hernias, as the inguinal canal is larger and shorter than males. Sex hormones have a role in the aetiology as the majority of inguinal hernias occur during oestrus or pregnancy. Lastly, metabolic diseases that weaken the abdominal wall, such as hyperadrenocorticism or obesity, which increases intra-abdominal pressure, may predispose animals to inguinal hernia formation.

Repair of inguinal hernias is as for other hernias. An incision is made over the hernia, the contents of the hernia sac reduced and the defect closed. In more complicated hernias in which strangulation or incarceration of contents has occurred then an approach through the ventral midline is performed first for exploration and repair of herniated organs prior to hernia repair (Fig 3.8).

Wound dressings and bandages are generally not indicated following routine inguinal hernia repair. Wound observation and limited exercise is advised for 14 days. Controlled exercise may help reduce seroma formation. Postoperative complications include haematoma formation, infection and reluctance to walk. If wound infection occurs, management should include opening the skin and subcutaneous tissue and providing local wound treatment measures.

Traumatic ruptures

Traumatic body wall ruptures with abdominal organ herniation are most frequently caused by blunt trauma. Traumatic hernias are more prone to organ strangulation and adhesion formation than true hernias due to the associated inflammation, tissue swelling and contraction of the hernia ring during healing. The initial management of traumatic hernias is to assess and treat the patient for life threatening problems that have occurred as a result of the trauma. The traumatic hernia is surgically repaired only once the patient is stable. In rare circumstances repair of the hernia may be required as an emergency procedure if vital abdominal organs have become incarcerated in the abdominal wall rupture, resulting in deterioration of a patient's condition.

The degree of complications is related to the amount and type of tissues traumatised. Severely traumatised animals require intensive care and monitoring. Strict rest until suture removal is essential following traumatic hernia repair to reduce tension and motion at the surgery site. Seromas, infection and haematomas are frequently seen after repair of traumatic hernias. Drainage of the surgical site is required and should be provided by drains placed within the surgical site during surgery. Active suction drains with one-way valves should be used to promote effective wound drainage. Compared with passive drains active drains have a reduced risk of introducing an ascending infection up the drain. All drains are handled using aseptic technique and should be protected from the environment with sterile dressings. The volume of effusion collected by active drains is recorded to aid decisions with regard to drain removal and wound healing progression. Passive drains, such as Penrose drains, should be covered with sterile dressings. These dressings are changed on a daily basis or when strike through is observed.

Acute abdominal diseases

Peritonitis

Peritonitis is inflammation of the peritoneum. In most cases peritonitis is secondary to another disease or a result of dehiscence of an intra-abdominal organ following surgery. Approximately 60% of animals with septic peritonitis have contamination from the gastrointestinal tract. Gastrointestinal tract leakage may be secondary to dehiscence of gastrointestinal surgery sites, gastric dilatation volvulus, neoplastic lesions, gastrointestinal ulceration, penetrating trauma, traumatic perforation or bowel strangulation. Other sources of contamination include abscess formation in or adjacent to many organs, e.g. pancreas, genitourinary tract (especially the uterus and prostate) and the hepatobiliary system. Occasionally migrating foreign bodies can cause peritoneal contamination and peritonitis. When an intra-abdominal source of contamination is not found the peritonitis is termed primary or spontaneous bacterial peritonitis. Spontaneous peritonitis is rare and such infections are usually monobacterial.

The hallmark clinical sign for peritonitis is vomiting and is of particular concern in patients who have undergone gastrointestinal surgery within the previous 5 days. Abdominal pain may be observed on abdominal palpation. Varying degrees of anorexia, lethargy and depression are observed. Cats tend to have few clinical signs compared with dogs and only develop signs when the disease is advanced.

The majority of patients with peritonitis have significant haemodynamic and electrolyte abnormalities on presentation. Careful patient evaluation including a complete history and physical examination, haematology and serum biochemistry, bacterial and cytological evaluation of abdominal fluid, abdominal ultrasonography, thoracic and abdominal radiographs is frequently required. In most patients stabilisation of haemodynamic abnormalities requires intravenous fluid therapy. Once the patient is stabilised surgical intervention is indicated. In rare circumstances stabilisation of the patient is not possible prior to surgery.

Due to the possibility of a large abdominal incision the surgical field that is prepared should be extensive and begin cranial to the xiphoid, extend caudal to the pubis and lateral to the skin folds of both the fore and hind limbs.

During surgical treatment of bacterial peritonitis the surgeon must identify the source of contamination or infection, reduce intra-abdominal bacterial burden, remove any foreign material and necrotic debris and prevent recurrent intra-abdominal contamination. Additional goals of surgery may be to provide drainage of the abdominal cavity and/or enteral access.

The identification of the source of intra-abdominal contamination requires a thorough and systematic exploration of the abdominal cavity. Prevention of recurrent intra-abdominal contamination is dependent on the original source of contamination. Consequently the surgical team must be prepared for a wide range of potential procedures. Removal of the septic focus frequently involves organ removal or abscess wall debridement. The placement of the omentum within the abscess cavities is advocated as a means of improving local drainage, facilitating phagocytosis and enhancing local blood supply.

Reduction of the intra-abdominal bacterial burden and removal of foreign material is largely achieved by copious peritoneal lavage. Abdominal lavage should be performed with warm isotonic saline solution and should be continued until the fluid removed with suction is clear. The addition of antibiotics or antiseptics to lavage solution is not necessary and may be detrimental. If the omentum has become grossly diseased, omentectomy may be indicated to prevent ongoing abdominal contamination.

Provision of abdominal drainage may be achieved by open peritoneal drainage or the use of intra-abdominal drains. Not all patients require abdominal drainage following abdominal lavage and correction of the underlying problem. The decision to manage a patient with primary celiotomy closure versus open peritoneal drainage or the implantation of peritoneal drains is dependent on the individual patient, the degree of contamination observed and the expected continued contamination after the initial surgery. The use of open peritoneal drainage is usually restricted to those patients with diffuse abdominal infection that cannot successfully be removed at the time of surgery.

Open peritoneal drainage facilitates continued drainage of necrotic debris from the peritoneal cavity and gives the surgeon the opportunity to re-explore the abdomen at the time of definitive closure. It is achieved by loose closure of the celiotomy with a continuous non-absorbable monofilament suture. A highly absorbent abdominal bandage protects the abdominal organs. A suitable abdominal bandage may consist of large sterile abdominal swabs as the primary layer followed by large quantities of cotton wool, an incontinence sheet and finally an outer protective layer. The bandage is changed daily in an aseptic manner or when 'strike through' is observed.

General anaesthesia on a daily basis for aseptic bandage change has been suggested but is generally not required. If appropriate analgesia is administered, patients tolerate bandage change, including breakdown of omental adhesions to the celiotomy site, without discomfort. The disadvantage of open peritoneal drainage is the additional resources required to manage the abdominal bandage. Inability to adequately manage the open peritoneal cavity can lead to either ascending nosocomial infections or abdominal organ herniation.

The use of peritoneal drains has been suggested as a method of overcoming the additional nursing requirement of open peritoneal drainage while continuing to obtain the benefits of postoperative drainage. If intra-abdominal drains are used then appropriate drain choice and placement is required for effective drainage to be achieved. Continuous closed suction drains, such as the Jackson Pratt, are ideal. Drains need to be positioned in the abdomen so as to avoid obstruction by the omentum. Two drains are placed in the cranial abdomen between the liver and the diaphragm and two in the caudal abdomen. The drains require bandaging postoperatively to prevent premature removal by the patient and to help reduce the risk of ascending infection. Additionally, drains are handled in an aseptic manner to reduce the risk of an ascending nosocomial infection.

Timing of closure of an open abdomen, or the removal of peritoneal drains, is based on the volume and character of the fluid retrieved from the abdomen. Weighing of the abdominal bandage before application and following removal provides an estimation of the volume of peritoneal exudate. A significant reduction in the volume of exudate, a change in its character from turbid to clear, plus the absence of bacteria and a decrease in toxic neutrophils on cytological examination are indications for either drain removal or abdominal closure. The exudation will never completely resolve especially if drains have been used, since they themselves incite an inflammatory reaction.

Haemoperitoneum

Splenic followed by hepatic masses are the most common source of intra-abdominal haemorrhage. Other causes of haemoabdomen are neoplasia in other organs, abdominal trauma, coagulopathy, splenic torsion, liver torsion, iatrogenic following diagnostic procedures or rupture of abdominal viscera.

Splenic masses are a frequent underlying cause of haemoabdomen in small animal patients. Gross inspection of the spleen is an unreliable method of differentiating neoplasia and nodular hyperplasia. In dogs approximately 50% of splenic masses are malignant, with 80% of malignancies being haemangiosarcoma. In cats approximately 37% of splenic masses are malignant, with 30% of these being lymphoma, mast cell tumor or myeloproliferative disorders.

Surgical intervention is indicated when the volume of haemorrhage is sufficient to affect peripheral packed cell volume (PCV), is progressive over time and where the source of the abdominal haemorrhage can be successfully ligated or resected. Rarely, masses in other organs such as the adrenals or haemangiosarcoma originating from the lumbar musculature are a source of intra-abdominal haemorrhage. In these cases advanced surgical procedures such as adrenalectomy may be required. Inspection of the liver is advised if a malignant neoplasm is suspected in the gastrointestinal tract or associated structures. It is common for large volumes of bloody fluid to be aspirated from the abdomen at surgery (Fig 3.9). Frequently the PCV of the bloody abdominal fluid is low due to dilution of the haemorrhage by a peritoneal effusion. The volume of fluid does not necessarily correlate with the severity of anaemia in the patient.

Uroperitoneum

Uroperitoneum is the presence of urine in the abdominal cavity and results from leakage of urine from any region of the urinary tract. Urine in the peritoneal cavity has severe metabolic consequences but induces minimal chemical peritonitis. If a concurrent urinary

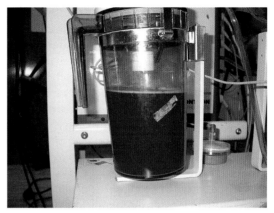

Figure 3.9   A typical volume of fluid aspirated from a medium sized dog with a haemoabdomen secondary to a splenic mass. Despite the fluid appearing to be blood the PVC of the abdominal fluid is typically substantially lower than that of the peripheral blood due to dilution of the haemorrhage by peritoneal effusion. Photograph © Arthur House.

tract infection occurs then bacterial peritonitis may develop. If evidence of bacterial peritonitis is observed then rapid surgical intervention is indicated.

Preoperative evaluations such as contrast radiographic studies and abdominal ultrasonography are essential to determine the location of the urine leakage. Any metabolic or haemodynamic abnormalities should be stabilised with intravenous fluid therapy prior to anaesthesia. Short-term management of an uroperitoneum without evidence of urinary tract infection, to allow stabilisation of a patient's metabolic status, can be achieved by drainage of the urine from the abdomen by abdominocentesis and the placement of a transurethral catheter.

Urine leakage following bladder surgery or cystocentesis will usually resolve after a short period of urinary diversion via a transurethral catheter. Rupture of the urinary tract following abdominal trauma usually requires exploratory celiotomy and definitive repair. Defects of the bladder wall may be closed with either a simple interrupted appositional suture pattern or a continuous double layer closure.

Monofilament absorbable sutures with a long lasting tensile strength, such as Polydioxanone or Glycomer 631, are ideal for bladder repair. Bladder tears secondary to urethral obstruction require removal of the obstruction, primary bladder repair and a period of urinary diversion. In most circumstances retrograde hydropulsion or passage of a urinary catheter is sufficient to relieve urethral obstruction. In some instances an urethrotomy may be necessary. Tube cystotomy can be used to provide either short- or long-term urinary diversion following any of these procedures.

Penetrating abdominal wounds

Damage to abdominal viscera frequently occurs following penetrating wounds of the peritoneal cavity. Consequently routine exploratory celiotomy is recommended for penetrating abdominal wounds, particularly bite wounds and gunshot wounds. The abdominal cavity should be systematically explored and surgical repair or removal of damaged organs undertaken.

Postoperative care of acute abdominal disease

Patients with peritonitis often require intensive postoperative care, with many patients remaining haemodynamically unstable postoperatively and at risk of postoperative complications, systemic inflammatory response syndrome or multiple organ failure. Maintenance of the patient's intravascular fluid volume with either crystalloid, colloid solutions or blood products is required to maintain cardiac output and peripheral perfusion.

The success of postoperative care is frequently due to careful patient monitoring with regular measurement and recording of parameters including heart rate, respiratory rate, urine output, central venous pressures and peripheral arterial pressure, packed cell volume, total protein, electrolytes and arterial blood gases. To facilitate patient monitoring jugular catheters, arterial catheters and urinary catheters are required. If arterial catheters and jugular catheters are not feasible, urine output provides a valuable estimation of renal perfusion. Urine output is expected to be above 1–2ml/kg/h – volumes lower than this indicate reduced arterial blood flow to the kidneys and hence the need for intervention. Trends in any parameter provide the clinician with information to maximise patient care.

In patients with peritonitis, fluid infusion rates must be tailored to the perceived needs of the individual patient based on changes in mucous membrane pallor, capillary refill time, peripheral arterial pulses, urine output, PCV/total protein and arterial blood gases. Crystalloid administration is the mainstay of fluid therapy. Colloids may be beneficial in patients who remain hypotensive despite crystalloid therapy and adequate volumes of plasma are not available. Disadvantages of colloids are the potential for development of coagulopathies, volume overload and the potential to exacerbate peripheral and pulmonary oedema if there is significant leakage of the colloid into the interstitial space. Fresh frozen plasma is the colloid of choice in patients with peritonitis. Plasma has several advantages including colloid support and supplementing plasma proteins such as clotting factors. Many patients with peritonitis are hypoproteinaemic due to the large amount of protein lost in the peritoneal exudate. Normalisation of serum protein levels, however, is not a realistic goal of plasma transfusions.

Animals recovering from peritonitis are suffering from bacterial sepsis and may have compromised immune function. Empirical antibiotic therapy should be administered initially but modified according to aerobic and anaerobic culture and sensitivity results. Typical antibiotic choices are second-generation cephalosporins or ampicillin + fluoroquinolone + metronidazole combinations.

GASTROINTESTINAL SURGERY

Tissue handling

In all surgery, exposure and handling of tissues results in desiccation and abrasion. Poor tissue handling skills in gastrointestinal surgery results in an increased degree of inflammation and a greater risk of adhesion formation, motility disorders and peritoneal fluid formation. Even minor procedures that involve minimal handling of the intestinal tract will decrease gastrointestinal motility for 24 hours postoperatively.

The use of stay sutures, moist swabs and appropriate instruments will decrease the effects of tissue handling. Stay sutures should be placed and used to mobilise organs in preference to instruments. Organs that need to be retracted or are within the surgical field should be protected with moist swabs at all times, particularly prior to retraction. Toothed forceps (e.g. Allis tissue forceps) should never be used on the gastrointestinal tract.

The least traumatic method of occluding bowel is by use of an assistant surgeon grasping the bowel between the index and middle finger. If an assistant surgeon is not available then an alternative is using atraumatic bowel forceps such as Doyen bowel forceps. The bowel is placed at the tip of the clamp and the clamp closed to one click. Crushing forceps should be only placed on bowel that is to be resected.

Surgical stapling devices

Surgical staples are becoming increasingly available in veterinary surgery and have many applications in intestinal surgery. Advantages of stapling equipment are that they decrease surgery and anesthesia time, decrease tissue handling, potentially decrease peritoneal contamination and lastly provide an accurate and consistent closure of tissue with evenly spaced staples that leads to increased bursting and tensile strengths when compared with conventional suturing. The disadvantages are the increased cost, limited availability, decreased flexibility of application compared to conventional sutures and the requirement of additional technical skills to operate the equipment. Stapling equipment is not a replacement for good basic surgical skills, with the rates of dehiscence between stapled and sutured intestinal anastomoses being similar.

Many types of staples are available and they are named based on their function:

- GIA 50, GIA 90 (gastrointestinal anastomosis 50 and 90mm long) – creates two double staggered lines of staples and cuts between them
- TA 30, TA 55, TA 90 (thoracoabdominal 30, 55 and 90mm long) – places 2–3 lines of staples without cutting (Fig 3.10)
- EEA (end-to-end anastomosis) – anastomoses two ends of bowel by inverting each end, placing a double layer of staples and resecting excess tissue beyond the staples
- LDS (ligate, divide and separate) – places two ligature staples and divides between them.

The stomach

The most common indications for gastric surgery are foreign body removal and correction of gastric dilatation and volvulus. Less frequently gastric surgery is performed for gastric outflow obstruction, neoplasia or gastric ulceration. In nearly all circumstances the stomach is approached through a ventral midline celiotomy. Vomiting with or without anorexia is the classical clinical sign associated with gastric disease and may lead to dehydration

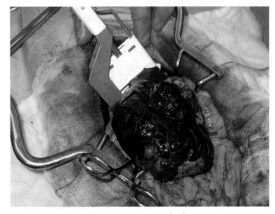

Figure 3.10   A transabdominal (TA) 55mm stapling device being used to resect a large hepatic mass. The stapling device fires a double row of staples, which provide haemostasis. The mass is excised with a scalpel blade using the edge of the stapler as a cutting guide. Photograph © Arthur House.

and electrolyte imbalances. Haematemesis can occur in erosive gastric diseases or in patients suffering from coagulopathies. Secondary conditions such as oesophageal ulceration and aspiration can occur in vomiting animals.

Preoperative evaluation of animals with gastric disease should include a minimum of haematology and serum biochemistry, thoracic and abdominal radiographs and abdominal ultrasound. In patients with haematemesis coagulation profiles should be performed. Prior to anaesthesia primary and secondary metabolic abnormalities should be managed. Electrolyte and haemodynamic abnormalities should be corrected with appropriate intravenous fluids and coagulopathies managed with blood product transfusions. Oesophageal ulceration will generally resolve once the underlying cause of vomiting is removed. Broad-spectrum systemic antibiotics, physical therapy such as coupage and nebulisation and, in severe cases, oxygen therapy should be administered if aspiration pneumonia is observed in a patient. Ideally, antibiotic therapy should be modified according to culture and sensitivity results obtained from a bronchoalveolar lavage if the patient is sufficiently stable to safely anaesthetise and evaluate with a bronchoscope.

Gastrotomy

A gastrotomy is an incision through the stomach wall into the stomach lumen. It is most commonly indicated for removal of gastric foreign bodies or full thickness biopsies of the stomach wall – these should be performed endoscopically in preference to a surgical approach, if possible. Stay sutures are used to manipulate the stomach in preference to instruments such as Allis forceps. The gastrotomy incision is made in an avascular portion of the stomach wall between the lesser and greater curvature away from the pylorus.

Gastrotomy incision can be closed as a single layer using a simple interrupted appositional suture pattern or as a two-layer inverting pattern. If a two-layer closure is performed the first layer includes the submucosal, muscularis and serosa in a Cushing or simple interrupted suture pattern, followed by a Lembert or Cushing suture pattern that includes the muscularis and serosal layers. Absorbable monofilament sutures with prolonged tensile strength such as Polydioxanone or Glycomer 631 are recommended for suturing the gastrointestinal tract. Poliglecaprone 25 has been described for suturing the gastrointestinal tract, though its rapid rate of absorption may increase the chance of surgical dehiscence if delayed healing occurs.

Partial gastrectomy

A partial gastrectomy is resection of a portion of the stomach and is indicated when ulceration, necrosis or neoplasia of the stomach wall occurs. The most common gastric necrosis is of the greater curvature of the stomach secondary to gastric dilatation volvulus (GDV). Partial gastric resection is required if gastric wall necrosis is suspected. The determination of gastric wall viability is based upon serosal colour, gastric wall thickness and pulsation of local vessels. When performing a partial resection the stomach should be isolated from the abdominal cavity using stay sutures and moist large abdominal swabs. Full thickness partial gastric resection is performed and the stomach closed in two layers – using a continuous layer in the mucosa/submucosa and either an interrupted appositional closure or continuous inverting closure of the seromuscular layer. Gastrointestinal stapling devices, particularly the GIA (gastrointestinal anastomosis) device may be used as an alternative to hand suturing the resected stomach. Invagination of the necrotic stomach wall and over sewing healthy serosa has been described as an alternative to partial gastrectomy for management of necrotic stomach wall secondary to GDV.

For resection of neoplasia or gastric wall ulceration located within the pylorus that cannot be managed by local resection, a pylorectomy is indicated. Following pylorectomy the junction between the stomach and the small intestine can be reconstructed by performing either a Billroth 1 or Billroth 2 procedure. When performing a Billroth 1 the stomach is anastomosed directly to the duodenum. For a Billroth 2 the distal stomach and proximal duodenum are sutured closed and a new communication is created between the jejunum and greater curvature of the stomach. For both procedures care must be taken to identify and preserve the common bile duct and the pancreatic ducts. If the common bile duct is damaged or involved in the disease then a cholecystoduodenostomy can be performed. Pylorectomies can be sutured by hand or with gastrointestinal stapling devices.

Gastrostomy

A gastrostomy is the creation of an artificial opening into the lumen of the stomach. The most common indication for a gastrostomy is for placement of a feeding tube – these should always be placed on the left within the fundus of the stomach. The creation of a temporary gastrostomy through the right paracostal abdominal wall has been described for temporary decompression of the stomach in patients with gastric dilatation and volvulus. This technique is no longer considered the optimum management for patients with GDV and hence is rarely performed. A right-sided tube gastrostomy into the antrum of the stomach is an alternative to performing a right-sided gastropexy in patients with GDV to prevent recurrent gastric torsion.

Gastropexy

A gastropexy is the creation of a permanent adhesion between the stomach and the body wall. The most common indication for a gastropexy is to prevent recurrence of gastric torsion that occurs in GDV. For most gastropexy techniques described, the adhesion is created between the pyloric antrum and the right body wall. Techniques for creation of an adhesion between the body of the stomach and the midline or the fundus and the left body wall are also described. The most commonly used gastropexies are an incisional gastropexy, a belt-loop gastropexy and a right-sided tube gastrostomy. Historically, circumcostal gastropexies were popular but this technique has been replaced by the simpler belt-loop.

Pyloromyotomy and pyloroplasty

Both pyloromyotomy and pyloroplasty are performed to increase the diameter of the pylorus. These procedures are indicated to correct gastric outflow obstruction, which in most cases is secondary to benign mucosal hyperplasia. As gastric outflow is an uncommon disease of both cats and dogs these procedures are rarely performed. A pyloromyotomy is performed by incising through the serosa and muscular layers over the pylorus, leaving the mucosa intact, which allows the pylorus to expand and the mucosa to bulge. A pyloroplasty is a full thickness incision over the pylorus with reconstruction of the incision that allows expansion of the diameter of the pylorus. The two most common pyloroplasties are a Heineke-Mikulics and a Y-U.

Gastric foreign bodies

The severity of clinical signs associated with gastric foreign bodies varies enormously and is dependent on the degree of gastric outflow obstruction. Most animals present with vomiting, anorexia and depression. Foreign bodies that obstruct gastric outflow can precipitate an acute abdominal crisis. Metabolic alkalosis, electrolyte abnormalities, dehydration and, less commonly, metabolic acidosis may develop following obstruction of the pylorus. Gastric foreign bodies can be an incidental finding on radiographs. They are easily retrieved via a gastrotomy as described above, if they are not retrievable by endoscopy.

Prior to anaesthesia and surgery any haemodynamic, acid–base and electrolyte abnormalities should be corrected. Food is withheld for 12 hours prior to anaesthesia to reduce the incidence of regurgitation. Broad-spectrum perioperative antibiotics such as second generation cephalosporins are indicated. There is no indication to continue antibiotics beyond 12 hours postoperatively. Multimodal analgesia, which includes both opiates and NSAIDs, is administered prior to and following surgery as required.

Gastric dilatation and volvulus

Gastric dilatation and volvulus is the disease complex in which gaseous distension and rotation of the stomach into an abnormal position occurs, resulting in occlusion of the duodenum and oesophagus. The hallmark presenting clinical sign is non-productive retching and abdominal distension. This distension and torsion of the stomach leads to compromise of both the gastric vascular supply and venous return to the heart. Patients rapidly develop haemodynamic shock and progress from alert and walking to recumbent and depressed or non-responsive. Patients with GDV suffer haemodynamic instability – this should be addressed with intravascular fluid therapy prior to general anaesthesia. Large volumes of crystalloid intravenous fluids are used in most patients. To facilitate administration of these fluids the largest catheters possible (usually 18 gauge) are placed in both cephalic veins. Preoperative stabilisation and postoperative care of the patient have the biggest impact on survival.

Decompression of the stomach can be performed by passage of an orogastric stomach tube, percutaneous drainage using a large-bore needle, or a combination of the two. Decompression of the stomach should be delayed until measures to improve the haemodynamic stability are well under way. The diagnosis of GDV is rarely challenging and is rapidly achieved from physical examination findings and plain abdominal radiography.

Following preoperative stabilisation, the patient can be prepared for surgery. Ideally following induction of anaesthesia, jugular catheters, arterial catheters and urinary catheters are placed to facilitate pre- and postoperative monitoring of the patient. A wide clip of the ventral abdomen is performed and the area prepared aseptically. The goals of surgery are to decompress the stomach, return it to its normal anatomical position, evaluate organs such as the stomach, spleen and pancreas for viability, and perform a gastropexy to prevent recurrence of GDV.

Return of normal gastric anatomy is achieved by determining the direction of the gastric rotation. In the majority of dogs a clockwise gastric rotation occurs and the stomach enters the omental bursa. The pylorus will be found in the craniodorsal left abdominal quadrant. Gastric repositioning is achieved by pushing the body of the stomach down to the left while pulling the pylorus and duodenum ventrally and to the right. Following derotation, an orogastric tube is advanced into the stomach to achieve complete decompression. Gavage is performed to remove liquid and solid contents from the stomach. Occasionally if large pieces of material remain in the stomach, gastrotomy is needed to facilitate their removal.

Necrosis of the gastric wall may be observed in patients with GDV (Fig 3.11). The determination of gastric wall viability is based upon serosal colour, gastric wall thickness and pulsation of local vessels. Black, green or grey discoloration of the serosal surface and a thin gastric wall are all indicative of gastric necrosis. Purple or deep red discoloration may be consistent with either severe gastric wall congestion or loss of vascular integrity. To assist decision making, small stab incisions into the serosa to assess for arterial bleeding are useful for determining gastric wall viability. Vascular integrity of the mucosa can be assumed to be adequate if bleeding of the serosal surface is seen.

Partial gastric resection is required if gastric wall necrosis is suspected. The diseased stomach should be isolated from the abdom-

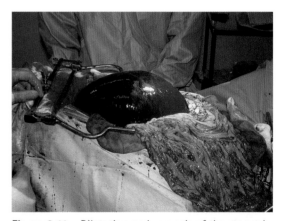

Figure 3.11   Dilatation and necrosis of the stomach secondary to GDV in a dog. Determination of gastric wall viability is based upon serosal colour, gastric wall thickness and pulsation of local vessels. Photograph © Arthur House.

inal cavity using stay sutures and moist large abdominal swabs. Full thickness partial gastric resection is performed and the stomach is closed in two layers, using a continuous layer in the mucosa/submucosa and either an interrupted appositional closure or continuous inverting closure of the seromuscular layer. Gastrointestinal stapling devices have simplified gastric resection and made it a more rapid procedure.

The spleen may also suffer irreversible ischaemia following GDV. The spleen is commonly engorged following correction of the gastric position and hence initial spleen size and colour is not a good indicator of viability. The spleen should be returned to its normal position for 5–10 minutes before re-evaluation. Evaluation of viability of the spleen is achieved by close examination of splenic arteries and veins. If the vascular integrity is intact, small foci of splenic discoloration will usually spontaneously resolve. The presence of major splenic artery or venous thrombi or avulsion warrants splenectomy. Again partial or complete splenectomy can be done by hand but is facilitated by stapling equipment.

A gastropexy should be performed to create adhesions between the pyloric antrum and the right body wall. Many techniques have been shown to achieve this – currently the author prefers either incisional or belt-loop gastropexy.

Postoperative care following gastric surgery
The postoperative care of patients following GDV is challenging and requires intensive monitoring. These patients are susceptible to poor perfusion and hypotension, cardiac arrhythmias, dehiscence of surgical sites and peritonitis. Despite the severity of the haemodynamic changes observed in patients with GDV, expected mortality rates should be approximately 10% for animals without gastric necrosis and 30% for animals with gastric necrosis requiring partial gastric resection. The postoperative care of animals following gastric foreign bodies is typically straightforward as the patients are frequently haemodynamically stable prior to surgery. The prognosis for these animals is generally considered excellent.

For all animals following gastric surgery the haemodynamic, electrolyte and acid–base balance should be closely monitored. Following GDV continuous ECG monitoring is advisable for the first 24–48 hours. Intravenous fluid therapy is continued until the animal is eating well and any preoperative haemodynamic, electrolyte or acid–base abnormalities are corrected. Bland food is fed 12–24 hours after surgery.

Surgical complications include postoperative wound infection, seroma formation, abdominal wall dehiscence, gastrotomy dehiscence and peritonitis, intestinal ileus and vomiting. If vomiting occurs the patient should be closely evaluated for the possible complication of peritonitis. If vomiting continues and is not a result of peritonitis then antiemetics such as metoclopramide can be administered.

Small intestine

The most common indications for small intestine surgery are foreign body removal and correction of intussusception. Less frequently small intestine surgery is performed for neoplasia or intestinal strangulation. Vomiting with or without anorexia secondary to gas and fluid distension of the intestine and voluminous diarrhoea are classical clinical signs associated with small intestinal disease. Vomiting may lead to dehydration and electrolyte imbalances. Small intestine obstruction interferes with myoelectrical activity and decreased intestinal activity or atony. This environment allows bacterial proliferation and endotoxins may be absorbed, leading to endotoxaemia.

Preoperative evaluation of animals with small intestinal disease should include a minimum of haematology and serum biochemistry, thoracic and abdominal radiographs, and abdominal ultrasound. Prior to anaesthesia primary and secondary metabolic abnormalities should be managed. Electrolyte and haemodynamic abnormalities should be corrected with appropriate intravenous fluids.

Enterotomy
An enterotomy is an incision through the intestine wall into the intestine lumen. It is

most commonly indicated for removal of foreign bodies. Enterotomy incisions are closed in a single layer typically using a simple interrupted appositional suture pattern. Absorbable monofilament sutures with prolonged tensile strength such as Polydioxanone or Glycomer 631 are recommended for suturing the small intestinal tract. Poliglecaprone 25 has been described for suturing the small intestinal tract though its rapid rate of absorption may increase the chance of surgical dehiscence if delayed healing occurs.

Resection and anastomosis

Indications for enterectomy include ischaemia, necrosis, neoplasia or irreducible intussusception. The arcadial vessels (from the mesenteric artery) supplying the area of intestine to be resected and the terminal arcadial vessels at the mesenteric border are ligated. The intestine is occluded approximately 1.5cm proximal and distal to the area to be resected using an assistant's fingers or bowel forceps (Fig 3.12). Crushing forceps are used to occlude the intestine to be resected. Typically some healthy intestine is resection along with the diseased intestine to ensure that the region of anasto-

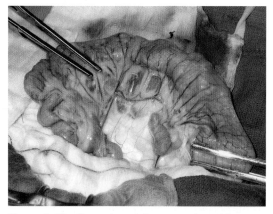

Figure 3.12   Doyen bowel forceps and crushing forceps in place prior to resection of the diseased bowel. The Doyen forceps (lateral forcep of each pair) have been placed so the tips are just protruding beyond the mesenteric border of the bowel and have been closed one 'click' of the ratchet. This cat has megacolon and is undergoing a subtotal colectomy. Photograph © Arthur House.

mosis is disease-free and has an adequate blood supply.

The anastomosis is closed in a single layer typically using a simple interrupted appositional suture pattern. Use of a simple continuous suture pattern, skin staples and TA (transabdominal) stapling devices are also described for anastomosis closure. Due to the omentum's rich vascular and lymphatic supply, it can be draped over an anastomosis site to improve vascular supply, lymphatic drainage and to help prevent leakage from the surgical site. Serosal patching (a technique that involves suturing the serosa of an adjacent piece of bowel across the anastomosis site) can also be used to reinforce an anastomosis. Unlike the omentum, serosal patching only provides structural support to the surgical site and provides minimal additional benefits to blood supply or lymphatic drainage.

Small intestine foreign bodies

The severity of clinical signs associated with small intestinal foreign bodies varies enormously and is dependent on the degree of intestine obstruction and chronicity of the obstruction. Most animals present with vomiting, anorexia and depression.

Pre- and postoperative care for small intestinal foreign bodies is similar to gastric foreign bodies. Prior to anaesthesia and surgery, any haemodynamic, acid–base and electrolyte abnormalities should be corrected. Food is withheld for 12 hours prior to anaesthesia to reduce the incidence of regurgitation. Broad-spectrum perioperative antibiotics such as second generation cephalosporins are indicated – there is no need to continue antibiotics beyond 12 hours postoperatively. Multimodal analgesia, including both opiates and NSAIDs, is administered pre- and postsurgery as required.

Foreign body removal may be as simple as performing an enterotomy through which to remove the obstructing foreign body. The enterotomy should always be performed in a region of healthy bowel, usually just aboral to the obstruction. Frequently the bowel in the region of the obstruction is devitalised from ischaemic necrosis secondary to the obstruction. In these cases resection of the devitalised bowel with anastomosis is performed.

More challenging are linear foreign bodies. These result in partial obstruction and commonly vague and chronic symptoms of gastrointestinal disease. They are more commonly observed in cats than dogs. In approximately 50% of cats the linear foreign body is anchored around the tongue, hence a careful oral examination should be performed. The peristaltic contractions of the intestine attempt to push the foreign body aborally. If a linear foreign body becomes anchored in the gastrointestinal tract and cannot move aborally the bowel becomes plicated around the foreign body. Eventually the foreign body may cut through the mesenteric border, leading to multiple perforations along large lengths of the bowel. Due to the length of linear foreign bodies and the risk of multiple perforations, surgical removal frequently involves multiple enterotomies and careful inspection of the entire gastrointestinal tract.

Intussusception

Intussusception is the invagination of one part of the intestine into another. The intussusceptum is the portion of bowel that invaginates into the adjacent bowel or intussuscipiens. Intussusceptions are classified according to site and are most common at the ileocaecocolic junction. Causes of intussusception are often idiopathic. Bowel hypermobility secondary to diseases including enteritis, intestinal parasites, intestinal foreign bodies, intestinal masses and previous surgery may also lead to the development of an intussusception.

The typical presentation is an animal less than one year of age with a history of vomiting, diarrhoea, weight loss, anorexia and a palpable abdominal mass. Less commonly melena, haematochezia, dehydration, abdominal pain, tenesmus and protrusion of the intussusceptum from the rectum may be observed. Preoperative care is the same as for small intestinal foreign bodies. At surgery attempts are made to manually reduce the intussusception by milking out the intussus-

ceptum. More commonly resection of the intussusception and anastomosis of the bowel is required.

Recurrence is seen in up to 25% of animals. An attempt to prevent recurrence can be made by performing an enteroplication – the creation of permanent serosal adhesions between loops of bowel from the duodenocolic ligament to the ileocolic junction. The loops of bowel are sutured together with sutures placed 6–10cm apart using a monofilament suture.

Intestinal strangulation

Strangulation is rare and occurs when portions of small intestine herniate through traumatic body wall ruptures or hernias. The clinical signs associated with small intestinal strangulation can be more severe than those observed with small intestinal obstruction. Animals may present with severe haemodynamic instability and metabolic abnormalities. Prior to anaesthesia and surgery attempts are made to stabilise haemodynamic, acid–base and electrolyte abnormalities. On occasion patients with small intestinal strangulation are poorly responsive to initial medical therapy and require emergency surgery to remove the affected bowel. The prognosis for these animals is dependent on the animal's cardiovascular status prior to surgery and the degree of intestinal compromise.

Postoperative care following small intestinal surgery

The intensity of the postoperative care for patients following small intestinal surgery is largely dependent on the patient's presurgical cardiovascular status, the extent of bowel devitalisation, and the percentage of bowel resected. However for most animals undergoing an enterotomy or resection anastomosis the prognosis is considered excellent. The prognosis worsens if more than 80% of the bowel is resected as animals may suffer from short bowel syndrome. As for animals undergoing gastric surgery, postoperatively the patient's haemodynamic, electrolyte and acid–base balance should be closely monitored. Intravenous fluid therapy is continued until the animal is eating well and any preoperative haemodynamic, electrolyte or acid–base abnormalities are corrected. Bland food is fed for 12–24 hours after surgery. If vomiting occurs the patient should be closely evaluated for the possible complication of peritonitis. If vomiting continues and is not a result of peritonitis then antiemetics such as metoclopramide can be administered.

Large intestine

Surgery of the large intestine is rarely indicated and is uncommon. The most common indication for large intestine surgery is in cats for management of megacolon. Due to the relatively high risk of postoperative dehiscence large bowel biopsies and large bowel foreign bodies are retrieved per rectum in preference to transabdominal/transcolon approaches.

Clinical signs associated with large bowel disease are haematochezia, constipation, tenesmus, dyschezia and diarrhoea. Diarrhoea of large bowel origin is typically high frequency, low volume with fresh blood and mucus within the faeces.

Preoperative evaluation of animals with large intestinal disease should include a minimum of haematology and serum biochemistry, thoracic and abdominal radiographs, abdominal ultrasound and colonoscopy. Colonoscopy is a powerful diagnostic tool for investigation of large bowel disease. Preparation of the large bowel is essential for effective evaluation and mucosal biopsy of the colon. Preparation of the large bowel requires fasting – 3 days is ideal, 2 days adequate and 1 day generally inadequate. Enemas or gastrointestinal lavage solutions can provide colonic cleaning. Gastrointestinal lavage solutions are the best (e.g. GoLYTEL, Endlaws Preps, NY; Braintree Labs) and contain replacement electrolytes and polyethylene glycol, which acts as an osmotic agent. Most regimes advise approximately 25ml/kg by stomach tube, two or three doses over a period of 12–24 hours prior to the procedure.

Warm water, mineral oil or lactulose can be used as enema solutions. Soap, hypertonic sodium phosphate (Fleet enemas) and bisacodyl laxatives all potentially result in colonic mucosal inflammation, which interferes with histopathological interpretation of biopsies and hence should be avoided. Hypertonic sodium phosphate enemas have been associated with fatal hyperphosphataemia and hypernatraemia in cats.

In veterinary surgery routine preparation of the bowel is performed prior to colonoscopy but not prior to surgery. Preparation of the bowel prior to surgery may convert 'manageable' faeces into faecal slurry that is more likely to contaminate the surgical field. If enemas are used it is recommended that they be given 2–3 days prior to surgery.

Patients with large bowel disease rarely have electrolyte and haemodynamic abnormalities unless profuse or chronic diarrhoea has been present. If electrolyte and haemodynamic abnormalities do exist they should be corrected prior to anaesthesia with appropriate intravenous fluids.

The use of preoperative antibiotics in veterinary colonic surgery has not been investigated. In human colonic surgery preoperative antibiotics combined with mechanical cleansing of the bowel has been shown to reduce postoperative infection rates. The use of preoperative antibiotics in veterinary surgery remains the opinion of the individual surgeon. Perioperative antibiotics are indicated and are administered intravenously at the time of surgery. Second generation cephalosporins are frequently used. No benefit has been demonstrated in continuing antibiotics beyond surgery. Postoperative antibiotics may be detrimental as normal bacterial flora enhances healing of intestinal anastomoses and prolonged use of antibiotics leads to bacterial resistance.

Healing of the colon is similar to the small intestine but delayed. Wound tensile strength in the colon lags behind the return of strength observed in the small bowel. Consequently the colon is more susceptible to dehiscence and leakage, with subsequent peritonitis, following surgery. Due to this delayed healing sutures or staples must maintain adequate strength for a minimum of 14 days. Poliglecaprone 25 and Polyglytone 6211 are not advised as they both have a rapid loss of tensile strength over the first 14 days following implantation. Polydioxanone and Glycomer 631 are suitable suture choices. A simple interrupted appositional suture pattern is advised as this is associated with the lowest reduction in tissue oxygen tension levels and highest gain in tensile strength over time when compared with continuous or inverting suture patterns. The strength of stapled anastomoses using an end-to-end anastomotic (EEA) stapling device is the same or greater than sutured anastomoses and is associated with significantly lower postoperative morbidity in human colorectal anastomosis.

Colotomy

A colotomy is an incision through the colon wall into the colon lumen. It is most commonly indicated for removal of foreign bodies or faeces that cannot be removed via the anus. This is rarely performed as most foreign bodies that reach the large bowel will pass unassisted. Colonic biopsy via a colotomy is rarely performed or indicated. Mucosal biopsies can be performed via endoscopy.

Colectomy

A colectomy is resection of a section of the colon followed by anastomosis. Indications for a colectomy include resection of neoplasia, removal of devitalised bowel secondary to irreducible intussusceptions or trauma, and the management of megacolon in cats. A colectomy is typically performed through a midline celiotomy, though 'pull through' colonic resection via a transanal approach is described. When resection of the colorectal junction or the distal aspects of the descending colon is planned a pubic symphysiotomy or pubic osteotomy may be required to improve surgical exposure. Anastomosis of the colon is performed using a monofilament suture material with a prolonged tensile strength such as Polydioxanone or Glycomer 631 with an appositional simple interrupted suture pattern. An alternative to sutures is the use of an EEA stapling instrument that creates a circular inverting anastomosis with a double row of stainless steel staples.

Typhlectomy

Typhlectomy is removal of the caecum and is indicated for treatment of caecal inversion, impaction or perforation and occasionally caecal neoplasia. The base of the caecum is clamped, the caecum resected and the stump over-sewn using a Parker-Kerr suture pattern.

Colopexy

A colopexy is the creation of a permanent adhesion between the descending colon and the left abdominal wall. It is most commonly indicated to prevent recurrent rectal prolapse. The technique is performed via a ventral midline celiotomy. Cranial traction is applied to the descending colon and the colon is sutured to the left abdominal wall using two rows of six to eight single interrupted non-absorbable monofilament sutures.

Colostomy

A colostomy is creation of a permanent artificial opening in the colon to the exterior through the body wall. Colostomies are created to allow passage of faeces when obstruction of the rectum exists. They are described in veterinary literature for the management of rectal or intrapelvic masses that cannot be managed by primary excision. Two techniques have been described, either creation of a side-to-side anastomosis of the colon to the body wall or an end-to-end anastomosis of the colon to the body wall. Colostomies are rarely performed in veterinary patients due to the demanding long-term postoperative management required.

Feline megacolon

Approximately 60% of feline megacolon is idiopathic, with the vast majority of the remainder of cases secondary to pelvic stenosis from pelvic fractures (25%) or nerve injury (5%). Management of feline megacolon is dependent on the severity and duration of the condition. Initial episodes or recurrent cases responsive to medical therapy are treated medically. Immediate relief of the constipation is provided by warm water enemas under general anaesthesia. Long-term management includes laxatives, prokinetics, and dietary modification. Lactulose appears to be the most effective laxative and is often combined with a bulk-forming laxative such as Peridale granules.

Widening of the pelvic canal is described as a management of megacolon that has occurred secondary to pelvic stenosis. This approach is typically reserved for those cases that have suffered constipation for less than 6 months. For cases of idiopathic megacolon not responsive to medical management or those cases secondary to pelvic stenosis with constipation greater than 6 months a subtotal colectomy is the management of choice.

Prior to anaesthesia and surgery, abdominal radiographs are used to assess the degree of colonic dilation and to rule out extraluminal compressive lesions. Haematology and serum biochemistry is indicated as chronic constipation may lead to electrolyte imbalances and dehydration. Any haemodynamic or electrolyte abnormalities should be corrected with intravenous fluid prior to anaesthesia. A subtotal colectomy is performed via a caudally positioned midline abdominal celiotomy. An enema is not performed prior to the surgery.

Postoperative complications included peritonitis secondary to dehiscence of the anastomosis, tenesmus, loose faeces, occasionally severe diarrhoea, stricture formation at the surgery site and recurrent megacolon. Loose faeces are observed in the majority of cases and should resolve within 3 months of surgery.

Postoperative care following large intestinal surgery

Postoperative care following large intestinal surgery is rarely demanding as the majority of patients are not critically ill and the surgery is performed as an elective procedure. Intravenous fluid therapy is continued until the animal is eating well and any preoperative haemodynamic, electrolyte or acid–base abnormalities are corrected. Animals are fed an appropriate diet for 12–24 hours after surgery. If postoperative tenesmus is observed then analgesia is provided. Severe tenesmus may require local anaesthetic or opiate epidurals to lessen the severity of straining. Topical local anaesthetic creams applied per rectum may control mild tenesmus. As with all bowel surgery if vomiting occurs the patient should be closely evaluated for the possible complication of peritonitis.

LIVER, SPLEEN AND PANCREAS

Liver

Symptoms of liver disease can vary tremendously from clinical jaundice, to cranial abdominal pain, to vague non-specific gastrointestinal disease. Liver disease can result in many metabolic abnormalities including hypoproteinaemia, ascites, abnormal clotting, fasting hypoglycaemia and electrolyte imbalances. Evidence of liver disease can be evaluated by measuring serum hepatic enzymes and bilirubin, performing functional biochemical tests including pre- and postprandial serum bile acids, abdominal radiographs and abdominal ultrasonography.

Prior to anaesthesia and surgery, attempts are made to correct any metabolic abnormalities using intravenous fluid therapy and appropriate medical therapy. As many drugs, including premedicants and anaesthetic agents, are metabolised by the liver, reduced doses of these drugs frequently have equivalent or increased effects compared with normal doses in healthy animals. All medications that are metabolised by the liver should be administered using reduced or conservative dosing regimes and preferably avoided if possible. Liver disease impairs protein synthesis and consequently the production of albumin and clotting factors. Evaluation of clotting profiles to detect coagulopathies secondary to the hepatic disease is performed prior to surgery in these patients.

The most common indication for liver surgery is to perform a biopsy or partial hepatectomy for removal of discrete hepatic masses and occasionally to occlude a portosystemic shunt. The liver is approached via a midline abdominal celiotomy. The skin is clipped and scrubbed for a midline celiotomy and the patient positioned in dorsal recumbency. Partial hepatectomies can be performed by hand using the 'finger fracture' technique combined with ligation of vessels with suture material or mechanically using a transabdominal (TA) stapling device.

Repeated evaluation of the patient's packed cell volume (PCV) may be required postoperatively as there is an increased risk of postoperative haemorrhage. If significant haemorrhage is observed then surgical exploration of the abdomen, to identify the source of bleeding, may be required. Repeated evaluation of blood glucose is indicated, as patients with liver disease are susceptible to hypoglycaemia postoperatively. Postoperative hypoglycaemia can be managed by administration of isotonic dextrose (5%) in water and encouraging the patient to eat. For patients with occlusion of a portosystemic shunt intensive care monitoring is required with regular evaluation of the cardiovascular system. Postoperative antibiotics are indicated in some patients following hepatic surgery, though this is dependent on the underlying disease process.

Spleen

The most common indication for surgery of the spleen is to perform a splenectomy to remove a splenic mass (Fig 3.13). Rarely a partial splenectomy is performed. Frequently the splenic masses rupture and the patient presents due to haemorrhage into the abdomen. Less common indications for splenic surgery are splenic torsions and severe trauma to the spleen.

Patients with a haemoabdomen secondary to a ruptured splenic mass or splenic trauma are evaluated for evidence of haemodynamic abnormalities and possible shock. Preoperative management is dependent on the severity of changes. In the majority of patients intravenous crystalloid fluid therapy will be sufficient to stabilise any haemodynamic

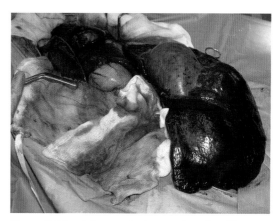

Figure 3.13 A large splenic mass in a dog. The spleen is engorged due to the dog having been administered a barbiturate anaesthetic agent. Despite the size of the mass it is still possible that it is not malignant as only 50% of splenic masses are malignant. Photograph © Arthur House.

abnormalities, though in rare cases whole blood transfusions or colloid infusions may be required.

Splenic neoplasia may be either malignant or a metastatic nodule rather than the primary tumour. The patient should be thoroughly evaluated for the primary mass or metastatic nodules at other sites in the body. Typical presurgical evaluation involves thoracic radiographs and abdominal ultrasound.

Postoperative haemorrhage is an uncommon complication following splenic surgery. Repeated evaluation of the patient's PCV may be required. If the surgery is successful at preventing further haemorrhage then the presurgical anaemia will be of limited duration and an increase in the PCV will be observed within days. If significant postoperative haemorrhage is observed then surgical exploration of the abdomen, to identify the continued source of bleeding, may be required.

Pancreatitis following splenic surgery is a rare complication and results from traumatic handling of the pancreas. Patients who develop vomiting postoperatively should be evaluated for development of either pancreatitis or peritonitis.

Pancreas

Surgery is infrequently performed on the pancreas, as most diseases of the pancreas are not amenable to surgical treatment. The pancreas is approached via a midline abdominal celiotomy. The skin is clipped and scrubbed for a midline celiotomy and the patient positioned in dorsal recumbency. Partial pancreatectomies are occasionally performed to remove discrete pancreatic masses such as insulinomas (Fig 3.14) or pancreatic abscess and cysts. Animals with severe pancreatic disease suffer significant metabolic abnormalities that require intensive medical therapy. Manipulation of the pancreas at surgery can result in increased inflammation of the pancreas and worsening of the underlying condition. All patients are monitored for development of pancreatitis following pancreatic surgery. The value of feeding animals with pancreatitis is presently disputed, though there is recent evidence to suggest that it is beneficial to feed dogs with pancreatitis. The decision to feed a patient is on an individual basis

Insulinomas result in recurrent episodes of hypoglycaemia. Medical management for hypoglycaemia involves frequent small meals and hyperglycaemic drugs. Dogs with insulinomas should not have prolonged periods of starvation prior to anaesthesia. Postoperative blood glucose levels are monitored as some animals develop hyperglycaemia following removal of an insulinoma.

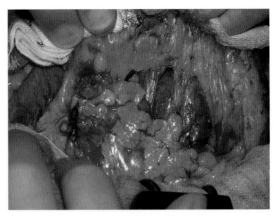

Figure 3.14   An insulinoma within the duodenal limb of the pancreas (left aspect of image, pink nodule adjacent to haemorrhage). Typically insulinomas are small nodules and can be difficult to image prior to surgery. Photograph © Arthur House.

ENTERAL ACCESS

The need for and the provision of enteral access should be part of the initial surgical plan. Enteral access can be achieved via oesophagostomy, gastrostomy or jejunostomy tubes. Tube placement is as orad as possible and is dictated by the disease process. Early and adequate nutritional support is essential in the critically ill patient to maintain the animal's defences to injury mechanisms and restore or maintain a positive nitrogen balance. Enteral feeding is associated with fewer complications and preferable to parenteral nutrition when possible. Alimentary nutrition (oesophageal, gastric or jejunal) has positive effects on enterocyte viability and intestinal wall integrity. Calorific requirements for each patient are calculated as a factor of resting energy requirement and are dependent on the disease process.

Further reading

Journal articles

Aronson L R, Brockman D J, Brown D C 2000 Gastrointestinal emergencies. Vet Clin North Am Small Anim Pract 30(3):555–579

Brockman D J, Mongil C M, Aronson L R, Brown D C 2000 A practical approach to hemoperitoneum in the dog and cat. Vet Clin North Am Small Anim Pract 30(3):657–668

Brockman D J, Holt D E 2000 Management protocol for acute gastric dilation – volvulus syndrome in dogs. Compend Contin Educ Pract Vet 24(8)1025–1034

Pavletic M M, Schwartz A 1994 Stapling
instrumentation. Vet Clin North Am Small Anim
Pract 24(2):247–278

Marks S L 1998 The principles and practical
application of enteral nutrition. Vet Clin North
Am Small Anim Pract 28(3):677–708

Textbooks

Slatter D 2003 Textbook of small animal surgery,
3rd edn. W B Saunders, Philadelphia

Fossum T W 2002 Small animal surgery, 2nd edn.
Mosby, St Louis

Borab J (ed) 1998 Current techniques in small
animal surgery, 4th edn. Williams and Wilkins,
Baltimore

Chapter 4

Urogenital Surgery

Alison Beck

CHAPTER OBJECTIVES

- Diagnosis of urogenital disease
  - History
  - Physical examination
  - Blood tests
  - Radiography
  - Ultrasonography
  - Advanced imaging techniques
  - Cystoscopy
  - Abdominocentesis
  - Biopsy techniques

- Preoperative considerations
  - Urinary obstruction
  - Fluid therapy
  - Anaesthesia

- General surgical principles for urogenital diseases
  - Classification of urogenital surgery
  - Preparation for surgery
  - Surgical instruments
  - Abdominal exploration
  - Suture materials and closure techniques
  - Lavage
  - Antibiotic use
  - Tissue healing
  - The assistant's role

- Diseases of the kidneys
  - Hydronephrosis and hydroureter
  - Renal neoplasia
  - Ureteronephrectomy

  - Renal biopsy techniques
  - Renal transplantation

- Diseases of the ureters
  - Ectopic ureters

- Diseases of the bladder
  - Urolithiasis
  - Bladder rupture
  - Bladder neoplasia
  - Cystotomy (including calculus removal)
  - Tube cystostomy

- Diseases of the urethra
  - Urethral sphincter mechanism incompetence
  - Colposuspension
  - Urethral obstruction
  - Urethral trauma
  - Urethrotomy and urethrostomy in male dogs
  - Perineal and prepubic urethrostomy in cats
  - Indwelling urinary catheters

- Diseases of the female reproductive tract
  - Pyometra
  - Vagina oedema and vaginal prolapse
  - Neoplasia
  - Neutering
  - Caesarean section
  - Episiotomy
  - Mammary neoplasia

continued

CHAPTER OBJECTIVES *(continued)*

■ Diseases of the male reproductive tract
    Prostatitis and prostatic abscesses
    Prostatic and paraprostatic cysts
    Prostatic neoplasia
    Prostatic omentalisation

■ Peri- and postoperative management
    Monitoring urine output
    Fluid therapy
    Wound management

Urogenital disease is commonly seen in companion animal practice. Obtaining an accurate and complete history, combined with a complete physical examination, provides the clinician with the ability to devise a problem list. This will influence further diagnostic tests that are performed and allow an accurate diagnosis to be made. Treatment options are then based on the disease process, its severity and the owner's wishes. Some urogenital diseases are incidental findings of no clinical significance. Failing to understand the owner's presenting complaint may cause the significant problem to be overlooked or inappropriate treatment to be given.

Signs of urogenital disease (Table 4.1) include:

- haematuria – macroscopic or microscopic blood in the urine
- anuria – absence of urine production
- dysuria/stranguria – difficulty or pain on urination
- pollakiuria – increased frequency of urination
- vaginal or penile discharge
- urinary incontinence.

DIAGNOSIS OF UROGENITAL DISEASE

More information on the diagnostic tests described here can be found in the *Textbook of veterinary medical nursing* (see Further reading).

History

The animal's history is obtained at the time of first consultation, and should be detailed and complete before further investigations are performed. Definitions may need to be explained to some owners, and it is worth noting that owners may mistake dysuria for constipation. Many owners will not know their pet's normal urination habits, particularly outdoor cats. Urogenital disease may reflect disease of a different organ system (e.g. urate urolithiasis in animals with portosystemic shunt, calcium urolithiasis in dogs with primary hyperparathyroidism), so careful questioning about all aspects of the animal's health is required.

Questions to ask the owner include:

- Is your dog continent?
  - Does it dribble urine when walking around?
  - Does it leave a puddle of urine when it has been lying down?
- Can the animal void urine normally?
- Does the dog urinate in the house or overnight?
- Does the cat use a litter tray?
- Does the animal strain to urinate unproductively?
- Does the animal strain to produce small quantities of urine or cry out when urinating?
- Does the urine smell?
- Has there been blood in the urine?
  - Is it throughout the stream?
  - Is it at the end of urination?
  - Does he drip blood from his penis?
- Is the urine discoloured?
- Is there a vaginal or penile discharge and what is its character?
- Is the animal urinating more frequently or larger volumes?
- Is the animal drinking more than normal?

Table 4.1   Diseases of the urogenital system

Kidney	Congenital	Agenesis
		Supernumerary
		Small kidney (hypoplasia/dysplasia)
		Ectopic kidney
		Fused kidneys
		Cysts
	Acquired	Trauma
		Idiopathic haematuria
		Urolithiasis
		Hydronephrosis
		Pyelonephritis
		Renal failure (acute, chronic)
		Neoplasia
Ureters	Congenital	Ectopic ureters
		Ureterocoele
		Agenesis
		Duplication
	Acquired	Trauma (rupture, crushing, urinoma)
		Obstruction (urolithiasis, stricture, fibrosis, blood clot)
Bladder	Congenital	Urachal anomalies
	Acquired	Trauma/rupture
		Urolithiasis
		Cystitis
		Neoplasia
Urethra	Congenital	Sphincter mechanism incompetence
		Hypospadias/epispadias
		Urethrorectal fistula
	Acquired	Sphincter mechanism incompetence
		Urethritis
		Prolapse
		Obstruction (urolithiasis, neoplasia, stricture)
		Urolithiasis
		Trauma
		Lower urinary tract disease in cats

Table 4.1   continued

Female reproductive tract	Congenital	Ovarian agenesis/ supernumerary ovary
		Vaginal aplasia/ hypoplasia
		Persistent hymen (vaginovestibular stenosis, vertical bands)
		Rectovaginal fistula
		Intersex
	Acquired	Pyometra
		Neoplasia
		Vaginal oedema
		Vaginal/uterine prolapse
Male reproductive tract	Congenital	Mono-/anorchism
		Cryptorchidism
		Persistent frenulum
		Phimosis
	Acquired	Orchitis
		Trauma
		Neoplasia
		Paraphimosis
		Priapism
		Benign prostatic hyperplasia
		Prostatitis and prostatic abscess
		Prostatic and paraprostatic cysts

- – If entire, when was the last season?
- Does the animal strain to pass faeces?
- What food does the animal eat?
  - – Wet or dry food?
  - – Prescription or commercially available diet?
- Has the animal had treatment for any other disease?
- Are these clinical signs recurrent?
  - – e.g. repeat episodes of urinary tract infection may occur in dogs with other urinary tract disease.

Physical examination

A routine physical examination including temperature, pulse and respiration, is performed in all animals. Concurrent diseases may be

- Is the animal neutered?
  - – When was it neutered?
  - – Had the bitch had a season before neutering?

present, particularly in older animals, and may influence the treatment of urogenital disease. Some animals may present in varying stages of shock and collapse. A brief physical examination is performed before emergency treatment such as fluid therapy is instituted, but it is important to complete a full examination, including rectal examination, when the patient is stable.

Examination of the urogenital system includes careful abdominal palpation, vaginal and rectal examinations, and examination of the external genitalia and mammary glands. Organomegaly may be apparent on abdominal palpation, including kidneys, ovaries, uterus and prostate. Pain may be elicited, especially with inflammatory or infectious conditions such as prostatic abscesses or peritonitis. Complete urethral obstruction leads to a distended bladder that is firm and painful even with gentle palpation. Care is taken when handling a turgid distended bladder as rupture may occur. Cystic uroliths are palpable in approximately 20% of affected animals.

The mammary chain is carefully palpated for masses and the inguinal and axillary lymph nodes are palpated for lymphadenopathy. Milk is examined in lactating bitches.

Vaginal examination may allow palpation of the urethra, urethral tubercle, vagina, vestibule and cervix. Abnormal findings may include masses, strictures or inflammatory lesions. Further investigation using vaginoscopy is usually performed under sedation or anaesthesia. The vagina and vulva are carefully examined for congenital anomalies, e.g. intersexuality, anorectal cleft.

The penis and prepuce are examined for congenital anomalies including hypospadias. The penis is extruded from the prepuce and examined for masses, trauma etc.

Rectal examination allows palpation of the vagina in females, urethra and prostate in males, and the medial iliac (sublumbar) lymph nodes. A normal prostate can be identified on either rectal or abdominal palpation, except in large dogs. It should be symmetrical, mobile and pain-free. In older entire males the gland may be enlarged and in an intra-abdominal position due to benign prostatic hyperplasia.

Blood tests

Biochemistry

Increases in urea and creatinine may occur with primary renal disease (e.g. acute renal failure), prerenal disease (e.g. dehydration) or postrenal disease (e.g. complete urinary tract obstruction, bladder rupture). Hyperkalaemia and metabolic acidosis may accompany complete urinary tract obstruction or renal failure.

Haematology

Animals with inflammatory disease may have leucocytosis (especially with prostatic and renal inflammation) or occasionally leucopaenia with toxic changes in severe cases. Anaemia may occur in chronic renal failure or with prolonged haematuria. The reader is referred to the *Textbook of veterinary medical nursing* for more information regarding interpretation of blood tests.

Urinalysis

Cystocentesis is the method of choice for obtaining a urine sample, particularly when bacteriological culture and sensitivity is required, or to differentiate bladder and prostatic disease. It can be performed with or without ultrasound guidance. It may be difficult to obtain a sample in dysuric or incontinent animals as the bladder may be empty. Collection by urethral catheterisation may also be performed, and in males the penis should be cleaned first. In male dogs catheter samples may contain prostatic fluid. Both the prepuce and vagina have normal commensal bacterial flora, so free-catch urine samples should be considered contaminated. The reader is referred to the *Textbook of veterinary medical nursing* for more information regarding technique. Urine is submitted for:

Specific gravity This should reflect the hydration status of the animal. A low specific gravity in the face of dehydration is suggestive of primary renal disease. The reader is referred to the *Textbook of veterinary medical nursing* for more information regarding interpretation of specific gravity.

Dipstik Haematuria may be seen with idiopathic haematuria, inflammation, bacterial infection, neoplasia or trauma.

Cytology

- *White blood cells* are increased in sediment with inflammation or infection.
- *Urinary crystals* are often present in normal urine, but in the presence of uroliths may give an indication of their composition.
- *Transitional epithelial cells* are a normal finding. However, it can be difficult to differentiate malignant from reactive epithelial cells. Fresh transitional cells can be obtained by flushing the bladder with sterile saline before collecting a sample.
- *Spermatazoa* may be seen in entire males.

Bacteriological culture and sensitivity The most commonly isolated bacterium from infected urine is *E. coli*. Bacteria are rarely identified on cytology.

Prostatic wash

Prostatic fluid is routinely obtained in the investigation of prostatic disease. The reader is referred to the *Textbook of veterinary medical nursing* for more information regarding technique.

Radiography

A well-performed radiographic study (Box 4.1) is fundamental for the diagnosis and treatment of urogenital disease. These techniques do not require specialist equipment, but do require planning and patience. Patients are starved for 24–36 hours. Removing residual faecal material from the colon allows better visualisation of the urinary tract, particularly the ureters. Soapy enemas are avoided as bubbles may cause artefacts. In medium and large dogs a single preparation of a phosphate enema (Fletchers enema, Forest Labs UK Ltd) can be given 6–12 hours before anaesthesia and the patient allowed outside to defecate. Small dogs should have warm water enemas only as phosphate enemas can cause hyperphosphataemia.

Radiographs are obtained under anaesthesia. A large bore intravenous catheter is placed to allow rapid injection of contrast, but intravenous fluids are withheld until intravenous urography is completed.

Plain orthogonal abdominal radiographs are always obtained before contrast studies. They are analysed for changes in size, shape, number and opacity. They are particularly useful for the recognition of radio-opaque calculi. Intravenous urography is indicated for investigation of renal and ureteric disease. Positive-, negative- and double-contrast retrograde studies are indicated for investigating urethral, bladder, prostatic and vaginal diseases.

Ultrasonography

Ultrasonography is routinely performed during the investigation of urogenital disease. It can give valuable information regarding the structure of the kidneys, ureters, bladder and prostate. It is particularly useful for the diagnosis of urolithiasis, mass lesions, inflammatory disorders, hydronephrosis and hydroureter, prostatic disease, and ectopic ureters. It is also beneficial in obtaining urine and tissue samples.

Advanced imaging techniques

Renal angiography, computed tomography and magnetic resonance imaging have been described but have limited availability. Nuclear scintigraphy is a specialised technique that allows assessment of individual renal function, and is useful before ureteronephrectomy to assess the function of the contralateral kidney.

Cystoscopy

Cystoscopy is a more specialised technique that allows examination of the urethra, bladder, ureters and vagina. It allows biopsy of mucosal lesions, identification of ectopic ureters and removal of small cystic uroliths.

Abdominocentesis

Diagnostic yield is increased if aspiration is made from four quadrants of the abdomen

Box 4.1   Performing a radiographic study

1. Plain radiographs

Obtain lateral and ventrodorsal radiographs of the cranial abdomen (kidneys), pelvis and penis in males. Pull the legs cranially for a second lateral radiograph in males to allow visualisation of the urethra without superimposition of the pelvic limbs.

2. Pneumocystogram

Catheterise and empty the bladder (submit the urine for urinalysis and culture). Instil 1ml/kg of air into the bladder and ensure the bladder is palpably full. The air will help to outline contrast in the ureter during later studies. Obtain a radiograph if required.

3. Intravenous urography (Fig 4.1)

Place the animal in dorsal recumbency with the beam centred over the kidneys. Perform a rapid intravenous injection of 700mg/kg aqueous organic iodide (e.g. Urografin 370mg/ml iodide, Schering).

Obtain two consecutive ventrodorsal radiographs immediately after contrast injection (the renal vasculature and the kidneys are outlined) and then at 5 and 10 minutes (the ureters and renal pelvis are outlined). Obtain a lateral radiograph centred over the caudal abdomen and pelvis at 15 minutes. Further radiographs are taken as needed.

Note changes in size, shape and position of the kidneys and renal pelves. Poor filling may occur with poor renal blood flow or hydronephrosis. Adverse reactions such as hypotension are rare.

4. Retrograde urethrocystography (male dogs) (Fig 4.2)

Place the dog in lateral recumbency with the beam centred on the pelvis and caudal abdomen. Fill a syringe with Urografin (diluted 50:50 with saline, 1ml/kg total dose) and prefill a dog urinary catheter (6–10Fr) to avoid air bubbles. Place into the tip of the penis and hold with tongue forceps.

Wearing protective lead clothing, inject the contrast and obtain a radiograph during the last part of the injection or sooner if resistance is felt. Repeat the study with the legs pulled forward to outline the distal urethra and penis if urethral disease is suspected. Repeat to obtain orthogonal views.

5. Retrograde urethrocystography (male cats) (Fig 4.3)

Place the cat in lateral recumbency. Extrude the penis and place a prefilled cat urinary catheter or sheath of an intravenous catheter into the tip of the penis. Hold in place with tongue forceps if necessary. Inject diluted contrast agent and obtain orthogonal radiographs as above.

6. Retrograde vaginourethrocystography (females) (Figs 4.4, 4.5)

Position the animal in lateral recumbency. Cut the tip off a Foley catheter without damaging the bulb. Place the prefilled catheter within the vestibule, place tongue forceps across the vulva and inflate the Foley balloon. Place caudal traction on the catheter so the bulb is caudal to the urethral tubercle.

Inject up to 2ml/kg of diluted contrast, or until resistance to the injection is felt, and obtain a radiograph during the last part of the injection. Repeat to obtain orthogonal views. The contrast will outline the vestibule, vagina, urethra and bladder. Do not perform when in oestrus or receiving exogenous oestrogens, as the vagina will over distend and the uretha will not fill with contrast or the vagina may rupture.

7. Double-contrast cystography

After positive contrast cystography, remove residual contrast from the bladder and instill 1ml/kg of air or until the bladder is palpable. Obtain orthogonal radiographs.

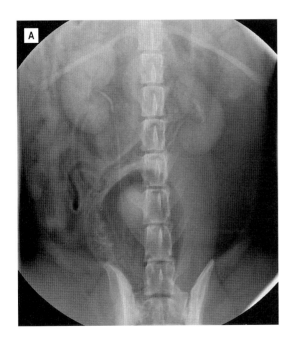

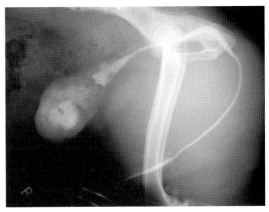

Figure 4.2   Positive contrast retrograde urethrocystogram (lateral projection) in a male dog. A radiolucent calculus is visible in the bladder, highlighted by contrast. The urethra is normal. Swirling of contrast in the bladder occurs due to injection of contrast whilst the radiograph is being taken. Photograph © Alison Beck.

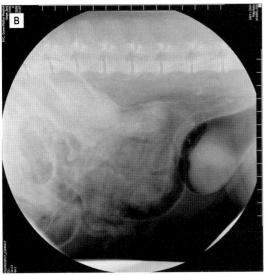

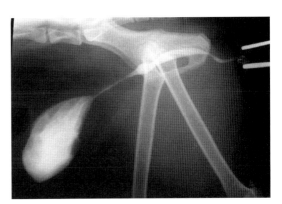

Figure 4.3   Positive contrast retrograde urethrocystogram (lateral projection) in a male cat. No abnormalities are noted. Photograph © Alison Beck.

Figure 4.1   Intravenous urogram: (a) dorsoventral and (b) lateral projections. Contrast highlights the renal silhouettes, renal pelves and ureters. Air and contrast are visible within the bladder. The left kidney is irregular in outline. Photograph © Alison Beck.

or by using ultrasonography to sample small volumes of fluid and avoid inadvertent puncture of abdominal organs. Fluid is submitted for cytology, bacteriological culture and sensitivity, and biochemistry where appropriate.

Urine may be present if there is rupture of the urinary system, particularly after abdominal trauma or urinary tract obstruction. The bladder is the most likely source. Urine is confirmed by the presence of higher concentration of creatinine in the fluid compared with serum sampled at the same time.

Exudate may be associated with rupture of a urogenital abscess or infected hollow viscus, e.g. pyometra, prostatic abscess.

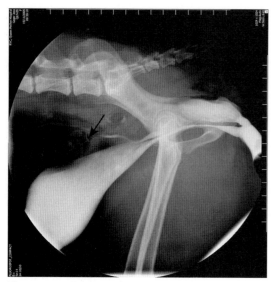

Figure 4.4   Positive contrast retrograde vaginourethrocystogram (lateral projection) in a female dog. An ectopic ureter enters the proximal urethra. Photograph © Alison Beck.

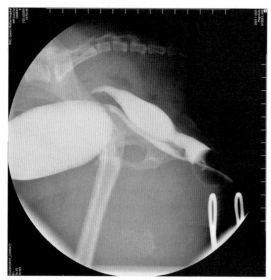

Figure 4.5   Positive contrast retrograde vaginourethrocystogram (lateral projection) in a female dog. The bladder is caudally positioned consistent with USMI. Photograph © Alison Beck.

Biopsy techniques

Tissue may be sampled for histopathology or for bacteriological culture and sensitivity. Methods for obtaining tissue include: fine needle aspirate; tru-cut biopsy; catheter biopsy; laparoscopic or surgical incisional/excisional biopsy techniques.

Fine needle aspirate

Although the sensitivity may be low, FNA is an easy, minimally invasive method of obtaining tissue or fluid. Ultrasound guidance is useful to allow aspiration of deeper tissues. Fluid, including pus, may leak into surrounding tissues when aspirating cystic masses so it is preferable to completely drain them if they are aspirated. Aspiration or biopsy may potentially seed malignant tumours along the needle tract, especially transitional cell carcinoma, but is uncommon. Aspiration has been described for:

- renal lesions e.g. lymphoma in cats
- prostatic cysts
- testicular masses
- inflammatory mammary lesions to differentiate non-malignant inflammation from inflammatory carcinoma.

Tru-cut biopsy

Tru-cut is performed similarly to aspiration but more tissue is obtained. Sedation is usually required. The reader is referred to the *Textbook of veterinary medical nursing* for more information regarding technique.

Catheter biopsy

Bladder and urethral mucosa can be biopsied by placing a side-hole catheter into an empty bladder or urethra and repeatedly sucking on a 20ml syringe attached to the catheter. Tissue or fluid that is collected can be sent for histopathology or placed on a slide for cytology. Grab biopsies using endoscopic forceps can be used to obtain biopsies and ultrasound guidance can improve accuracy.

Laparoscopic or surgical incisional/excisional biopsy techniques

These are performed if other biopsies have been inconclusive or if they are considered dangerous to perform, e.g. for prostatic abscess. All tissue removed during surgical exploration of the urogenital tract should be sent for histopathology to confirm the diagnosis and to rule out neoplasia.

PREOPERATIVE CONSIDERATIONS

Urinary obstruction

Prolonged urinary tract obstruction will lead to dehydration, uraemia, hyperkalaemia and metabolic acidosis. Left untreated, death will occur within 3 days. Treatment of the metabolic abnormalities is mandatory before sedation or anaesthesia is performed. Intravenous fluid therapy is often all that is required, but marked hyperkalaemia may need specific treatment to avoid potentially fatal arrhythmias. A severely distended bladder can be decompressed by cystocentesis, but this should not be performed repeatedly and is not as a substitute for relieving the site of obstruction.

Fluid therapy

Intravenous fluid therapy is indicated for all animals undergoing surgery or prolonged anaesthesia. The recommended fluid therapy rate is 10ml/kg/h but is adjusted depending upon preoperative assessment of dehydration or hypovolaemia, intraoperative fluid losses, haemodynamic status, and cardiac and renal disease. A balanced electrolyte solution is used, e.g. Hartmann's. Synthetic colloids and blood products may be indicated in certain circumstances.

Anaesthesia

Routine anaesthesia (Table 4.2) can be used in animals with urinary tract disease. This may include premedication with an opioid and/or acepromazine before induction with thiopental or propofol. Cats can be safely sedated with a benzodiazepine and ketamine, especially for urethral obstruction. Analgesia is mandatory for surgical treatment of urogenital disease. Opioids are given peri- and postoperatively for 1–5 days depending upon the disease and surgical treatment. Non-steroidal anti-inflammatory drugs (NSAIDs) are given to dogs unless contraindicated, e.g. gastric disease, renal insufficiency, but are used with care in cats. The reader's attention is drawn to different licensing of NSAIDs in cats. Epidural and regional local anaesthesia techniques can be considered.

Table 4.2   Anaesthesia/analgesia in the treatment of urinary tract disease

Stage	Drug used	Dosage
Premedication	Acepromazine Pethidine Morphine	0.01–0.03mg/kg* 2–5mg/kg* 0.2–0.4mg/kg*
Induction	Thiopental Propofol	25mg/kg to effect 10mg/kg to effect
Maintenance	Halothane or isoflurane	
Sedation	Diazepam or midazolam with ketamine	0.2mg/kg 5mg/kg iv
Opioid analgesia	Morphine Buprenorphine	0.2–0.4mg/kg q4h for first 12–48h 0.01–0.03mg/kg q6–8h for 1–5 days
Non-steroidal anti-inflammatory drugs	Carprofen Meloxicam	4mg/kg sid (dogs) 0.2mg/kg day 1 then 0.1mg/kg sid (dogs)

*Higher dose rates can be used with caution

GENERAL SURGICAL PRINCIPLES FOR UROGENITAL DISEASES

Classification of urogenital surgery

See Table 4.3.

Preparation for surgery

As with all surgical procedures, a wide area of hair is clipped, so that the incision can be extended if necessary. It is better to prepare a larger area than is needed than to find the surgical wound impinges on hair.

If the surgical wound is close to the urethra, e.g. during colposuspension or prostatic surgery, the urethra is catheterised preoperatively to minimise inadvertent damage. Catheterisation is also useful to identify the urethral lumen during urethral surgery. Catheterisation may be required intraoperatively, e.g. to flush the urethra when removing uroliths via cystotomy, so the prepuce in males should be lavaged with an antiseptic during the surgical preparation. Females are catheterised with a silicone Foley catheter. Males can be catheterised with either a Foley catheter or a male urinary catheter – the latter is stiffer and ideal during urethral surgery.

Routine draping using impermeable drapes is optimal. Large amounts of lavage fluids are often used during urogenital surgery and strike through may occur with cotton drapes.

Surgical instruments

See Box 4.2 for details of the instruments used. Magnifying equipment, e.g. loupes and operating microscopes, are available in larger institutions and are invaluable for ureteric surgery, particularly in cats. Laparoscopy allows less invasive procedures, e.g. biopsy, to be performed.

Abdominal exploration

An incision of sufficient size for the surgical procedure should be planned. Complications can occur due to performing surgery through an incision that is too small. Laparotomy incisions should be large enough to allow complete abdominal exploration, and may need to extend from the xiphisternum to the pubis. For bladder exploration only, the incision may extend from the umbilicus to the pubis. A pubic osteotomy or symphysiotomy may be required to examine the urethra and prostate and is not associated with high morbidity. Self-retaining abdominal retractors are mandatory.

Table 4.3 Classification of urogenital surgery	
Classification	Description
Clean	Urogenital tract not entered
Clean contaminated	Vaginal or other urogenital surgery in the absence of infection
Contaminated	Urogenital tract entered in the presence of urinary infection
Dirty	Traumatic wounds more than 4 hours old or infected tissues

Box 4.2   Surgical instruments used in urogenital surgery

1. Fine tissue forceps e.g. Debakey
2. Metzembaum and mayo scissors for cutting fine tissues (e.g. urethra) and fibrous tissue (e.g. linea alba) respectively
3. Fine mosquito forceps for dissection
4. Separate mosquito forceps for stay sutures
5. Lavage fluids and suction apparatus with a Poole or Yankauer tip
6. Cotton buds for haemostasis or dissection of delicate tissues, e.g. during ectopic ureter surgery
7. Surgical swabs (small and large) with radio-opaque markers
8. Self-retaining abdominal retractors, e.g. Balfour
9. Synthetic absorbable monofilament suture material with swaged on needles

The urinary tract is explored from the kidneys distally. Exceptions to this rule occur when a defined procedure is being performed, e.g. colposuspension, or when urogenital disease has been localised to one anatomical area by preoperative imaging, e.g. cystotomy for removing cystic uroliths. The kidneys, ureters and reproductive organs can be visualised by displacing the descending colon and descending duodenum towards the midline (Fig 4.6). Peristalsis can be seen in normal ureters.

Large moistened laparotomy sponges are used to isolate the urinary tract from the rest of the abdominal cavity to avoid contamination and to increase exposure. The urinary tract is susceptible to trauma from surgical instruments – it should be handled with smooth-tipped instruments. Using the fingers and thumbs is a more gentle way to handle the kidneys and bladder. Stay sutures are placed in the bladder or urethra and on incision edges to allow manipulation without trauma from surgical instruments, and to improve visualisation (Fig 4.7). Oedema and erythema can occur with excess manipulation, especially in the young dog, and may lead to urinary tract obstruction. Dissection is avoided on the dorsal aspect of the bladder neck and urethra to avoid damaging neurovascular structures.

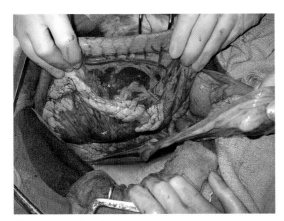

Figure 4.6 Duodenal manoeuvre in a dog. The duodenum, with the pancreas seen in the mesoduodenum, is reflected medially, to allow visualisation of the right kidney, ovary and uterine horn. Photograph © Alison Beck.

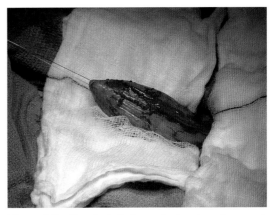

Figure 4.7 Surgical photograph showing placement of a stay suture in the apex of the bladder. Note the placement of laparotomy swabs to isolate the bladder from the abdomen. Photograph © Alison Beck.

Care is taken to identify the ureters and reproductive tract to avoid inadvertent damage, particularly during resection of prostatic and bladder neck masses.

Incisions are made with a scalpel blade or fine Metzembaum scissors. Excess electro-coagulation is avoided in tissues susceptible to trauma such as the bladder and ureter. Laser surgery has been reported.

Suture materials and closure techniques

Absorbable, synthetic, monofilament sutures are mandatory. Braided sutures potentiate infection and non-absorbable sutures act as a nidus for urolith formation. All sutures rapidly lose strength in infected, alkaline urine. The ideal suture material is polydioxanone (PDS, Ethicon). Catgut is not recommended due to poor knotting characteristics and unpredictable breakdown. Small suture size is selected (1–1.5 metric) for the bladder and urethra. Smaller suture for ureteral surgery may require the use of magnification.

Cystotomy incisions can be sutured using simple interrupted or continuous sutures that do not include the mucosa to decease the risk of urolith formation, or with a double layer inverting pattern (Fig 4.8). The bursting

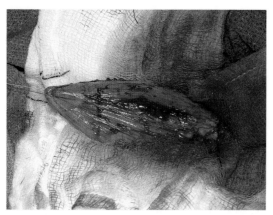

Figure 4.8 Surgical photograph showing simple interrupted closure of a cystotomy incision with a monofilament absorbable suture material. Photograph © Alison Beck.

taminated procedures or when surgical time is likely to exceed 2 hours. Therapeutic antibiotics are given when there is evidence of infection, e.g. urinary tract infection, pyometra, prostatic abscess. Antibiotics are administered intravenously at anaesthetic induction and every 2 hours until the end of surgery. Postoperative antibiotics are only indicated when known infection is present. Use of antibiotics other than by this regime, e.g. subcutaneous injection postoperatively, may actually increase the rate of infection. The most common bacteria in urogenital infections are *E. coli* and *Staphylococcus* species. Antibiotics effective against these bacteria include cephalosporins e.g. cefuroxime (Zinacef; Glaxo Smith Kline 20mg/kg) and amoxicillin-clavulanate (Augmentin; Glaxo Smith Kline 20mg/kg).

strength of the bladder is similar after both techniques.

Urethrostomy incisions are sutured with simple interrupted sutures of polyamide (Ethilon, Ethicon) no larger than 1–1.5 metric. Sutures are removed 10–14 days postoperatively, usually under sedation.

Ligation of vessels uses a suture material with good knot security e.g. polyglactin 910 (Vicryl, Ethicon) or Polydioxanone (PDS). Some surgeons prefer to double ligate arteries, particularly the renal artery.

Lavage

Lavage solutions are required if the urogenital tract has been opened or if there is contamination of the wound. The amount of lavage solution varies depending upon the disease process and surgical procedure. Rupture of a uterus with pyometra or treatment of a prostatic abscess will require lavage with large volumes, e.g. 4–8 litres of a warmed, physiological solution. All lavage solution must be removed with suction.

Antibiotic use

Prophylactic antibiotics are not indicated for short procedures such as neutering, but are indicated for clean-contaminated and con-

Tissue healing

Healing of the bladder is rapid, with the normal bursting strength achieved within 14–21 days, and complications following bladder surgery are rare. The urethra can re-epithelialise denuded areas in 7 days. Ureteral and urethral surgeries carry the risk of wound dehiscence or stricture formation, especially if there is excess tension on the wound. Alternatives to ureteral and urethral surgery, including cystotomy or pyelotomy (incision into the renal pelvis) are performed in preference wherever possible. Urinary diversion with nephrostomy and cystostomy tubes is considered during healing of the ureter or urethra.

Renal surgery is not associated with a decrease in renal function in normal animals. Extravasation of urine may occur if a suture line is not secure, and can lead to inflammation and tissue necrosis. This is avoided with careful placement of sutures. Cystotomy closure may leak if there is continued urethral obstruction.

The assistant's role

Urogenital surgery is easier with an experienced assistant. Retraction of abdominal organs with moistened swabs or malleable retractors aids visualisation, particularly for deep structures such as kidneys and ureters. Traction on bladder stay sutures allows better visualisation of the urethra. A good assistant can decrease surgical time by anticipating the need for surgical instruments, stay sutures, lavage solutions etc.

DISEASES OF THE KIDNEYS AND SPECIFIC SURGICAL PROCEDURES

Hydronephrosis and hydroureter

Hydronephrosis and hydroureter (Fig 4.9) occur secondary to partial or complete urine outflow obstruction, usually due to renal pelvis or ureteral calculi. Other less common causes include ectopic ureters, ureteral neoplasia, ureteral stricture, inflammation or fibrosis, inadvertent ligation of the ureter during ovariohysterectomy and disease of the bladder trigone. Obstruction leads to progressive dilation of the ureter and renal pelvis and atrophy of the renal parenchyma. Pyelonephritis may accompany hydronephrosis. Bilateral complete obstruction is rapidly fatal. Unilateral hydronephrosis and hydroureter may be clinically silent or may be accompanied by vague clinical signs. Abdominal distension or an abdominal mass may be noted.

Diagnosis is on the basis of imaging studies including plain radiography, intravenous urography (Fig 4.10) and ultrasonography. If the dilation is recent, not advanced and the obstruction can be relieved, some renal function can be maintained. If it is advanced, ureteronephrectomy is required.

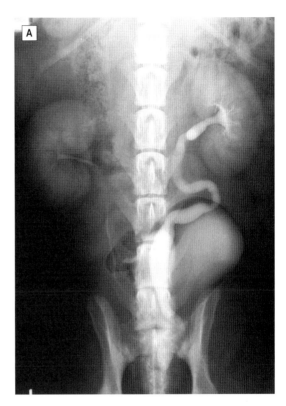

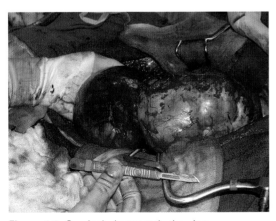

Figure 4.9 Surgical photograph showing hydronephrosis (kidney is on the right) adjacent to the bladder (left). Photograph © Alison Beck.

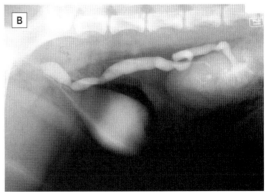

Figure 4.10 Intravenous urogram: (a) dorsoventral and (b) lateral projections. There is hydronephrosis and hydroureter involving the left kidney and ureter. The left ureter is ectopic. Photograph © Alison Beck.

Renal neoplasia

Carcinomas are the most common tumour in dogs. Clinical signs include haematuria and a palpable abdominal mass, as well as vague signs such as weight loss and decreased appetite. Pulmonary metastasis at diagnosis is present in half of dogs and bilateral neoplasia is common. Diagnosis tests include imaging studies and histopathology. Treatment by ureteronephrectomy is performed if there is unilateral disease and no evidence of metastatic disease. Lymphoma is the most common renal tumour in cats and is often confined to the kidneys. One-third of cats have bilateral disease. Clinical signs are those of renal failure. Feline lymphoma is treated with chemotherapy.

Ureteronephrectomy

Indications include renal neoplasia, hydroureter and hydronephrosis, renal trauma, chronic pyelonephritis, idiopathic haematuria and ureteral abnormalities. The presence of a normally functioning contralateral kidney is necessary. Confirmation of this can be difficult, but is suggested if urea, creatinine, urine specific gravity and intravenous urography are within normal limits.

Ureteronephrectomy is performed via a midline laparotomy. The kidney is isolated from the rest of the abdominal organs using laparotomy sponges. It is freed from the peritoneum and reflected medially to locate the hilus. The renal artery and vein are ligated close to the aorta and caudal vena cava, as some animals have multiple renal arteries or veins, using polyglactin 910 or polydioxanone. In intact animals, the left testicular or ovarian vein drains into the left renal vein and should not be ligated. The ureter is ligated and transected adjacent to the bladder. An assistant is useful to retract other organs, and to hold the kidney during its removal.

Renal biopsy techniques

Renal biopsy is performed to identify the cause of renal failure, haematuria or proteinuria. It can be performed by percutaneous or ultrasound guided needle or Tru-cut biopsy. Contraindications include renal cysts, abscesses, renal outflow obstruction or bleeding disorders. Laparoscopic biopsy or surgical wedge biopsy provides more tissue for histopathology.

Renal transplantation

Renal transplantation in cats is widely reported for the treatment of renal insufficiency. Ethical considerations remain the major obstacle for renal transplantation in the UK.

DISEASES OF THE URETERS AND SPECIFIC SURGICAL PROCEDURES

Ectopic ureters

Ectopic ureters are a congenital anomaly in dogs. Females are over-represented, probably due to subclinical disease in males. Breed predispositions include the Labrador and Golden retrievers, poodle, West Highland white terrier and Newfoundland. Most cases in dogs are bilateral and intramural, with the ureter entering the bladder wall at the normal position, and opening at a more distal site (bladder neck, urethra, vagina or uterus). Different anatomical variations have been described. Clinical signs are of incontinence (include dribbling of urine) or signs referable to urinary tract infections. Ureters may be dilated due to functional obstruction.

Diagnosis (see Fig 4.4) can be made by intravenous urography, positive contrast retrograde studies and ultrasonography.

Surgical treatment is by neoureterostomy. A ventral cystotomy and proximal urethrostomy are performed and stay sutures placed to minimise oedema from handling tissues. An incision is made through the bladder and ureteral mucosa into the lumen of the ectopic ureter, close to its entry into the bladder wall. The ureteral and bladder mucosa are sutured together to create a new stoma. The distal segment of the ureter is ligated or resected.

Dogs are observed closely postoperatively for stranguria. Urethral obstruction is rare but may occur with tissue oedema. Dogs are assessed for continence after 4–6 weeks. Half of animals remain incontinent due to congenital urethral sphincter mechanism incompetence, bladder hypoplasia or other causes.

DISEASES OF THE BLADDER AND SPECIFIC SURGICAL PROCEDURES

Urolithiasis

Formation of uroliths depends upon many factors including mineral supersaturation of urine, urinary tract infection and metabolic disease. Struvite uroliths (magnesium ammonium phosphate) are most common in the UK, although oxalate uroliths are more prevalent in the USA. Silicate and cysteine uroliths are rare. Breed predispositions exist for many urolith types. Some predisposing causes of urolith formation are shown in Table 4.4.

Most uroliths are located in the bladder and urethra. Renal and ureteral uroliths are rare and often incidental, although treatment is required if they cause obstruction. Clinical signs of cystic uroliths include haematuria and stranguria. Diagnosis is made by diagnostic imaging. Struvite and calcium oxalate uroliths are radio-opaque and are visible in the bladder or urethra on plain radiographs. Identification of radiolucent calculi (urate, cysteine, silicate) requires positive and double-contrast urethrocystography or ultrasonography (see Fig 4.2).

Radiographic appearance, urine pH, presence of bacteria, serum biochemistry and crystalluria give an indication of the urolith composition. Struvite and urate uroliths are amenable to medical dissolution. All other uroliths, or those causing obstruction or severe clinical signs, are removed surgically. A ventral midline cystotomy is performed with a large enough incision to allow visualisation of the whole bladder lumen. Visible uroliths are removed with a curette or forceps (Fig 4.11). Small uroliths tend to be displaced into the urethra, so a catheter is placed in the distal penile urethra and uroliths are flushed into the bladder from where they are removed. Failure to do this may result in residual urethral uroliths that may cause urethral obstruction and continuing clinical signs.

Uroliths are sent for mineral composition analysis and culture. Based on urolith composition, minimising recurrence will require a change in diet. Animals are fed a diet formulated to prevent the formation of struvite and calcium oxalate uroliths whilst awaiting results. Antibiotics are given if a urinary tract infection is suspected pending urine culture. Despite medical management, uroliths may still recur. The management of uroliths causing urethral obstruction is described on pages 103–4.

Bladder rupture

Bladder rupture may occur following blunt abdominal trauma. Rupture of the remainder of the urinary system is uncommon. Rupture

Table 4.4	Predisposing causes of urolith formation
Urolith	Predisposing factor
Struvite	Urinary tract infection
Calcium oxalate	Hypercalcaemia (cats)
Urate	Metabolic defects e.g. Dalmatians Hepatic disease e.g. portosystemic shunts

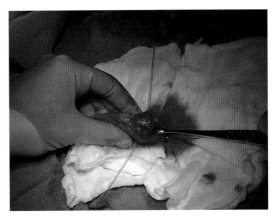

Figure 4.11 Surgical photograph showing removal of a large urolith via a ventral cystotomy. Note the stay sutures on the edge of the incision. Photograph © Alison Beck.

can also occur during palpation or expression of a bladder with urethral obstruction, or naturally with prolonged bladder distension from obstruction. Many animals are able to urinate normally, with no evidence of haematuria, so urinary tract rupture should be considered in any animal with a history of trauma.

Clinical signs are related to the presence of uroabdomen causing a chemical or septic peritonitis, if the urine is sterile or infected, respectively. Animals develop uraemia and hyperkalaemia over 2–3 days with signs of depression, anorexia and vomiting. Some animals are dysuric, haematuric or anuric.

Plain radiography usually demonstrates peritoneal fluid, which is confirmed as urine by abdominocentesis. The diagnosis is confirmed by positive contrast cystography showing leakage of contrast into the peritoneal cavity.

Following a period of fluid therapy to correct the azotaemia and electrolyte and acid–base disorders, laparotomy is performed. The rupture is identified, usually near the apex, and repaired primarily. Urinary tract diversion is not usually required.

Bladder neoplasia

The bladder is the most common site of urinary tract neoplasia, although tumours are rare, especially in cats. Transitional cell carcinomas are most common, and usually arise at the trigone. Clinical signs include haematuria, dysuria, incontinence, and occasionally obstruction. Radiography and ultrasonography reveal a mass but confirmation of the diagnosis requires biopsy. Cytology of urine is often unhelpful in differentiating malignant cells from normal epithelial cells.

Partial cystectomy can be performed, but will require ureteral diversion if the tumour is at the trigone. This is associated with many complications and is rarely performed. Many tumours are not resectable, but placement of a cystostomy tube may give palliation of clinical signs. NSAIDs, e.g. Meloxicam (Metacam, Boehringer Ingelheim, UK), has some anti-tumour activity, and can provide palliation of

clinical signs and analgesia. Although long-term prognosis is poor, palliative care can be successful for many months.

Cystotomy (including calculus removal)

Cystotomy is performed for the treatment of ectopic ureters, removing cystic uroliths and biopsy of masses. Cystotomy incisions are performed on the ventral midline of the bladder away from large blood vessels. A stab incision can be enlarged with Metzembaum scissors. The incision should be long enough to allow visualisation of the bladder lumen and mucosa, and may extend from close to the bladder apex into the urethra. Urine is removed via suction. Mucosa may be submitted for bacteriological culture and is more sensitive at identifying urinary tract infection than culture of urine. Cystotomy closure has been described.

Tube cystostomy

Tube cystostomy is used as a urinary diversion technique. Indications include diverting urine away from urethral surgical sites, palliation of urinary obstruction due to bladder or urethral neoplasia and detrusor atony. It can be performed at the time of urinary tract surgery or as a separate procedure. It is well tolerated by both dogs and cats, and cystostomy tube care is easily taught to owners.

A purse string suture is placed in the bladder and a Foley or mushroom tip catheter is placed through a stab incision in the middle of the suture. The suture is tightened. The catheter is passed through an incision in the lateral abdominal wall, and four mattress sutures are placed between the bladder and abdominal wall to create a cystopexy. The catheter is sutured to the skin with a Chinese finger trap suture. The tube must be kept in place for 7 days before removal to allow a fistula to form and prevent intra-abdominal leakage of urine. Catheters can be maintained long-term and replaced as necessary with Foley catheters or a low-profile gastrostomy tube (Fig 4.12). Urinary tract infection is com-

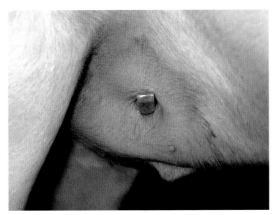

Figure 4.12   A low profile gastrostomy tube used as a permanent cystostomy tube in a dog. Photograph © Alison Beck.

mon, but is only treated when clinical signs are present to avoid the development of antibiotic resistant bacteria.

DISEASES OF THE URETHRA AND SPECIFIC SURGICAL PROCEDURES

Urethral sphincter mechanism incompetence

Urethral sphincter mechanism incompetence (USMI) is seen mainly in female dogs, especially Old English sheepdogs, Doberman pinschers, Springer spaniels and miniature poodles, and may present at any age. It has also been reported in cats and male dogs. Risk factors for development of USMI include neutering, obesity, tail docking, congenital abnormalities and an intra-pelvic bladder. Animals are predisposed to urinary tract infection, which may exacerbate the incontinence.

Diagnosis is made on the basis of radiographic studies after ruling out other causes of incontinence, and may identify an intrapelvic bladder and short urethra (see Fig 4.5). Dogs should not be under the influence of endogenous or exogenous oestrogens, as urethral filling during vaginourethrocystography may not occur.

Medical treatment with phenylpropanolamine (Propalin, Vetoquinol) and/or estriol (Incurin, Intervet) to increase urethral smooth muscle tone may improve or cure incontinence. Surgery (colposuspension) can be considered in bitches that remain incontinent or suffer side effects of medical therapy. Animals should not be overweight before surgery is considered. Colposuspension leads to a cure or improvement in 90% bitches. Some animals may require concurrent medical therapy.

Colposuspension

The aim of surgery is to move the bladder neck and proximal urethra into an intra-abdominal position and lengthen the urethra. A caudal laparotomy is performed. The vagina is pushed cranially by inserting a finger into it, and sutures are placed between the vaginal wall and prepubic tendons to hold the vagina, and therefore the urinary tract, in a more cranial position.

Postoperatively bitches are monitored for signs of obstruction or stranguria. The effects of surgery on continence may take 4 weeks to become apparent due to postoperative discomfort. Animals must be strictly rested in this time to avoid suture failure.

Urethral obstruction

Obstruction is most common secondary to urolithiasis, but may also occur secondary to neoplasia, trauma or stricture. Obstruction is more common in males due to a small urethral diameter but rare in females. In male dogs uroliths are most likely to obstruct at the ischial arch or caudal to the os penis. Obstruction in cats usually occurs in the distal third of the urethra, and is due to mucus and debris associated with lower urinary tract disease.

Complete obstruction results in azotaemia, hyperkalaemia and metabolic acidosis, which is fatal if untreated. Many animals present with a history of stranguria, progressing to vomiting and collapse. Emergency management includes intravenous fluid therapy and treatment of hyperkalaemia. Anaesthesia at this stage is usually fatal.

Male cats

Obstruction is usually with a mucus plug and can usually be relieved with urethral flushing. Under sedation the penis is straightened using fingers or forceps and a lubricated urinary catheter is inserted into the end of the penis. The urethra is flushed with saline until a catheter can be passed into the bladder. The catheter is left in place for 2–4 days whilst the cat is maintained on intravenous fluid therapy to 'flush out' the bladder. Failure to relieve a distal obstruction, or recurrent episodes of obstruction, may necessitate perineal urethrostomy. Iatrogenic urethral rupture may occur if the penis is not straightened and the catheter is placed forcefully.

Male dogs

Most uroliths can be flushed into the bladder by retrohydropropulsion and then removed by cystotomy. A catheter is placed just distal to the urolith and the urethral opening held closed. An assistant occludes the urethra proximally using a finger in the rectum. Saline is instilled via the catheter to dilate the urethra, and then the assistant releases the proximal urethra to allow the urolith to be flushed proximally. Several attempts may be required but is usually successful, so this technique should be exhausted before resorting to urethrotomy.

Urethral trauma

Trauma is more common after failed attempts to catheterise an animal than secondary to pelvic fractures. Clinical signs are due to urine leakage into the abdomen, pelvis or subcutaneous tissues, including bruising, pain and tissue necrosis, uraemia and hyperkalaemia. Animals may urinate normally. Diagnosis can be made by positive contrast urethrography.

Partial tears can be treated conservatively by diverting urine with an indwelling urethral catheter or a cystostomy tube. Damage to the distal urethra in male cats may make catheter-

isation impossible and the site of urethral damage can be removed by perineal urethrostomy. Prepubic urethrostomy may be required if trauma to the mid or distal urethra is extensive. Repair of urethral transection is rarely performed and requires laparotomy and/or pubic symphysiotomy to perform debridement and anastomosis.

Urethrotomy and urethrostomy in male dogs

Urethrotomy is performed to remove uroliths, usually close to the os penis, that cannot be retrohydropropulsed to the bladder. Cystotomy is preferred as urethrotomy carries the risk of postoperative stricture formation and recurrent obstruction. A ventral midline incision is made over a catheter located in the urethra. Prescrotal urethrotomy requires lateral retraction of the retractor penis muscle before the urethral lumen is entered. Primary closure of the mucosa will reduce the postoperative haemorrhage, but the incision can be left to heal by second intention. Haemorrhage from the wound and during urination can be profuse and last for several days. Perineal urethrotomy is rarely performed in the dog.

Urethrostomy may be performed in dogs that suffer recurrent episodes of urethral obstruction e.g. Dalmatians with urate urolithiasis, to produce a wider orifice that is less prone to obstruction. Other indications include urethral stricture or neoplasia. Scrotal urethrostomy is preferred as the urethra is wider, in a more superficial location and suffers less haemorrhage than either a prescrotal or perineal urethrostomy. Entire males are castrated. A 4cm incision is made into the urethra as described for urethrotomy. The urethral mucosa is sutured to the skin using non-absorbable simple interrupted sutures. Haemorrhage is profuse but will subside as sutures are placed. Postoperative haemorrhage, usually during urination, will decrease over 3–7 days.

Perineal and prepubic urethrostomy has been described in male and female dogs for the treatment of stricture, trauma and neoplasia that is located more proximally.

Perineal and prepubic urethrostomy in cats

Urethrostomy is indicated in cats with recurrent episodes of urethral obstruction due to feline lower urinary tract disease, urethral stricture or severe iatrogenic urethral damage following attempts at catheterisation.

Perineal urethrostomy is performed in preference over prepubic urethrostomy. An incision is made around the penis and scrotum. The penis is dissected free from the surrounding tissues. The bulbourethral glands are identified and an incision made in the dorsal urethra from the distal third to a point cranial to the glands. The distal one-third of the penis is ligated and transected. The urethral mucosa is sutured to the surrounding skin to create a stoma 1–1.5cm long (Fig 4.13).

Postoperatively cats wear a buster collar to prevent self-trauma and are provided with a litter tray containing shredded paper. Haemorrhage is usually mild and sutures can be removed under sedation in 10–14 days. Complications include stricture if the stoma is too

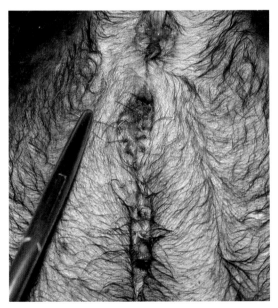

Figure 4.13   A healed perineal urethrostomy in a cat 14 days after surgery. Note the use of size 1 metric suture. Photograph © Alison Beck.

small and leakage of urine if suture placement is not accurate. Bacterial cystitis is common postoperatively but clinical signs are rare. Clinical signs of feline lower urinary tract disease will still occur and should be treated accordingly, but the risk of stoma obstruction is low.

Indwelling urinary catheters

Urinary catheters are placed postoperatively after major surgical procedures where animals are unlikely to be ambulatory, and to assess urine output. The routine use of catheters after surgery allows easy nursing in the first 12–24 hours, avoids urine soaking of the animal, and avoids distress in animals that need to urinate but are unable to go outside. They may be placed in animals with spinal disease that are unable to urinate, to divert urine after urethral surgery or trauma, and after an episode of urethral obstruction in male cats.

Catheters are placed aseptically and can be performed conscious in males and some females. Sedation is preferred to catheterise an animal with urethral obstruction. Females can be catheterised with the aid of a vaginoscope. Foley catheters are checked before use and are filled with saline rather than air after placement to avoid inadvertent balloon let down. Catheters in cats can be sutured to the prepuce. The reader is referred to the *Textbook of veterinary medical nursing* for more information on performing catheterisation.

Closed collection systems are used to minimise ascending urinary tract infections, or are capped and drained intermittently. Commercially available collection systems can be used for dogs and cats or can be modified from a giving set and fluid bag. Animals wear a buster collar to avoid chewing out catheters (as they may leave a catheter bulb in the bladder) and the cage is kept clean.

Catheters are kept in surgical patients for the minimum time necessary. Long-term use of catheters will invariably lead to urinary tract infection, but antibiotics are not given prophylactically as they promote growth of antibiotic resistant bacteria. It is better to treat the infection after the catheter is removed, unless clinical signs are present.

DISEASES OF THE FEMALE REPRODUCTIVE TRACT AND SPECIFIC SURGICAL PROCEDURES

Pyometra

During dioestrus in bitches, increased release of progesterone from the corpus luteum leads to an increase in uterine secretions, poor uterine muscle contraction and closure of the cervix. Development of inflammatory infiltrates of the uterine wall and pyometra may subsequently develop, and are usually associated with cystic endometrial hyperplasia. Under the influence of progesterone the uterus is more susceptible to infection, usually from vaginal bacteria (especially *E. coli*). The risk of pyometra increases with each episode of dioestrus, thus it is more common in middle aged and old bitches. Pyometra is rare in cats, as they do not ovulate spontaneously and are not under the influence of progesterone for as long. Pyometra is usually seen 4–8 weeks after oestrus in the bitch and 1–4 weeks in the cat.

Pyometra is usually accompanied by systemic changes secondary to inflammatory disease and occasionally bacteraemia. Clinical signs include vaginal discharge, polyuria, depression, anorexia, vomiting and collapse. More severe clinical signs may be seen if the cervix is closed. Left untreated, bitches may die from endotoxaemia. Uterine rupture is rare.

Some animals may present with clinical signs of shock and endotoxaemia. Other physical examination findings include abdominal distension and a palpably enlarged uterus.

Laboratory tests demonstrate leucocytosis and hyperglobulinaemia, although leucopaenia may occur in severe cases. Other changes include anaemia, azotaemia, and low urine specific gravity. Concurrent urinary tract infection is common.

Diagnosis is based on history, physical examination findings and laboratory data, and confirmed with diagnostic imaging. A fluid filled uterus is seen on plain radiography or ultrasonography.

Ovariohysterectomy is the treatment of choice. Animals should receive intravenous fluid therapy and antibiotics before anaesthesia and prompt surgical treatment. Care is taken to avoid inadvertent uterine rupture by gentle manipulation of the friable uterus. The uterus is isolated from the rest of the abdomen using laparotomy sponges. Ovariohysterectomy is performed routinely. The uterine stump is not over-sewn to avoid the development of a stump abscess or granuloma. Early diagnosis and prompt surgical treatment will usually ensure survival.

Medical treatment with prostaglandins has been described, but is not currently recommended.

Some bitches will continue to show signs of oestrus if ovarian tissue remains following ovariohysterectomy. Abdominal exploration in the region of the ovary can be performed at any time of the oestrus cycle to remove residual tissue. Stump pyometra may occur concurrently and surgical treatment also involves removing the uterine stump.

Vagina oedema and vaginal prolapse

Brachycephalic dogs are prone to both conditions. Oedema of the vaginal and vestibular mucosa is normal in bitches during the follicular phase of the oestrus cycle. This may occasionally become extreme, usually during the first oestrus, and the mucosa is seen protruding from the vulva. It will spontaneously resolve at the start of the luteal phase, but is likely to recur at subsequent oestrus. Clinical problems occur if the mucosa becomes traumatised or if the bitch becomes pregnant, when dystocia may occur. Surgical resection of redundant mucosa via episiotomy is performed only if the mucosa is traumatised. Otherwise ovariohysterectomy is performed at a later date.

Prolapse is less common than oedema. The vagina, including the urethral tubercle, protrudes from the vulva, and complete prolapse including the cervix. This is differentiated from vaginal oedema where the mucosa arises from the vestibular floor cranial to the urethral tubercle. Prolapse may occur from excess straining related to the gastrointestinal or urogenital tracts or secondary to a difficult mating. Mild prolapse will regress during dioestrus. More severe prolapse may require manual reduction with lubrication and possible episiotomy, followed by placing sutures across the labia. Recurrent prolapse may require uterus or broad ligament pexy to the abdominal wall, or ovariohysterectomy. If the vagina has become traumatised, surgical resection via episiotomy is required.

Neoplasia

Ovarian and uterine tumours are rare in dogs and cats. Vaginal and vulval tumours are more common, and tend to be seen in older, intact females. Most are benign and may become quite large before presentation. Benign tumours are differentiated from malignant tumours by biopsy. Benign masses are excised, via the vulva if the mass is on a pedicle, or via episiotomy. Care is taken to avoid urethral damage. Ovariohysterectomy decreases the incidence of tumour recurrence.

Neutering

Bitches can be neutered by ovariectomy or ovariohysterectomy. Ovariectomy is quicker and less invasive. There are no advantages to removing the uterus; however, ovariohysterectomy is more commonly performed in the UK. Neutering is performed to avoid the inconvenience of oestrus and pregnancy, avoid pyometra and reproductive neoplasia, and decrease the risk of mammary neoplasia. Neutering before the first oestrus decreases the risk of mammary neoplasia to less then 0.5% of that seen in entire females. The protective effect decreases after each oestrus, until no protection against mammary neoplasia occurs after 2.5 years. Neutering before the first season may, however, be associated with the

development of USMI. At-risk breeds should therefore be allowed to have one oestrus before neutering. Early-age neutering at 8–16 weeks can be performed safely in male and female dogs and cats with no difference in complication rates compared to neutering at 7 months old.

In bitches, a midline laparotomy is made with an incision large enough to visualise the ovaries and the uterus. The ovaries are isolated and ligated using a three-clamp method. Suture material with good knot security is used, e.g. polyglactin 910. Catgut is avoided due to poor knot security and unpredictable breakdown. The uterine arteries are individually ligated at the cervix before the uterus is ligated and transected. In cats, ovariohysterectomy can be performed similarly or through a left flank incision.

The most common complication is haemorrhage. This is usually due to poor operative technique, including making too small an incision so tissues are stretched or torn, failure to place secure ligatures and improper suture material selection. Operative haemorrhage may require the laparotomy incision to be enlarged. Reflecting the mesoduodenum or mesocolon towards the midline and locating the caudal pole of the kidney helps isolate the ovarian stump. A bleeding vessel can be clamped and ligated. An animal with postoperative haemorrhage may present with collapse and pale mucous membranes. Abdominocentesis will usually reveal blood. Intravenous fluid therapy, and possibly blood products, are required for cardiovascular support. Surgical exploration is required to identify and ligate the vessel.

Other complications include ovarian remnant syndrome, stump pyometra or granuloma, fistulous tracts and inadvertent ligation of a ureter.

Caesarean section

Caesarean section is required for dystocia, defined as a prolonged interval between puppies (>4 hours), weak or strong straining for more than 2 hours or 30 minutes respectively, abnormal vaginal discharge or distress of the dam. Elective caesarean is sometimes performed in brachycephalic breeds, although many can deliver puppies normally.

Care is taken when handling the uterus during laparotomy. An assistant may be useful to support the uterus if there are a large number of foetuses. After isolating the uterus with laparotomy sponges, an incision is made over the ventral aspect of the uterine body, large enough to remove the foetuses without tearing the uterus. Each foetus is 'milked' towards the incision and removed by applying gentle traction. The foetus is removed from the sac with the placenta unless the placenta is stuck or bleeds. The foetus is handed to an assistant for resuscitation. It is helpful to have several assistants receiving puppies/kittens as they are removed relatively fast, as well as an assistant monitoring anaesthesia. Both horns of the uterus and the vagina should be checked for remaining foetuses. The uterus is sutured with a single or double layer continuous pattern. Uterine involution will be observed during closure.

If the dam is very weak or showing signs of shock, ovariohysterectomy can be performed instead of caesarean section, with similar neonatal survival. Ovariohysterectomy may also be performed in animals that are not intended for breeding at a later date.

Episiotomy

Episiotomy is a simple technique to perform, and mandatory for vaginal surgery unless lesions are located at the vulva. The bitch is placed in sternal recumbency with the pelvic limbs elevated. Doyen clamps are placed on either side of the vaginal midline, with one arm in the vagina, to minimise haemorrhage. The skin, subcutaneous tissues and vaginal wall are incised on the midline to just ventral to the anal sphincter. Stay sutures or self-retaining retractors improve exposure. Closure of the episiotomy is in three layers, starting at the vulva. Haemorrhage associated with vaginal surgery may be brisk, but is usually controlled with direct pressure or iced saline. Suturing vaginal tissues should stop further haemorrhage.

Mammary neoplasia

Mammary tumours are the most common tumour seen in female dogs and the third most common in female cats. Most occur in middle aged or old animals. Breed predispositions include poodles, spaniels and terrier breeds. As mentioned previously, ovariohysterectomy before the third oestrus will decrease the incidence of tumours in bitches.

In bitches, half of tumours are malignant. Half of these have metastatic disease at the time of diagnosis. Multiple masses are seen in one in four dogs. Most tumours are found in the caudal mammary glands. Dogs are presented due to the presence of one or more masses in the mammary chain, or they may be an incidental finding.

Inflammatory carcinomas should be differentiated from mammary inflammation or infection by fine needle aspiration. The prognosis is grave.

Mammary masses are removed surgically. Fine needle aspiration is not usually performed, as it is inaccurate in determining malignancy and tumour type, due in part to the mixed nature of many tumours. Tumour staging includes thoracic radiography or computed tomography to identify thoracic metastasis.

Surgical treatment is defined by the size of the tumour. Small masses are removed by mammectomy including a 2cm margin of normal tissue. Removal of adjacent glands (regional mastectomy) is performed for multiple masses in adjacent glands. In bitches, glands 1–3 and glands 3–5 are removed together based on the lymphatic drainage of the glands. Radical mastectomy is performed for multiple masses that cannot be removed by regional mastectomy. Masses in both mammary chains are removed by radical mastectomy of one side followed by the other side 2–4 weeks later. Bilateral radical mastectomy can be performed, but closure of the resultant skin deficit can be problematic. There are differences of opinion as to whether concurrent ovariohysterectomy improves survival. All masses are sent for histopathology, as a number of tumour types, including benign and malignant, may be present.

Negative prognostic indicators for canine mammary tumours include large size (>3cm), adherence to underlying tissues, ulceration, histological type and degree of differentiation and lymph node involvement. Type of surgical procedure performed does not influence survival, except where lymph node metastasis has occurred. Adjuvant therapy is poorly described for canine mammary neoplasia.

Feline mammary tumours are more likely to be malignant (80%), ulcerated (25%) and multiple (50%) than canine tumours. More then 80% have metastasised at the time of diagnosis. Radical mastectomy is indicated, and staged bilateral surgery is often required. Prognostic indicators in cats include tumour size and degree of differentiation. Cats with tumours less than 2cm have a median survival of 3 years. Overall median survival is 1 year.

DISEASES OF THE MALE REPRODUCTIVE TRACT AND SPECIFIC SURGICAL PROCEDURES

Prostatitis and prostatic abscesses

Clinical signs of prostatic disease include dyschezia, dysuria, haematuria, pyuria, anorexia, weight loss and depression. Despite protective mechanisms, the prostate can become infected with bacteria of urethral origin, and abscesses can develop. Clinical signs can range from vague signs of prostatic disease, to purulent discharge and pelvic limb lameness. Collapse and shock may be seen if an abscess ruptures into the abdominal cavity.

Identifying bacteria or degenerate neutrophils in the urethra, a prostatic wash, or a fine needle aspirate, combined with diagnostic imaging, confirms the diagnosis. Prostatitis can be treated with antibiotics on the basis of culture and sensitivity for 4–6 weeks. Castration minimises the risk of recurrence.

Abscesses can be surgically drained and omentalised. Rapid surgical intervention is required if an abscess has burst with signs of septic peritonitis.

Prostatic and paraprostatic cysts

Cysts may arise from the prostatic parenchyma or from embryological remnants of the male urogenital tract. They may increase to a large size before clinical signs of obstruction occur, or may be associated with inflammation and infection causing vague clinical signs. Diagnosis is based upon identifying a fluid filled structure in the vicinity of the prostate and aspirating fluid. Treatment has been successful using repeated ultrasound guided drainage or surgical drainage, local resection and omentalisation. Care must be taken to avoid excess dissection, especially dorsal to the urinary tract and prostate, to avoid damaging the neurovascular structures.

Prostatic neoplasia

Prostatic tumours are uncommon but are seen most commonly in elderly male entire or neutered dogs. Clinical signs include signs of prostatic disease, and dogs may have lameness due to skeletal metastasis. Diagnosis is based on imaging studies and biopsy. Surgeons should be aware that prostatic neoplasia may be clinically similar to other prostatic diseases, and histopathology should be performed on any prostatic tissue removed at surgery.

Prognosis is poor. Prostatectomy is difficult to perform, may lead to incontinence and many animals will already have metastatic disease at diagnosis. Palliative care can be provided by the placement of a cystostomy tube in animals with severe dysuria, and can be combined with prostatic biopsy to confirm the diagnosis.

Prostatic omentalisation

Surgery of the prostate gland, other than omentalisation, carries a high morbidity rate. Omentalisation is indicated for the treatment of prostatic and paraprostatic cysts, prostatitis unresponsive to medical therapy and prostatic abscesses. The omentum can either be passed through the prostate or sutured to the remaining lining of cysts or abscesses after resection. Omentalisation of prostatic diseases is associated with a low risk of recurrence.

PERI- AND POSTOPERATIVE MANAGEMENT

Monitoring urine output

Urine output is important in animals undergoing major surgery, animals with renal disease and animals at risk of urinary tract obstruction. Urine output should equal or exceed 2ml/kg/h and can be measured accurately via a urinary catheter. Decreased urine output may reflect hypovolaemia and if it is noted fluid therapy should be reassessed. Anuria may represent renal dysfunction, hypovolaemia or obstruction. Dysuria or stranguria may represent urinary obstruction.

Abdominal ultrasonography can help to differentiate anuric animals form those that are unwilling or unable to urinate. If there is the risk of obstruction, animals noted to have bladder distension should be allowed an opportunity to urinate and then be catheterised to assess urethral patency. A decision should be made as to whether an indwelling urinary catheter is to be used. Further surgical intervention may be required in some cases, e.g. repeat surgery to remove suture if there is obstruction following colposuspension.

Fluid therapy

Fluid therapy should be assessed for each individual animal, depending upon the level of dehydration, maintenance requirements and ongoing losses. Animals with renal dysfunction are less able to concentrate urine in the face of dehydration. Following urinary tract obstruction, hyposthenuric urine is produced for several days, and fluid therapy should be increased to accommodate this. High fluid levels are useful in cats with feline lower urinary tract disease and in animals following urinary tract surgery, to produce dilute urine that will minimise the formation of mucus plugs and blood clots. Regular assessment of degree of dehydration, PCV, total solids and electrolytes is recommended for animals with severe urogenital tract disease or a recent episode of obstruction.

Wound management (with specific reference to urethrotomies and urethrostomies)

All surgical wounds are monitored for signs of inflammation, discharge and swelling. Urethrostomy and urethrotomy incisions are prone to marked haemorrhage, especially in the first 2–3 days, but this should resolve over 5–7 days. Incisions are not handled, as this may exacerbate haemorrhage. Bruising around the incision may suggest extravasation of urine that may lead to tissue necrosis. Surgical wounds should be examined under sedation if there is doubt regarding the integrity of the wound.

Further reading

Bass M, Howard J, Gerber B, Messmer M 2005 Retrospective study of indications for and outcome of perineal urethrostomy in cats. J Small Anim Pract 46(5):227–231

Bowden C, Masters J (eds) 2003 Textbook of veterinary medical nursing. Butterworth-Heinemann, Edinburgh

Collins R L, Birchard S J, Chew D J, Heuter K J 1998 Surgical treatment of urate calculi in Dalmatians: 38 cases (1980–1995). J Am Vet Med Assoc 213(6):833–838

Cornell K K 2000 Cystotomy, partial cystectomy, and tube cystostomy. Clin Tech Small Anim Pract 15(1):11–16

Heuter K J 2005 Excretory urography. Clin Tech Small Anim Pract 20(1):39–45

Holt P 1983 Urinary incontinence in the dog. In Pract 5(5):162–164, 169–173.

Holt P E 1990 Long-term evaluation of colposuspension in the treatment of urinary incontinence due to incompetence of the urethral sphincter mechanism in the bitch. Vet Rec 127(22):537–542

Holt P E, Moore A H 1995 Canine ureteral ectopia: an analysis of 175 cases and comparison of surgical treatments. Vet Rec 136(14):345–349

Johnston G R, Walter P A, Feeney D A 1986 Radiographic and ultrasonographic features of uroliths and other urinary tract filling defects. Vet Clin North Am Small Anim Pract 16(2):261–292

McLoughlin M A, Chew D J 2000 Diagnosis and surgical management of ectopic ureters. Clin Tech Small Anim Pract 15(1):17–24.

Osborne C A, Lulich J P, Polzin D J et al 1999 Medical dissolution and prevention of canine struvite urolithiasis. Twenty years of experience. Vet Clin North Am Small Anim Pract 29(1):73–111

Perez Alenza M D et al 2000 Factors influencing the incidence and prognosis of canine mammary tumours. J Small Anim Pract 41, 287–291

Silverman S, Long C D 2000 The diagnosis of urinary incontinence and abnormal urination in dogs and cats. Vet Clin North Am Small Anim Pract 30(2):427–448

Smith C W 2002 Perineal urethrostomy. Vet Clin North Am Small Anim Pract 32(4):917–925

White R A 2000 Prostatic surgery in the dog. Clin Tech Small Anim Pract 15(1):46–51

Chapter **5**

Thoracic surgery

Stephen J Baines

ANAESTHESIA AND PERIOPERATIVE CARE FOR THORACIC SURGERY

Preoperative period

Preoperative evaluation and preparation

Patients undergoing thoracic surgery are likely to have abnormalities of the cardiopulmonary system, and general anaesthesia and thoracic surgery are likely to place additional stresses on these systems. A good working knowledge of cardiopulmonary physiology and the pathophysiology of disorders of the thorax is essential.

It is important to have an accurate diagnosis prior to instituting any surgical procedure and any pathophysiological changes should be corrected before anaesthesia. For patients with cardiac disease, preanaesthetic therapy is aimed at improving cardiac output and treating congestive failure and arrhythmias. For patients with respiratory disease, preanaesthetic therapy is aimed at restoring the efficiency of ventilation and producing an unobstructed airway.

Other problems should also be corrected before the additional stresses of anaesthesia are induced, such as pericardiocentesis for pericardial effusion and pleurocentesis for pleural effusion or pneumothorax. Open chest wounds should be covered with an appropriate dressing, converting the open pneumothorax to a closed pneumothorax, and the pleural space evacuated of air.

Animals with clinical signs of respiratory distress, or where blood gas analysis indicates hypoxaemia, should be given supplementary oxygen via mask, nasal catheter or oxygen cage. All patients, particularly those involved in trauma, should be evaluated for shock and cardiovascular collapse. Appropriate fluid therapy, consisting of crystalloids, colloids or blood, and positive inotropes may be needed. Many anaesthetic agents result in cardiovascular depression and any pre-existing cardiovascular compromise may lead to profound collapse.

Anaesthetic principles

Animals with cardiopulmonary disease have a reduced oxygen reserve and should be preoxygenated with 100% oxygen, e.g. via face mask or nasal catheter, for 2–5 minutes before induction. A smooth, stress-free induction is desirable for the patient with cardiovascular compromise and rapid control of the airway is of the utmost importance in any patient with respiratory compromise. Hence, the use of a rapid induction technique which allows prompt endotracheal intubation is indicated.

These comments should be borne in mind when selecting a suitable technique and drug protocol. However, the careful use of a familiar drug is more likely to be successful than the use of an unfamiliar drug which may have theoretical advantages.

Premedication

Premedication is indicated to calm the patient, to ensure a smooth induction and to reduce the requirement for other anaesthetic drugs. The selection of a protocol which minimises cardiopulmonary depression is important. In the compromised patient, premedication may not be required, but care should be taken to avoid stress.

Acepromazine may calm the patient, may reduce afterload by causing vasodilation and may provide an anti-arrhythmic effect. However, it should be avoided in animals with hypotension, cardiac hypertrophy or seizures. Alpha-2 agonists (e.g. medetomidine) induce bradycardia and reduce cardiac contractility, and should be avoided in patients undergoing thoracic surgery.

Opioids may be used to provide pre-anaesthetic sedation and analgesia. The co-administration of a sedative or tranquilliser (e.g. acepromazine or diazepam) will prevent dysphoria. All opioids may produce dose-dependent respiratory depression and, in animals with respiratory disease, should be used at low doses or withheld until the trachea is intubated and ventilation can be supported. They may also induce bradycardia due to increased parasympathetic tone, which may be reversed with anticholinergics (e.g. atropine or glycopyrrolate).

Fentanyl and buprenorphine have minimal effects on the cardiovascular system. Fentanyl has a short duration of action and is used primarily as a continuous rate infusion intra-operatively or postoperatively. It may also be used postoperatively using transdermal administration from a patch. Morphine may be useful in patients with heart failure as it increases the capacitance of the large veins.

Benzodiazepines (e.g. diazepam, midazolam) have minimal effects on the cardiopulmonary system, but, as a sole agent, they may induce excitement and agitation in non-compromised individuals. They can be combined with opioids to produce a greater degree of sedation and may be given immediately prior to an induction agent to decrease the requirement for that drug.

Anticholinergics (e.g. atropine, glycopyrrolate) are indicated to prevent or treat sinus bradycardia during anaesthesia and should be considered whenever an opioid is used as part of the anaesthetic protocol. Atropine should not be given intravenously, to avoid the centrally-mediated parasympathomimetic effect of this drug. Glycopyrrolate has a longer duration of action, produces less tachycardia and has fewer ocular and gastrointestinal side-effects.

The routine use of anticholinergics is controversial. Atropine results in more viscous respiratory secretions, which may predispose to occlusion and collapse of the small airways, and also increases anatomic dead space. Atropine also causes tachycardia, which increases myocardial work and oxygen demand, and increases the incidence of arrhythmias.

A combination of agents for the premedication is generally the most suitable. Neuroleptanalgesic combinations such as a low dose of acepromazine (0.01–0.03 mg/kg IM) combined with an opiate such as morphine or pethidine, will give satisfactory sedation with mild haemodynamic effects.

Induction of anaesthesia

The careful administration of the induction agent and the monitoring of the effect of this drug are more important than the actual choice of drug. Most induction agents will result in dose-dependent respiratory depression. However, patients undergoing thoracic surgery will be intubated and ventilated, so this is a relatively minor concern. Induction agents which increase the heart rate and reduce contractility should be avoided in patients with cardiac disease. A rapid induction, which allows prompt endotracheal intubation, is desired.

Thiobarbiturates (e.g. thiopentone) are commonly used in non-compromised patients, but will reduce cardiac contractility and increase heart rate and should be avoided in patients with cardiac disease.

Propofol has less effect on the myocardium but it may cause hypotension (because of vasodilation) and reflex tachycardia. These effects may be ameliorated by administering the drug slowly, but then the benefits of a rapid induction are lost.

Ketamine is often used in compromised patients in combination with a benzodiazepine, e.g. diazepam. Diazepam has little cardiopulmonary depressant effect, and it offsets the detrimental effects of ketamine, such as muscle rigidity, excitement and seizures. In addition, ketamine provides sympathetic stimulation, thus maintaining or increasing cardiac contractility. However, the rate of induction is slower than with thiobarbiturates. Diazepam has minimal cardiopulmonary effects and helps to offset the negative effects of ketamine, such as muscle rigidity and a potential for seizures. Ketamine stimulates the sympathetic nervous system and thereby maintains or increases cardiac contractility, blood pressure

and heart rate. The induction is slower than with thiobarbiturates.

Opioids, such as fentanyl, may be used for induction of compromised patients. However, they induce profound sedation and analgesia rather than anaesthesia, and alert individuals may be difficult to intubate. These drugs have minimal effects on cardiac contractility, but may cause bradycardia. Opioids are given slowly in incremental doses, which delays control of the airway.

Induction with an inhalant agent (e.g. mask or induction chamber) allows a hands-off approach and may be considered in stressed patients, particularly cats with respiratory distress. However, some patients will not tolerate the presence of the mask and it is a relatively slow technique. The addition of nitrous oxide to the inhalant will increase the speed of induction, but will lower the inspired oxygen concentration, so should not be used in hypoxaemic patients.

Maintenance of anaesthesia

Anaesthetic agent Many anaesthetic agents are arrhythmogenic, particularly in the presence of catecholamines. This may be avoided by using a low concentration of inhalant anaesthetic (e.g. by using other agents such as opioids) and by reducing the level of circulating catecholamines (e.g. by achieving an adequate depth of anaesthesia and maintaining a satisfactory blood pressure).

Isoflurane is recommended for compromised patients. It is very insoluble, which allows rapid induction, recovery and change in depth of anaesthesia, and has less of a depressant effect on the myocardium than other agents, such as halothane. However, isoflurane will produce dose-dependent hypotension because of vasodilation and negative inotropic effects. Positive inotropes may therefore be needed to maintain adequate cardiac output.

Nitrous oxide may be used with any of the inhalant anaesthetics to decrease the amount of inhalant required. It is contraindicated in pulmonary disease, pneumothorax, anaemia or when hypoxaemia is present.

Intubation and ventilation   Intubation with an appropriate sized cuffed endotracheal tube should be performed as soon as possible after induction. A cuffed tube is necessary to ensure a good fit to enable efficient positive pressure ventilation. Thoracic surgery always requires controlled ventilation. However, the presence of adequate ventilation does not necessarily mean than there is adequate gas exchange, and both these parameters should be monitored individually. Controlled ventilation may be achieved by manually squeezing the reservoir bag of the breathing circuit or by using a mechanical ventilator.

Intraoperative concerns

Monitoring of the patient   Continuous, regular and detailed assessment of the patient is important. The presence of pre-existing disease and the adverse effects of anaesthesia and surgery may cause profound physiological abnormalities – rapid changes in the patient's status are possible.

An oesophageal stethoscope provides information on heart rate and rhythm and lung sounds. Pulse rhythm and quality should be monitored by palpating a peripheral pulse. Core temperature should be monitored and oesophageal thermistor probes are preferred to thermometers inserted per rectum.

Arterial blood pressure should be monitored, ideally directly via arterial catheterisation, and a central line should be placed to measure central venous pressure and monitor the adequacy of fluid therapy, as well as to provide a route for the rapid administration of fluids. Arterial blood gas analysis is the most useful means to monitor oxygenation and adequacy of ventilation. Pulse oximetry will monitor blood saturation and pulsatile blood flow.

Once the thorax is open, the following information may also be gained:

- confirmation of expansion of the lungs with each breath
- assessment of cardiac rhythm and contractility
- examination of the degree of filling of the venae cavae, which gives some indication of the venous return.

Support of the cardiovascular system   The rate of fluid therapy during anaesthesia will depend on:

- the nature of the pre-existing disease process
- the preoperative hydration status, electrolyte and acid–base balance
- the nature of the surgical procedure, particularly the presence or absence of significant bleeding.

Crystalloids are generally given at 10ml/kg/h. Fluids low in sodium (e.g. 5% dextrose or 2.5% dextrose with 0.45% saline) may be of benefit in the patient with cardiovascular disease since the reduced sodium load will reduce sodium and water retention. Patients in need of more profound volume support may benefit from the infusion of colloids, and blood products may be required if there is significant haemorrhage.

Pharmacological support of the cardiovascular system may also be required. The goals of drug therapy are to:

- maintain cardiac output
- maintain normal sinus rhythm and rate
- maintain normal tissue perfusion.

Bradycardia may result in reduced cardiac output and anticholinergic (e.g. atropine) therapy may be required. Tachycardia increases myocardial workload and oxygen demand and may also be detrimental to cardiac output since diastolic filling may be reduced. Sympatholytics (e.g. propranolol) may be required to reduce the heart rate.

Positive inotropic support may be required if hypotension occurs due to poor cardiac output. A continuous infusion of dobutamine or dopamine is most commonly used to improve contractility. Arrhythmias may adversely affect stroke volume and cardiac output. Ventricular premature contractions (VPCs) is one of the most common arrhythmias noted during anaesthesia. Isolated VPCs do not need to be treated but runs of VPCs or ventricular tachycardia may need to be treated with lignocaine.

Intraoperative analgesia   In compromised patients, supplementary analgesia should be used to reduce the level of inhalant anaesthetic agent. This includes the preoperative administration of an opioid (e.g. morphine) and, where not contraindicated, a NSAID (e.g. carprofen or meloxicam). This may be supplemented by other drugs, e.g. fentanyl, given by additional boluses or constant rate infusion.

Prevention of hypothermia   Any animal undergoing anaesthesia may become hypothermic – this is particularly true for those animals undergoing thoracotomy. Hypothermia has profound side-effects:

- accentuation of CNS depression caused by inhalant agents
- reduction in myocardial contractility
- predisposition to arrhythmias
- shifting of the oxygen–haemoglobin dissociation curve to the left
- increasing blood viscosity.

Heat loss should be minimised by:

- ensuring a warm environment
- eliminating draughts
- applying surface warming techniques (heating blankets)
- providing passive insulation (bubble wrap, foil blankets)
- avoiding excessive clipping or wetting of the skin
- warming and humidifying inspired gases
- warm-water lavage of thoracic cavity
- covering and moistening exposed serosal surfaces
- avoiding a deep plane of anaesthesia
- reducing surgery time.

Co-ordination between anaesthetist and surgeon   Close co-operation and communication between the anaesthetist and surgeon during the procedure will improve the success of the procedure and reduce the incidence of complications. Specific instances include:

- allowing the lungs to deflate before the thorax is opened
- ensuring the lungs are deflated when sharp instruments are used in the thorax
- timing the use of sharp instruments with lung inflation

- assessing integrity of the pulmonary parenchyma by applying high inflation pressures while the lungs are held under saline to identify leaks
- assessing the degree of inflation of the lungs with each ventilation.

Potential adverse effects of surgery   It is important to realise that the surgical procedure itself may have adverse effects on the cardiopulmonary system. These changes include:

- occlusion of the great vessels, e.g. vena cava, resulting in reduced venous return
- stimulation of the vagus nerves, resulting in bradycardia
- direct stimulation of the epicardium, resulting in arrhythmias, e.g. VPCs
- haemorrhage from laceration of a vessel or failure of haemostasis
- hypotension from reduced venous return or reduced heart contractility
- cardiac arrest as an iatrogenic event or end-stage of severe cardiac disease.

Recovery

The goal of recovery from anaesthesia is the prompt restoration of normal respiratory function and oxygenation in a rapid and comfortable manner.

Restoration of respiratory function

Re-expansion of the lungs and restoration of normal ventilation   Atelectic lung should be expanded before the thorax is closed, to ensure that there is adequate ventilation from this portion of the lung and to eliminate foci for bacterial growth. This requires removal of all of the air from the pleural space, which may be achieved by the following methods:

- inflating the lung maximally at the point of closure of the chest wall
- evacuating the air after closure of the chest by thoracocentesis
- placing a large-bore thoracostomy tube and evacuating the chest after closure.

Inflating the lungs maximally to inflate all collapsed lung and expel all residual air will not remove all of the intrapleural air. In addition, high inflation pressures of up to 30–40cmH$_2$O may be necessary to do this. The inspiratory pressure is increased gradually over a series of breaths. At the point of chest wall closure, when the final suture is tied or when the chest tube is sealed, the lungs are fully expanded to expel any residual pneumothorax. However, this procedure has a number of potential complications:

- abrupt re-expansion may open previously collapsed vessels, resulting in hypotension
- application of excessive inflation pressures may result in barotrauma
- expansion of chronically collapsed lung may result in diffuse pulmonary oedema.

The necessity for placing a thoracostomy tube after surgery in all patients following thoracic surgery is the subject of debate. It has been suggested that otherwise healthy animals undergoing elective thoracotomy for a brief procedure (e.g. ligation of patent ductus arteriosus) need only to have the pleural air removed by suction following closure of the thoracic cavity and do not require an indwelling tube. It is obvious that animals with more long-standing disease (e.g. ruptured diaphragm) will benefit from the presence of a thoracostomy tube to maintain the negative intrapleural pressure while the lung lobes gradually re-expand. A suitable compromise is to place a tube in all patients, but to remove it within 1–2 hours of recovery for those patients with no significant pulmonary compromise. When there is an injury to the lung which could cause an air leak or where there is any possibility of continuing haemorrhage or effusion, then a chest drain must be placed.

Once the tube is placed, it should be left open to the atmosphere until the thorax is closed, to avoid respiratory compromise from pneumothorax. Once the chest is closed, the pleural space is evacuated while the remainder of the wound is closed. At the end of surgery, the patient is moved into sternal recumbency and aspiration of the pleural cavity is repeated.

Spontaneous ventilation should be restored as soon as the chest is closed and the pleural cavity evacuated. However, a number of factors may delay the onset of normal respiration, including hypocapnia, hypothermia and residual anaesthetic drug activity (e.g. neuromuscular blocking agents).

The presence of a tube also allows for the monitoring of blood or fluid within the pleural space and allows supplemental local anaesthetic agent to be administered. However, it must be realised that the presence of a tube in the pleural cavity will induce the production of up to 2–10ml/kg/day of pleural fluid and allowing the tube to remain in place until no fluid is recovered is not a rational idea.

Management of the chest tube   The chest drain may be suctioned intermittently or continuously. The most informative procedure is to use an underwater drainage system. The drain tube is connected, via a flexible pipe, to a tube which enters a sealed bottle containing water. This acts as a non-return valve and allows air or fluid to be expelled from the pleural cavity, but prevents air from being drawn into the chest on inspiration. The tube attached to the chest drain dips about 2.5cm below the level of the water and should have an internal diameter of 0.5cm. The bottle should have an internal diameter of not less than 15cm. When the chest is closed, air is forced out of the pleural cavity whenever the intrapleural pressure is greater than 2.5cmH$_2$O (the depth to which the tube dips below the surface of the water). As long as the bottle is kept at least 80cm below the level of the animal's body, water cannot be aspirated into the chest. The large diameter of the bottle ensures that however high the water level rises in the tube, the tip will always sit underwater.

When the animal breathes spontaneously, the water level in the tube rises on inspiration and falls on expiration. When the pleural space is evacuated and the lungs occupy the whole of the pleural space, the meniscus does not show marked fluctuations during the respiratory cycle. However, if the lung is not completely expanded, large variations in pressure occur and the level of water in the tube swings from high to low – the greater the amplitude of the swing, the poorer the expansion of the lung.

If there is any doubt about the state of expansion of the lung lobes, chest radiographs should be taken. The radiographs will:

- confirm full expansion of the lungs
- identify pneumothorax if present
- show the position of any chest tubes
- serve as a reference for films taken later on.

Postoperative analgesia

Analgesia helps to restore normal ventilatory function and minimise complications associated with the cardiopulmonary system by:

- allowing normal respiratory patterns without splinting (limiting expansion of the thoracic wall to avoid pain)
- permitting normal minute ventilation volumes, thus allowing efficient gas exchange
- allowing large tidal volumes to be inspired, which are required to re-expand atelectic lung
- enabling coughing to allow the animal to expel material (e.g. blood, secretions) from the airway
- permitting animals to rise, walk and reposition themselves for optimum breathing comfort
- preventing excessive sympathetic tone and the detrimental effects associated with it (e.g. tachycardia, hypertension, increased myocardial oxygen demand).

Abnormalities in the rate and pattern of breathing may result in retention of airway secretions and poor expansion of atelectic lung, which increases the risk of pneumonia. If efficient respiration does not occur, the work of breathing is increased and hypoxia may result.

Techniques for analgesia following thoracotomy Many techniques are described and the most appropriate protocol depends on the patient, the procedure performed and the analgesic therapy given as part of the premedication or intraoperatively. The most effective analgesia will result from a combination of two or more of the following six techniques.

1. Systemic opioids Parenteral opioids may be given as part of the premedication. Although opioids are associated with respiratory depression, this may be avoided by using low doses or by using a mixed agonist/antagonist drug. In the postoperative period, opioids may actually increase ventilatory performance by preventing splinting and by producing slow, deep breathing. The full agonists, morphine, methadone and pethidine are the best choice. Repeated doses should be given as required. Opioid analgesia is generally indicated for the first 24–72 hours.

2. Non-steroidal anti-inflammatory drugs Non-steroidal anti-inflammatory drugs, such as carprofen, meloxicam or ketoprofen, are useful when given preoperatively, with opioids, as part of a multimodal analgesic strategy. They are continued in the postoperative period as required, e.g. for 5–7 days.

3. Intercostal nerve blocks Intercostal nerve blockade (Fig 5.1) is a simple technique, with minimal cardiopulmonary effects, which is performed immediately before closure of intercostal thoracotomies, or preferably, before the intercostal incision is made. Bupivicaine or ropivicaine are the local anaesthetics of choice, giving approximately 6–8 hours of analgesia. The intercostal nerves should be blocked two intercostal spaces cranial and two spaces caudal to the incision. The nerves run along the caudal border of the respective rib and local anaesthetic is deposited at the head of the rib, on its caudal aspect, taking care to avoid the associated intercostal artery and vein. A total dose of 2mg/kg, divided between the sites, should not be exceeded.

4. Intrapleural local anaesthetic Intrapleural local anaesthesia will provide analgesia for thoracic and cranial abdominal procedures. Its mode of action is uncertain, although it may relate to blockade of spinal nerves as they enter the spinal cord in the thorax or local blockade of the incision site. Intrapleural local anaesthetics or opiates may be administered via the thoracostomy tube or via a catheter placed into the pleural space. A dose of 1.5mg/kg bupivicaine or ropivicaine is given. The advantages are its simplicity, ease of

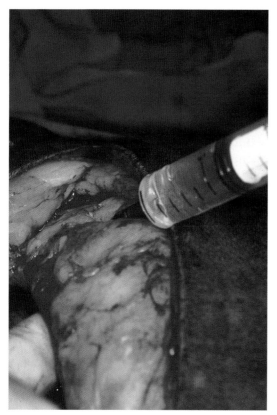

Figure 5.1   Intraoperative intercostal nerve block.

re-dosing and minimal cardiovascular effects. In the conscious patient, bupivicaine may be instilled through the thoracostomy tube. It is recommended that the patient should then be positioned in dorsal recumbency for 5 minutes to allow bilateral penetration of the spinal nerves, or should be positioned with the thoracotomy incision dependently.

5. Epidural opioids   Epidural opioids, such as morphine, may be given at the lumbosacral junction and have a duration of 6–24 hours with minimal cardiovascular depression. A dose of 0.1 mg/kg dissolved in 0.2 ml/kg saline is given and will provide analgesia for about 24 hours. Potential disadvantages include the risk of nerve or spinal trauma, delayed respiratory depression and urinary retention. In addition, some degree of technical skill is required. The epidural route is contraindicated in the presence of septicaemia, coagulopathies or local infection at the puncture site.

6. Local infiltration   Analgesia for sternotomy incisions may be provided by placing bupivicaine-soaked swabs on the retracted sections of the sternebrae during surgery and infiltration of the incision line immediately before closure.

Postoperative care

Pleural drainage   Residual pneumothorax, inflammatory exudate and blood should be removed via the chest tube. Suction may be applied continuously or intermittently. Evacuation of the pleural space will assist re-expansion of chronically collapsed lung.

Suction of the airway   The presence of intraluminal blood and secretions will contribute to obstruction and collapse of the smaller airways. This effect is exacerbated if coughing and deep breathing is suppressed in the postoperative period. Preoxygenation, the use of a low pressure vacuum and suction episodes of short duration (e.g. less than 10 seconds) will reduce the risk of suction-induced airway collapse and hypoxaemia.

Oxygenation   Supplementation with oxygen in the postoperative period will minimise the risk of hypoxaemia. In addition, increasing the inspired oxygen concentration will aid the evacuation of residual pneumothorax, by increasing the arteriovenous gas tension difference. Oxygen administration may continue via the endotracheal tube, until it is removed, and then via nasal catheter, face mask or oxygen cage.

Positioning   The patient should ideally be placed in a position which allows optimum ventilation, minimises patient discomfort and facilitates nursing care. Sternal recumbency allows optimum expansion of both lungs, thus maximising oxygenation, but may not be tolerated following sternotomy. In left lateral recumbency, the larger right lung remains uppermost and well-expanded. Following intercostal thoracotomy, animals should be allowed to recover with the affected side uppermost. This facilitates management of the chest drain, is less painful and promotes re-expansion of the affected lung. However, periodic re-positioning is useful, since this allows bilateral lung expansion and causes intrapleural pockets of gas or fluid to shift, where they might be removed more easily by the drain, and reduces the likelihood of pressure sores.

Continued patient monitoring Intensive monitoring of the patient should be continued in the immediate postoperative period, until it is apparent that the animal is making an uncomplicated recovery from anaesthesia and surgery. Appropriate monitoring includes:

- clinical signs (mucous membrane colour, chest wall excursion)
- breathing rate and pattern
- pulse oximetry
- arterial blood gas analysis
- arterial blood pressure measurement
- ECG monitoring
- measurement of peak negative inspiratory pressure.

Re-warming Hypothermia will delay recovery from anaesthesia, will heighten the sensitivity to painful stimuli and increases the oxygen demand at a time when respiratory performance may be impaired. Passive re-warming should consist of drying the animal, insulating it from cool surfaces and providing a blanket. Active surface re-warming is indicated using infra-red lamps and hot-water bottles, circulating warm-water blankets or forced air re-warming (e.g. Bair Hugger). Topical heat production must be supplied with caution, since poor cutaneous blood flow increases the likelihood of burns.

Urine output Postoperatively, the patient may not urinate because of urinary retention or reduced urine production. Consideration should be given to placing a urinary catheter prior to recovery to allow urine production to be measured and to prevent discomfort from retention.

Postoperative pain, hypotension and opioid use may contribute to urine retention, which may cause the animal considerable discomfort. The patient should be given opportunity to urinate once it has recovered. A urinary catheter should be placed in those animals which have a large bladder but show urinary retention.

The urine output should be approximately 0.5–1ml/kg/h – careful monitoring of the urine output is required. Adequate renal perfusion should be ensured by maintaining hydration status and administering intravenous fluids and, where necessary, frusemide (2–5mg/kg IV) and dopamine (1–2.5µg/kg/min IV).

Nutrition Postoperative caloric requirements will be increased following surgery. The animal should be encouraged to eat as soon as possible after recovery. Enteral tube feeding may be required in anorexic animals.

Postoperative problems

Postoperative care is particularly important for the first 24–48 hours. The problems which may arise following thoracotomy are:

- hypoventilation
- hypoxaemia
- hypothermia
- acid–base disorders
- hypotension
- shock
- oliguria.

Ventilation may be depressed by anaesthetic drugs, pneumothorax, pain and restrictive bandages. Hypoventilation causes hypoxaemia, hypercapnia and respiratory acidosis. A tidal volume of less than 10ml/kg, measured with a Wright's respirometer, suggests inadequate ventilation. This is confirmed by a $PaCO_2$ of more than 50mmHg.

Hypoxaemia may also arise from inadequate pulmonary gas exchange because of shunting or V/Q mismatching. This is most likely to be caused by atelectasis, particularly in the dependent lobes. For this reason, animals should be turned every 2 hours as long as they remain laterally recumbent. A PaO_2 of less than 60mmHg while breathing room air suggests that gas exchange is impaired – the patient should be given supplemental oxygen. The chest tube should be aspirated to remove any residual air in the pleural space. If there is any doubt about the presence of a pneumothorax, chest radiographs should be taken. This is particularly important following lobectomy, when the seal may not be airtight.

Animals which are hypothermic should be slowly warmed by the application of surface heat with warm water bottles or a circulating warm-water blanket and should be covered with a blanket.

Hypotension may be caused by hypothermia, hypovolaemia, anaesthetic drugs or pain. Therapy with intravenous fluids is required and may be titrated to maintain a normal CVP, if a central line is present. A minimum urine output of 1ml/kg/h should be obtained to ensure adequate renal function. Animals should also be assessed for acid–base and electrolyte disorders.

Chest bandages may help to protect the thoracotomy incision, but care should be taken to avoid placing them too tightly and restricting breathing. A bandage will also help to prevent the patient from dislodging a chest tube. As a guide, the chest tube should be aspirated every hour for 4 hours and then every 2–4 hours as appropriate until it is removed.

SURGERY OF THE THORACIC CAVITY

Instrumentation

A few specialised instruments are desirable for thoracic surgery. The most useful item during thoracic surgery is an assistant to help with the surgical procedure. The standard self-retaining retractor is the Finochietto retractor (Fig 5.2). This is of particular use for large dogs, and two sizes will help accommodate a range of patient sizes. For small dogs and cats, other self-retaining retractors such as Gelpis or Weitlaners may be used.

A set of long-handled instruments, comprising thumb forceps, scissors and straight and angled tissue forceps will aid manipulation of tissues deep in the chest. DeBakey forceps have a longitudinal row of very fine teeth and are particularly suited to atraumatic handling of delicate intra-thoracic structures. Long-handled angled tissue forceps (e.g. Lahey or Mixter) are of use in dissecting round

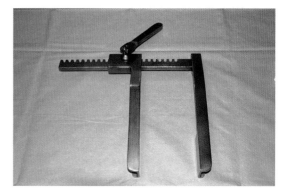

Figure 5.2   Finochietto retractor.

large vessels and for passing ligatures around vessels and pedicles. Ribbon malleable retractors (Fig 5.3) may be of use for retracting structures deep within the thorax. Saline-soaked swabs may also be used to pack-off structures, such as a lung lobe, and leave the surgical field free of other instruments. Tangential vascular clamps (e.g. Satinsky or Cooley) may be needed for lobectomy, excision of the right atrial appendage or repair of lacerated vessels. These instruments have rows of fine teeth which allow a secure but atraumatic grip to be achieved.

An oscillating saw (Fig 5.4) is used for median sternotomy. The use of surgical stapling equipment, primarily linear or thoraco-abdominal (TA) staplers (Fig 5.5), will reduce surgery time, since there is reduced dissection and no need to place sutures. However, they are associated with increased expense.

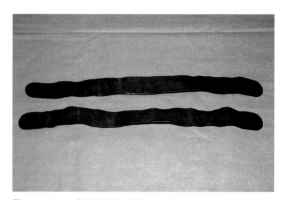

Figure 5.3   Malleable ribbon retractors.

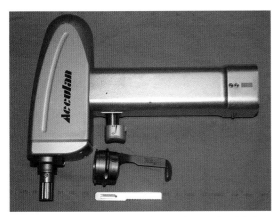

Figure 5.4   Sternal saw, with a reciprocating blade and guard.

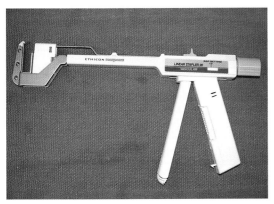

Figure 5.5   Thoracoabdominal (TA) or linear stapler.

Basic surgical techniques

All the principles of good surgical technique apply to thoracic surgery. However, thoracic surgery does differ in some respects. The consequences of poor surgical technique in the thoracic cavity (e.g. haemorrhage from a major vessel, air leakage from a surgical wound in the trachea or lung parenchyma) may be devastating. Continuous movement of the heart and lungs may interfere with surgery. Surgical procedures may have to be performed deep within a cavity, e.g. ligation of the hilar vessels during lobectomy via median sternotomy in a deep-chested dog. The ability to hand-tie knots under these circumstances is essential. Closure of various structures must be meticulous to avoid leakage of blood or air.

Surgical approaches to the thoracic cavity

Two approaches are commonly used, the intercostal approach and the median sternotomy (Fig 5.6). Rib resection or trans-sternal thoracotomy is used less often. Minimally invasive surgery (thoracoscopy) may be used in certain circumstances. The choice of surgical approach depends on the location of the lesion and the type of procedure to be carried out.

Intercostal thoracotomy

Intercostal thoracotomy (Fig 5.7) is indicated when exposure to a specific region of the thoracic cavity is required. This approach provides good access to structures in the immediate vicinity of the surgical site, but access to other structures is limited. As a general rule, this approach will provide access to one-third of the ipsilateral thoracic cavity and mediastinal structures. Access to structures in the contralateral hemithorax is severely limited. The exposure may be increased by performing a dorsal and ventral osteotomy on a rib immediately cranial or caudal to the surgical site, but this is not frequently performed. A caudal intercostal approach may be combined with an incision in the diaphragm to provide access to the cranial abdomen.

The location of the incision may be from the 3rd to the 10th intercostal space, depending on the structure being exposed (Table 5.1). The intercostal spaces normally used to approach various intercostal structures are listed in the table. A lateral thoracic radiograph may be useful to determine the intercostal space which best exposes a desired structure. However, the nature of the intended procedure as well as the location of the lesion will affect the choice of approach. For instance, a lung tumour may lie at the 10th intercostal space on a lateral thoracic radiograph. However, if a lateral thoracotomy is to be performed with a view to lobectomy of the caudal lobe, then this should be performed at the 6th intercostal space, since

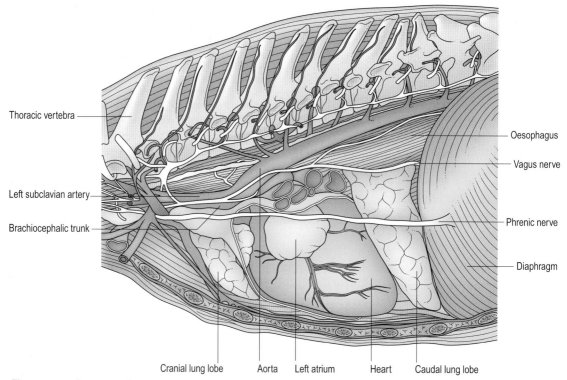

Figure 5.6 Anatomy of the thorax.

Thoracic vertebra

Left subclavian artery

Brachiocephalic trunk

Oesophagus

Vagus nerve

Phrenic nerve

Diaphragm

Cranial lung lobe   Aorta   Left atrium   Heart   Caudal lung lobe

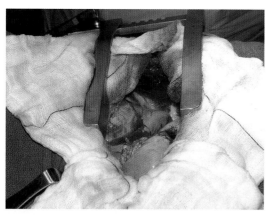

Figure 5.7 Intercostal thoracotomy.

this will give the best access to the hilus of the lobe for ligation of the vessels and bronchus.

Surgical approach for intercostal thoracotomy The animal is placed in lateral recumbency. A small sandbag or roll placed

Table 5.1 Access to thoracic structures via intercostal thoracotomy

Structure	Left	Right
Heart		
PDA	4 (4,5 cat)	
Pulmonic stenosis	4	
Pericardiectomy	5	
Lungs		
Cranial lobe	4,5	4,5
Middle lobe		5
Caudal lobe	5,6	5,6
Oesophagus		
Cranial	3,4	3–5
Caudal	7–9	7–9
Vessels		
Caudal vena cava		7–9
Thoracic duct (dog)		8–10
Thoracic duct (cat)	8–10	

underneath the thorax will tend to arch the uppermost thoracic wall and open the intercostal spaces. The forelimbs should be tied well forward. The approximate location of the chosen intercostal space is determined by counting the ribs from the first or last rib. This may be difficult in obese animals, and the first rib may be difficult to palpate in many animals. An incision is made in the skin, subcutaneous tissue and cutaneous trunci muscle, from the head of the rib to the sternum. The latissimus dorsi muscle dorsally and the pectoral muscle ventrally are incised along the same line. Alternatively, the latissimus dorsi muscle may be retracted dorsally without incision.

This procedure exposes the ribs and the chosen intercostal space is then easier to identify. In addition, the fifth rib may be identified by the caudal insertion of the triangular scalenus muscle and the cranial origin of the external abdominal oblique muscle. Either of these two muscles is elevated from the fifth rib, depending on the location of the thoracotomy. The serratus ventralis muscle is separated between its muscle bellies to expose the desired intercostal space.

The intercostal muscles are incised midway between the ribs to avoid the intercostal vessels. The parietal pleura is penetrated, during maximum expiration, and incised along the same line to immediately below the head of the rib dorsally and to the costal arch ventrally, taking care to avoid the internal thoracic vessels ventrally, which run parallel to the sternum. Saline-soaked swabs are placed over the wound edges and a retractor used to expose the thoracic structures.

If a chest tube is to be used, it is placed immediately before closure under direct visualisation. The tube is inserted through the skin at the 10th to 12th intercostal space, tunnelled subcutaneously for two intercostal spaces, before entering the thoracic cavity at the 8th to 10th intercostal space. The free end of the tube is then advanced to lie at the level of the first rib.

The intercostal wound is closed with simple interrupted sutures of a large gauge (3.5–4 metric) synthetic monofilament suture material (e.g. polydioxanone) passed around the ribs immediately cranial and caudal to the intercostal incision. The needle is passed blunt end first through the intercostal muscle to avoid lacerating the intercostal vessels. All the sutures are pre-placed, which allows the surgeon to close the wound whilst an assistant approximates the ribs with the other sutures. The ribs should not be over-riding or tightly apposed.

The incisions in the other muscles are closed with a simple continuous pattern using a synthetic absorbable suture material. Skin closure is routine.

Median sternotomy

This is the only thoracic approach which allows access to the entire thoracic cavity (Fig 5.8) and is therefore indicated when exploration of the thoracic cavity is required, such as in cases of spontaneous pneumothorax, or when access to the mediastinum is required, e.g. for masses in this location. However, structures in the dorsal thorax are more difficult to reach. This approach may be combined with a ventral midline laparotomy or cervical incision if access to the cranial abdomen or caudal neck is required.

It is important to leave either the manubrium or xiphisternum, or both, intact. This greatly improves the ability to achieve a stable closure, which reduces the risk of complications.

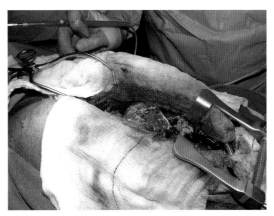

Figure 5.8   Median sternotomy.

Provided that good surgical technique is used and a secure closure obtained, postoperative pain and complication rates are no greater with this approach than for the intercostal thoracotomy. The degree of cardiopulmonary impairment produced by the two approaches is comparable, and hence the choice of approach should be based on the type of access to the thoracic cavity required.

Surgical approach for median sternotomy
The animal is placed in dorsal recumbency with the forelimbs secured cranially. The skin and subcutaneous tissues are incised in the ventral midline from the manubrium to the xiphisternum. The pectoral musculature is elevated from the ventral surface of the sternebrae. Haemorrhage may be brisk and the use of cutting diathermy simplifies the procedure. The sternebrae are then divided in the midline with an oscillating saw or mallet and osteotome. Care should be taken to stay in the midline. Depending on the access required, either the manubrium or xiphisternum, or both, are left intact. The edges of the wound are protected by saline-soaked swabs and Finochietto retractors used to increase exposure.

The sternotomy wound is closed with figure-of-eight sutures around adjacent sternebrae, incorporating a costosternal junction within each suture. Synthetic absorbable monofilament suture material (e.g. polydioxanone) or orthopaedic wire may be used. The former is easier to handle but the latter provides more stable closure. The incisions in the pectoral muscles and subcutaneous tissue are closed with a simple continuous pattern using synthetic absorbable suture material. Skin closure is routine.

Thoracoscopy

Minimally invasive surgery may also be used for exploration of the chest and biopsy of structures under direct visualisation, and for certain defined procedures (e.g. pericardectomy).

The usual approach for exploration is to insert the thoracoscope in a subxiphoid position (Fig 5.9) to view one hemithorax. An instrument portal is then placed in one hemithorax under direct visualisation. Instruments placed via this portal may be used to break down the mediastinum between the two hemithoraces and another instrument portal is placed in the contralateral hemithorax, opposite the first. A third instrument portal may be placed cranial or caudal to the first instrument portal in either hemithorax. Alternatively, the thoracoscope may be placed in an intercostal position (e.g. at the 6th–7th intercostal space) and instrument portals placed in the ipsilateral hemithorax cranial to this (e.g. 2nd–3rd intercostal space) and in the contralateral hemithorax at the 6th–7th intercostal space.

This technique allows direct visualisation of structures within the thorax and provides a magnified view. However, some structures, particularly dorsally, may still not be visible. Biopsies may be taken with grasping forceps and scissors or stapling instruments.

Complications of thoracotomy

- Haemothorax may occur intraoperatively or postoperatively if a vessel such as an intercostal or internal thoracic artery is damaged during closure, or if intraoperative haemostasis was inadequate. Exploration of the wound and ligation of the vessel is required if the haemorrhage is significant.
- Pneumothorax may be caused by inadequate closure of a tracheobronchial or pulmonary wound, laceration of a lung lobe by an instrument or needle, entrapment of the periphery of a lobe during closure or

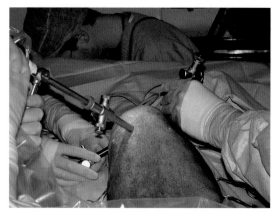

Figure 5.9 Thoracoscopy from a subxiphoid approach.

overzealous thoracostomy tube aspiration. Intermittent or continuous aspiration of the tube will allow most small leaks to heal spontaneously.

- Subcutaneous emphysema may result from escape of free air from the pleural space into the subcutaneous space, if the closure of the soft tissues is inadequate. This is generally a minor and self-limiting problem.
- Rib fractures or costovertebral luxations may occur if excessive rib retraction is used. Supportive bandaging and adequate analgesia is indicated.
- Wound complications, in some form, are seen relatively frequently, though major complications are uncommon. These include oedema, seromas or haematomas, wound discharge and dehiscence. Non-union of the sternotomy incision, sternal osteomyelitis and fracture of the sternebrae have been reported.
- Lameness in the ipsilateral forelimb following lateral thoracotomy is not uncommon, but is usually transient.

SURGICAL DISEASES OF THE THORAX

The lungs

Anatomy
The bronchial tree (Fig 5.10) begins at the tracheal bifurcation, which is dorsal to the heart at approximately the 5th intercostal space. The trachea divides into two principal bronchi which supply each lung. Within each lobe, lobar bronchi divide into segmental bronchi, subsegmental bronchi, terminal bronchioles and respiratory bronchioles. Each bronchus is accompanied by a pulmonary artery and vein, and a smaller bronchial artery. The pulmonary veins lie caudoventrally and the arteries craniodorsally relative to the bronchi. The bronchial arteries are usually single, but may be double in up to 10% of animals.

The left lung is divided into cranial and caudal lobes, and the cranial lobe is further divided into cranial and caudal portions. The right lung is divided into cranial, middle, caudal and accessory lobes. The accessory lobe

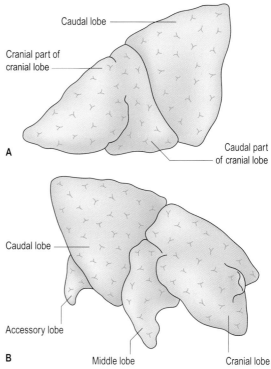

Figure 5.10   Anatomy of the lung lobes.

passes dorsal to the vena cava and is separated from the rest of the right lung lobes by the pleural reflection of the caudal vena cava. The right lung represents approximately 60% of the total lung volume and the left lung 40%. The lung lobes are spongy and provide little grip for sutures.

Surgical procedures
Partial lobectomy   Partial lobectomy is indicated in the management of:

- cysts, blebs and bullae
- lacerations
- biopsy of focal or diffuse lesions
- small abscesses
- small tumours.

For focal lesions, partial lobectomy is generally only indicated if they are located in the peripheral third of the lobe. The latter two conditions may be managed better by complete lobectomy.

Surgical technique The affected lobe is exteriorised and the affected area isolated by placing crushing forceps across the lung. A continual horizontal mattress suture using synthetic absorbable suture material is placed 0.5cm proximal to the forceps. The affected portion of lung is resected by cutting immediately proximal to the forceps but distal to the suture line. This leaves a small edge of lung tissue which is undamaged and may be over-sewn. The affected area may also be removed by using a line of staples with a linear stapler proximal to the lesion. The pleural cavity is then flooded with warm sterile saline and the lung examined for the presence of leaks under positive pressure ventilation. Additional sutures should be placed if leaks are apparent.

Complete lobectomy Complete lobectomy is indicated in the management of:

- large bullae
- tumours
- abscesses
- lung lobe torsion
- bronchial foreign bodies
- bronchiectasis
- pulmonary trauma.

Normal animals can tolerate removal of up to 50% of the normal lung capacity. However, the presence of generalised pulmonary disease decreases this figure substantially. The cranial and caudal portions of the left cranial lobe share a lobar bronchus and are removed together. The right accessory lobe is incompletely divided from the right caudal lobe and is generally removed with the right caudal lobe. The other lobes may be removed singly.

Surgical technique Lobectomy is easier to perform from an intercostal thoracotomy, but a median sternotomy allows exploration of the entire thoracic cavity. The approach depends on the lung lobe or lobes to be resected and the disease process present.

The non-affected lobes are retracted from the surgical field with moist swabs. The affected lobe is manipulated as little as possible to minimise the spread of pus or neoplastic cells through the airways or vessels. The lobe is retracted ventrally and the pleura and perihi-

lar connective tissue are dissected dorsally to identify the pulmonary artery. The artery is double ligated and a transfixing ligature is placed between the first two ligatures. The artery is divided between the distal two ligatures. The lobe is then retracted dorsally to expose the medial aspect of the lobe and the pulmonary vein, which is ligated and divided. The bronchus is cleared of any residual connective tissue and divided. The lumen of the bronchus is closed by placing horizontal mattress sutures through bronchial rings. The free edge of the bronchus is then over-sewn. The repair is examined for the presence of leaks as above. The surrounding pleura and connective tissue at the hilus may be closed over the bronchial stump.

Lung lobectomy via median sternotomy does not allow easy access for individual isolation and ligation of the vessels and bronchus. All three structures may be bunch ligated and then over-sewn after resection of the lobe.

A linear stapler (Fig 5.11) may be used for lobectomy, with or without prior ligation of the pulmonary vessels. The bronchus may then be over-sewn following resection of the lobe.

In patients with pulmonary abscesses or bronchiectasis, care should be taken to prevent any spillage of infected material from the cut surface of the bronchus. In patients with torsion of a lobe, the entire twisted pedicle is clamped and the lobe excised without untwisting it to avoid the release of toxins and inflam-

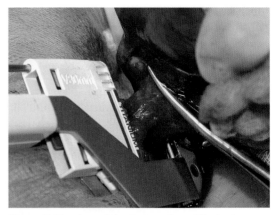

Figure 5.11   Lung lobectomy using a TA stapler.

matory mediators from the necrotic tissue into the systemic circulation. The pedicle is then divided into its anatomical structures and ligated as above.

Pneumonectomy   This involves removal of all the lung lobes in one hemithorax. The indications are similar to those for complete lobectomy, but where the disease is more widespread. This reduces the lung capacity severely, and the presence of normal lobes on the contralateral side should be ensured.

Diseases of the lungs

Lung tumours   Primary lung tumours are uncommon, representing approximately 1% of all canine tumours. However, they are the most common indication for lobectomy. A presumptive diagnosis may be made on the basis of the radiographic or CT signs. A fine needle aspirate may be taken prior to surgery, but generally lobectomy is performed without prior biopsy and histological examination of the excised lobe is performed. Excisional biopsy of the hilar lymph nodes, for staging purposes, is indicated if they are enlarged. Almost all lung tumours are malignant, and most are of epithelial origin. Histological types include:

- adenocarcinoma:
  - bronchial
  - bronchoalveolar
- carcinoma:
  - epidermoid
  - squamous cell
  - anaplastic.

Clinical signs include coughing, dyspnoea, haemoptysis, cachexia, pyrexia and exercise intolerance. Associated findings include aspiration pneumonia, hypercalcaemia and hypertrophic osteopathy. Radiography may reveal solitary or multiple nodules, consolidation of one or more lobes, diffuse infiltration of one or more lobes, hilar lymphadenopathy and pleural effusion. Skeletal metastases may occur.

Surgical excision is the primary mode of treatment. A partial or complete lobectomy may be performed. The former is only suitable for peripheral lesions and is associated with increased surgical time if stapling equipment is not used.

The mean survival time for dogs with non-metastasised lung tumours treated by lobectomy is approximately 11–13 months. The survival time of dogs with lymph node metastasis is 2 months. Prognostic indicators include involvement of hilar lymph nodes, histological type, tumour size and presence of pleural effusion.

Lung lobe torsion   This is a rare condition which usually occurs in deep-chested dogs. The condition may develop secondarily to several predisposing causes:

- thoracic trauma
- pleural effusion
- diaphragmatic rupture
- pneumothorax
- thoracic surgery.

The right middle lobe and the left cranial lobe are most commonly affected. Clinical signs include acute depression, weakness, dyspnoea, tachypnoea, cyanosis, cough and haemoptysis. Radiographs may reveal isolated collapse of the affected lobe, which may be displaced, and pleural effusion. The lobe fails to expand following thoracocentesis. Surgical treatment consists of lobectomy, without prior derotation of the lobe.

Pulmonary abscess   Pulmonary abscesses occur secondary to severe pulmonary infections, which are not cleared, or foreign bodies, which may enter via inhalation, migration through adjacent tissues or penetration of the thoracic wall. Pyothorax may be seen concurrently. The presence of a pulmonary abscess is suggested by persistent atelectasis and signs of pneumonia, which fail to resolve on antibiotic therapy.

Lobectomy is indicated, and should be performed with caution to prevent the extrusion of purulent material into the bronchial tree and adjacent lobes. During the surgery, the end of the resected bronchus may be unclamped and the adjacent large airways suctioned to remove any purulent debris. If the animal has active diffuse pneumonia, then surgery should be delayed if possible, until this has been controlled by medical therapy.

The pleural space

Anatomy
The thoracic cavity is lined by the serous pleural membranes (Fig 5.12). The visceral pleura covers the lungs and the parietal pleura covers the remaining thoracic cavity, and is divided into the parietal pleura, which lines the thoracic wall, and mediastinal pleura, which abuts the mediastinum.

Surgical procedures
The pleural space and mediastinum are potential spaces which may become occupied by air (pneumothorax), effusions (hydrothorax, haemothorax, chylothorax, pyothorax), or abdominal contents (ruptured diaphragm, pleuroperitoneal hernia). Surgery is indicated for management of diseases of the pleural space and mediastinum in order to:

- remove the effusion by tube thoracostomy
- transfer the effusion to another anatomic compartment by shunting
- obliterate the pleural space by pleurodesis
- ligate the thoracic duct in idiopathic chylothorax
- remove the affected lobes where pleural disease results from pulmonary disease
- repair the ruptured diaphragm.

Thoracic drainage The pleural cavity is a potential space between the visceral pleura on the surface of the lungs and the parietal pleura

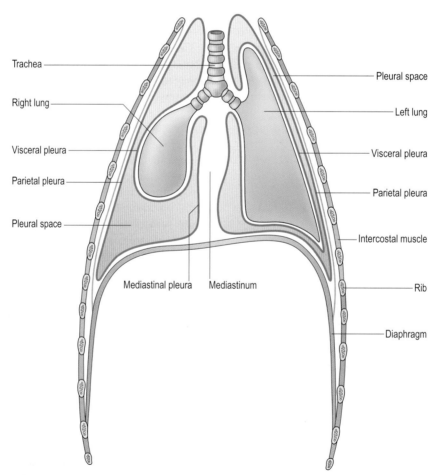

Figure 5.12 Anatomy of the pleural space. The left lung is expanded and the right lung is collapsed.

lining the thoracic cavity. This cavity requires drainage when it becomes occupied by gas or fluid. Indications include:

- diagnostic thoracocentesis
- relief of pleural effusion
- post-thoracotomy or thoracoscopy
- pleurodesis.

The pleural space may be sampled or drained on a single occasion by thoracocentesis. Long-term pleural drainage requires an indwelling chest tube. Once a chest tube is placed, drainage can be achieved by continuous or intermittent suction.

Thoracocentesis This may be performed as a diagnostic step or as a therapeutic measure if only a single episode of drainage is required, e.g. removal of air following acute, mild to moderate, closed, traumatic pneumothorax (Fig 5.13). There is a risk of lung laceration, which is minimised by careful technique.

The site for thoracocentesis is the 4th to 7th intercostal space. With the animal standing or in sternal recumbency, thoracocentesis is performed in the dorsal third of the chest if air is to be retrieved, or in the ventral third if fluid is to be retrieved. In lateral recumbency, the needle is introduced in the mid third of the chest.

Local anaesthetic is infiltrated into the skin directly over the proposed intercostal space and then into the intercostal muscles. Care is taken to avoid contact with the periosteum,

which may be painful, and the neurovascular bundle, which runs along the caudal aspect of the rib. If a needle is used, it should be directed parallel to the ribcage after penetrating the pleura, with the bevel facing the lung, to avoid lacerating the pulmonary parenchyma. The use of a large bore catheter avoids this complication. Advancing the needle while applying negative pressure to a syringe attached to it will help to identify when the needle enters the pleural space. The use of an extension tube and three-way tap between the needle or catheter and the syringe allows the syringe to be manipulated while minimising the risks of lung laceration or needle dislodgement.

Tube thoracostomy If repeated episodes of drainage are likely to be required, then a large bore chest tube should be used (Fig 5.14). This may be placed with the chest closed or open, as at the end of thoracotomy. Closed chest insertion may be performed in the conscious, sedated animal, under local anaesthesia, or under general anaesthesia, following therapeutic thoracocentesis. Placing the tube under general anaesthesia is simpler and less stressful for the animal and the operator.

Tubes are available in sizes from 14 to 40 French gauge and the diameter should approximate that of the mainstem bronchus. The tube is introduced using a central trochar or using forceps to force the tube through a bluntly dissected hole in the intercostal muscles. Smaller diameter tubes may be placed using the Seldinger guide wire technique.

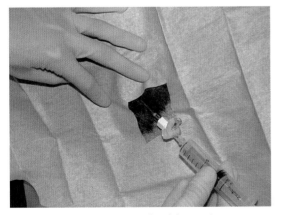

Figure 5.13 Thoracocentesis with a catheter.

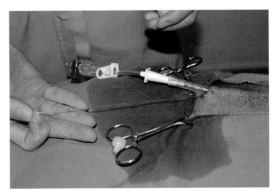

Figure 5.14 Closed chest placement of a chest tube.

The skin is clipped and aseptically prepared. Local anaesthetic is infiltrated into the intercostal muscles at the proposed site of entry into the chest and into the skin at a point two intercostal spaces caudally. A small incision is made in the skin two intercostal spaces caudal to the proposed site of drain insertion. The drain is inserted through the skin, tunnelled subcutaneously to the proposed site of insertion and then introduced into the chest.

The tube is secured to the skin with a Chinese Finger Trap friction suture or a tape butterfly. A purse-string suture is placed loosely in the skin around the entry point of the tube and the ends tied in a loose knot. This suture will be tightened on removal of the tube. When not being suctioned, the tube should be capped and the end folded over and secured with a gate clamp. The drain is then secured against the animal and prevented from being dislodged with a light bandage.

Pleural drainage Suction may be applied continuously or intermittently.

Intermittent suction Intermittent drainage is applied by aspirating the pleural space with a syringe attached via a three-way tap to the chest tube. Intermittent pleural drainage is generally adequate when the accumulation of pleural fluid or air is not life-threatening. Intermittent pleural drainage allows measurement of the volume of air and fluid removed and allows the tube to be incorporated into a bandage to reduce the risk of removal by the patient.

Continuous suction Continuous closed suction is indicated when the rate of accumulation of air or fluid becomes life-threatening or exceeds the limits of intermittent drainage. Continuous suction is likely to be more successful in removing all of the air or fluid from the pleural space and allows the pleural surfaces to remain in contact, which can aid in sealing a pneumothorax or bleeding lesion. However, this is cumbersome and requires that the animal is monitored continuously. In addition, the amount of air removed from the pleural cavity cannot be measured. Continuous suction may be applied using an external vacuum source and one, two or three bottles.

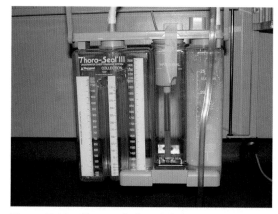

Figure 5.15   Thoraseal pleural drainage system.

Commercial units are available which are based on this system, but are presented as a single unit (Thoraseal; Fig 5.15).

The *one-bottle* system (Fig 5.16) is simply an underwater seal that acts as a one-way valve. Suction can be applied to the chest tube but air cannot enter the pleural space. The thoracostomy tube is attached to an extension tube, which is in turn attached to a tube whose end is submerged in 5cm of water in the bottle. Another tube enters the bottle (but does not enter the fluid) and is open to the atmosphere. Air is expelled from the pleural space whenever the intrapleural space becomes positive. The water seal prevents air or fluid from being aspirated into the pleural cavity as long as the bottle is kept more than 20cm below the patient.

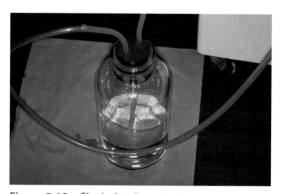

Figure 5.16   Single-bottle water-trap.

The *two-bottle* system adds another bottle between the single bottle and the source of suction and allows regulation of suction. This sealed bottle contains an ingress and an egress tube (like the first bottle) and a third tube, which is submerged below water at one end and open to the air at the other. The amount of negative pressure is regulated by submerging the end of the tube to varying depths. The absolute negative pressure applied is calculated as the difference between the depths of the submerged tubes in the two bottles, measured in centimetres of water. A negative pressure of 10–20cm of water is recommended for continuous pleural drainage.

The *three-bottle* system (Fig 5.17) adds an additional bottle between the patient and the water seal. This bottle is used to collect fluid from the pleural space so that it does not collect in the water seal bottle and reduce the negative pressure applied to the pleural space.

Continuous evacuation of air from the pleural space may be achieved with a Heimlich valve (Fig 5.18). This is a rubber one-way valve in a rigid plastic container and is attached to the end of the chest tube. On expiration, the intrapleural pressure increases and air is forced out of the valve. On inspiration, air cannot enter the pleural space because of the one-way valve. Use of this valve is limited to dogs of medium size and above, since smaller animals cannot generate the intrapleural

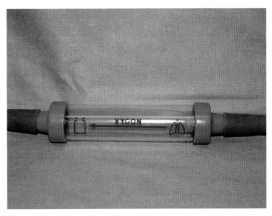

Figure 5.18   Heimlich valve.

pressures required to expel air through the valve. This is a simple technique, but may not provide complete evacuation of the pleural space. In addition, the pleural space is effectively open to the atmosphere and detachment of the valve will lead to air entering the thoracic cavity.

The tube should be removed as soon as possible. The exact timing depends on the disease process for which drainage was required. It is usually removed once the rate of fluid accumulation is less than 4ml/kg/day, although monitoring the falling trend of fluid production may be more informative. The presence of a tube in the pleural space will elicit an inflammatory response and may be associated with the production of an effusion of the order of 2–4ml/kg/day, and waiting until no fluid is produced is fruitless. The Chinese Finger Trap suture is removed and the drain is withdrawn whilst tightening the pre-placed purse-string suture around the skin entry point.

The most important complication is pneumothorax, which may occur if the end of the tube becomes open to the atmosphere, if the fenestrated part of the tube is not entirely within the thoracic cavity at the time of tube placement or becomes dislodged subsequently, or if air leaks alongside the tube. Damage to intrathoracic structures with the trochar may occur if great care is not taken.

Pleural shunts   Pleural shunting relieves the dyspnoea by transferring the effusion into

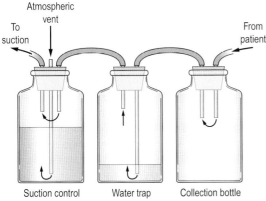

Figure 5.17   Three-bottle system for pleural drainage.

the peritoneal cavity or directly into the circulation. Diversion of the effusion into the peritoneal cavity has two benefits:

- the peritoneal cavity has a larger surface area and absorption of the fluid is likely to be more efficient
- animals can tolerate larger fluid volumes in the peritoneal cavity compared with the pleural cavity.

Shunting is indicated to treat intractable pleural effusion, such as refractory chylothorax, non-septic inflammatory effusions or persistent transudates. It is contraindicated for septic effusions.

Passive pleuroperitoneal shunting This is accomplished by implanting transdiaphragmatic silastic catheters or placing fenestrated silastic sheeting in a defect created in the diaphragm. The pleural fluid is then free to diffuse through these openings. However, the long-term results are not good and adherence of the liver or omentum with subsequent failure of drainage is common. An omental pedicle implanted in the thoracic cavity may also be used as a physiological pleuroperitoneal drain.

Active pleuroperitoneal shunting This requires the use of a double-valve Denver peritoneal-venous catheter or Hakim-Cordis ventricular-peritoneal catheter. These devices are designed for human surgery and are expensive. One end of the catheter is placed in the pleural space and the other end is placed in the peritoneal cavity. The pump, which is situated between these two ends, is fixed in position over the 9th rib. External compression of the pump moves fluid from the pleural cavity into the peritoneal cavity. The pump is compressed twice daily. Ascites may occur for 1 or 2 weeks postoperatively, but does not require treatment.

Pleurovenous shunting This technique uses a similar catheter, but the venous portion of the catheter is introduced into the thoracic vena cava or the azygos vein and advanced to the level of the right atrium. This technique is more demanding, and may be complicated by fatal haemorrhage or thrombosis.

Pleurodesis Pleurodesis involves obliterating the pleural space by inducing adhesions between the visceral and parietal pleurae. Pleurodesis is generally used as a last resort for chronic diseases such as refractory chylothorax, neoplastic effusion and recurrent spontaneous pneumothorax when other methods of therapy have failed. Pleurodesis may be performed chemically, by instilling an irritant (such as tetracycline or talc) into the pleural space via chest tubes, mechanically (by abrading the pleural surfaces with a dry gauze swab) and by pleurectomy (excision of the parietal pleura). However, pleurodesis is much less successful in small animal medicine compared with human medicine and this technique is not commonly performed.

Thoracic duct ligation for chylothorax Thoracic duct ligation is indicated for treatment of idiopathic chylothorax. Chylothorax associated with trauma should be managed medically with thoracostomy tube drainage. Chylothorax associated with thoracic neoplasia or cardiac disease requires correction of the underlying disease, and possibly thoracic duct ligation or pleuroperitoneal shunting.

The thoracic duct is made easier to visualise by cannulating an abdominal lymphatic vessel and injecting 1% methylene blue. The lymphatics are more easily identified if the animal is given a high fat meal (e.g. corn oil or cream), approximately 2ml/kg every hour, starting 3 hours before the surgery. A lymphatic vessel between the caecocolic lymph nodes and the cisterna chyli is cannulated.

The thoracic duct may be approached via a median sternotomy or via a 10th intercostal thoracotomy, on the right for dogs and on the left for cats. The duct is identified dorsolateral to the aorta and ventrolateral to the azygos vein, isolated and ligated. Alternatively, all of the structures in the caudal mediastinum dorsal to the aorta may be ligated *en bloc*. This technique should eliminate the development of lymphatic anastomoses around the ligated duct, but the success rate for this procedure is not reported.

It is recommended that lymphangiography is performed before and after duct ligation to ensure that ligation is complete. Ligating the duct with metal clips allows the site of ligation in relation to the patent lymphatics to be identified on the lymphangiogram. The chylous effusion may persist for up to one week postoperatively. The presence of a chylous effusion beyond this time necessitates lymphangiography and ligation of any unligated branches of the duct or new anastomoses, or selection of an alternative procedure such as pleuroperitoneal shunting or pleurodesis.

Additional procedures may also be carried out at the same surgery. Pleural omentalisation may be performed to provide increased drainage of the pleural space. Pericardectomy may be performed to remove the potential restrictive effect of a thickened pericardium on the heart, thus reducing right heart pressures and reducing any back pressure on the thoracic duct.

The most common complication is failure to resolve the chylothorax. Subcutaneous and peritoneal accumulation of chyle may occur after thoracic duct ligation. Another serious complication is fibrosing or constrictive pleuritis, which restricts lung lobe expansion. Decortication, which consists of peeling the dense fibrous tissue from the surface of the visceral pleura, is recommended to treat this problem. However, this is associated with a high risk of pneumothorax or haemorrhage.

Diseases of the pleural space

Pneumothorax   This is accumulation of air in the pleural space caused by:

- penetrating trauma to the thorax
- rupture of the trachea, bronchi or lungs
- oesophageal perforation.

The pneumothorax is open if associated with a penetrating thoracic injury and closed if not. Tension pneumothorax occurs when the pressure in the pleural space exceeds atmospheric pressure, when the site of leakage allows air into the pleural space on inspiration, but does not allow equilibration on expiration (e.g. a flap-like tear of the visceral pleura). Pneumothorax causes the lung lobes to collapse (Fig 5.19), thus reducing the functional

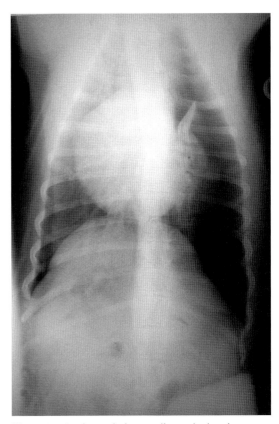

Figure 5.19   Lateral chest radiograph showing pneumothorax. The left lung is markedly collapsed.

lung volume. Tension pneumothorax will also impair venous return to the heart, reducing cardiac output, and may be rapidly fatal.

The patient displays a rapid shallow breathing pattern. Auscultation of the chest reveals muffled heart and lung sounds and the chest is hyper-resonant on percussion. Rupture of a large airway may also produce subcutaneous emphysema (Fig 5.20). Radiography will show elevation of the heart shadow from the sternum and retraction of the lung lobes from the chest wall. Thoracocentesis confirms the diagnosis and allows relief of respiratory distress.

Therapy for pneumothorax depends on whether it has a traumatic or spontaneous aetiology. Management of traumatic pneumothorax depends on the source and flow of air into the pleural space. An open pneumothorax is sealed with an occlusive dressing, convert-

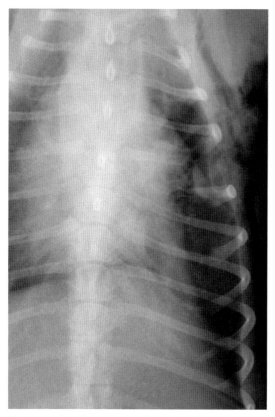

Figure 5.20 Dorsoventral thoracic radiograph showing fracture of the 5th rib and subcutaneous emphysema.

ing it into a closed pneumothorax, and the pleural space evacuated of air. Definitive repair of the wound is performed following stabilisation of the patient. This may be accompanied by exploration of the thoracic cavity if damage to intrathoracic structures is suspected.

Mild closed pneumothorax may be managed conservatively, allowing the air to be absorbed. Evacuation of air from the pleural space is indicated if respiratory distress is present. Placement of a thoracostomy tube is indicated if there is accumulation of air after thoracocentesis. Intermittent or continuous drainage should be performed. However, continual drainage of a traumatic pneumothorax may encourage air to accumulate in the pleural space and, in some cases, where respiratory distress is absent or mild, it is better to accept

a small volume pneumothorax and allow the lungs to be relatively under-inflated, which may allow the defect in the visceral pleura to heal. Exploratory thoracotomy is usually not indicated for closed traumatic pneumothorax, unless the accumulation of air in the pleural space exceeds the capacity of the pleural drainage technique. This may arise with rupture of a mainstem bronchus or extensive parenchymal damage.

Spontaneous pneumothorax occurs in animals with no evidence of trauma and is classified as primary, if there is no evidence of pulmonary disease, or secondary, when pulmonary disease is apparent. Primary spontaneous pneumothorax results from rupture of pulmonary blebs (air-filled spaces immediately beneath the visceral pleura) or bullae (air-filled spaces in the pulmonary parenchyma). Secondary spontaneous pneumothorax may result from:

- bacterial pneumonia
- pulmonary abscessation
- chronic obstructive lung disease
- pulmonary neoplasia.

Spontaneous pneumothorax generally requires a thoracostomy tube for effective drainage. If secondary pneumothorax is present, then therapy should be directed at the underlying cause, and lobectomy should be performed if a localised disease is identified. Primary spontaneous pneumothorax often fails to resolve with conservative management and surgical intervention is indicated to explore the thorax, to resect all lesions via partial or complete lobectomy. Mechanical pleurodesis may be considered if the lesions are too numerous, or no lesions are found, but as indicated above, this is not an effective technique.

Hydrothorax This results from an imbalance in the Starling forces (hydrostatic pressure and colloid osmotic pressure in both the vessels and tissues) responsible for fluid formation and resorption. It may be caused by:

- hypoalbuminaemia (reduced intravascular colloid osmotic pressure)

- congestive heart failure (increased intravascular hydrostatic pressure)
- venous or lymphatic obstruction, e.g. lobe torsion (increased intravascular hydrostatic pressure).

The fluid is generally a transudate, although long-standing effusions will contain degenerate mesothelial cells and neutrophils and have the characteristics of a modified transudate. Treatment is directed at correcting the underlying cause, with pleural drainage to relieve signs associated with pleural fluid accumulation.

Pleuritis and pyothorax Pleuritis may be caused by viruses such as hepatitis, distemper, FIP and upper respiratory tract viruses. It results in a virus-induced vasculitis and serofibrinous or pyogranulomatous inflammation of the pleura, and other serosal membranes, and pleural effusion. Purulent pleuritis, or pyothorax or empyema, is caused by bacteria or fungal infection of the pleural space. These micro-organisms may gain access to the pleural cavity via:

- penetrating thoracic trauma
- extension of bacterial pneumonia or pulmonary abscessation
- migrating foreign bodies
- oesophageal perforation
- extension of cervical, mediastinal or retroperitoneal infection
- haematogenous spread.

In cats, bite wounds are commonly implicated and *Pasteurella multocida* and anaerobes are most commonly isolated. In dogs, inhalation and migration of a grass awn is often suspected in working dogs, and *Nocardia asteroides*, Actinomyces spp. and anaerobes are commonly isolated. The disease may be insidious in onset and the patient may exhibit systemic signs of depression, anorexia and pyrexia at presentation. The effusion is an exudate, containing neutrophils and bacteria.

Treatment should be prompt and aggressive. Thoracocentesis is used to relieve respiratory distress and to obtain a sample for analysis and culture. Antibiotic therapy is started with intravenous antibiotics to achieve high levels in the pleural space, and because many patients have bacteraemia or septicaemia at presentation. Once the patient is stable, thoracostomy tubes are placed bilaterally. The pleural space is drained and then lavaged with approximately 20ml/kg warmed sterile saline once or twice daily. The fluid should be introduced slowly and discontinued if the animal develops respiratory distress. The fluid is allowed to remain in the pleural space for 30–60 minutes, and then removed. At least 25% of the initial volume will be absorbed by the patient. This therapy should be continued for at least 3–5 days, and certainly until the systemic signs resolve and the numbers of bacteria and degenerate neutrophils in the fluid resolve. This therapy will resolve approximately 50–60% of cases of pyothorax.

Surgical exploration of the thoracic cavity is indicated if:

- there is insufficient clinical improvement within 2–3 days
- undrained, encapsulated fluid is identified by radiography or ultrasonography
- there is radiographic evidence of a ruptured pulmonary abscess or other lesion.

Exploratory thoracotomy via median sternotomy is performed. Adhesions and loculated pockets of fluid are broken down with care. Mediastinectomy may be required if the ventral mediastinum is thickened or abscessed. Lung lobes which are consolidated or abscessed should be resected. Intraoperative lavage is performed before closure. Closed pleural drainage and lavage as above is continued for a few days postoperatively.

Constrictive pleuritis is a serious complication of chronic pyothorax and is manifest by an inability to expand the lungs after evacuation of the pleural space. Surgical removal (decortication) of the fibrous covering of the lungs may be performed, but is a difficult surgical procedure and associated with a high rate of morbidity and mortality from haemorrhage and pneumothorax.

Chylothorax This occurs when chyle from the thoracic duct/cisterna chyli system gains access to the pleural space. The thoracic duct courses dorsal and to the right of the aorta, lateral to the intercostal arteries and ventral to the azygos vein. At the level of the 5th thoracic vertebra it crosses to the left side of the aorta and continues cranioventrally along the left side of the oesophagus to empty at the junction of the left jugular vein and caudal vena cava. Although this is the classic anatomical description, most dogs will exhibit at least some anatomical variation. The aetiology of chylothorax is poorly understood, but includes the following.

Rupture of the thoracic duct:
- blunt or penetrating trauma to the chest
- ruptured diaphragm
- iatrogenic damage during surgery
- episodes of severe coughing or vomiting

Exudation of chyle through the duct:
- lymphangiectasia
- obstruction of the cranial vena cava, elevating systemic venous pressure:
  - thrombosis of the cranial vena cava
  - invasion or obstruction by tumours
  - right-sided heart failure:
    - cardiomyopathy
    - restrictive pericarditis
    - tricuspid dysplasia.

It is recognised that trauma and rupture of the duct is a relatively rare cause of chylothorax. If the duct is breached in some way, it will generally heal.

The accumulation of chyle within the pleural space will cause respiratory distress. The debility associated with chronic chylothorax is associated with the removal of the chyle, which contains lipid, protein and electrolytes – effectively depriving the patient of these substances.

Chylous effusions are typically opaque and milky white, creamy or yellow in colour. On standing, the effusion will retain its opacity and may form a creamy top layer. Biochemically, the effusions are similar to a modified transudate which contains lymphocytes and chylomicrons. Chylous effusions demonstrate triglyceride levels that are 10–100 times greater than in serum, but contain cholesterol levels similar to serum. Pseudochylous effusions are high in cholesterol or lecithin–globulin complexes and appear grossly similar to chylous effusions. The opacity of pseudochylous effusions is due to the presence of degenerating cells from an inflammatory or neoplastic lesion.

Radiography and ultrasonography should be undertaken to confirm the presence of an effusion and to examine for the presence of a mass or right-sided heart failure. Often, no definitive cause is found and a diagnosis of idiopathic chylothorax is made.

Therapy may be medical or surgical. Medical therapy is aimed at pleural drainage and reducing the formation of chyle. Low-fat diets reduce the triglyceride content of chyle, but there is little evidence to suggest they reduce its volume. The patient should be supplemented with fat-soluble vitamins and medium chain triglycerides, which are absorbed directly from the intestine into the blood and do not enter the cisterna chyli. Rutin, a benzopyrone drug which increases proteolysis by macrophages and increases the number of macrophages at the site of oedema, has been used for the treatment of lymphoedema in man. There is some evidence to suggest it may have some benefit in treating animals with chylothorax.

Surgical intervention may consist of:

- ligation of the thoracic duct, with or without pleural omentalisation and pericardectomy
- pleuroperitoneal shunting
- pleurodesis.

Surgery is recommended if:

- the flow of chyle does not diminish after 5–10 days of medical therapy
- loss of chyle exceeds 20ml/kg/day over a 5-day period
- there is protein-calorie malnutrition.

It must be realised that despite vigorous medical and surgical intervention, a significant number of animals will fail to respond to therapy.

Haemothorax   This may be caused by:

- trauma
- iatrogenic damage following surgery
- coagulopathies
- neoplasia.

Blood within the pleural space does not generally clot because of the mechanical defibrination and the activation of fibrinolytic mechanisms. Animals with significant haemothorax usually show clinical signs of hypovolaemia rather than dyspnoea, since it requires approximately 30ml/kg of fluid (approximately one-third of the circulating blood volume in a dog) within the pleural space before dyspnoea is evident. Clinical signs of marked hypovolaemia will develop before this volume is lost.

Mild haemothorax of traumatic origin which does not induce respiratory distress will resolve and should be managed conservatively. Pleural drainage is required in those animals with respiratory distress. Continuing haemorrhage necessitates exploratory thoracotomy to identify and ligate or repair the bleeding vessel.

Laboratory analysis of the components of the clotting cascade and a search for a primary tumour are indicated in animals with haemothorax and no history of trauma.

Neoplastic effusion   This may arise from primary or metastatic neoplasia such as:

- lymphosarcoma
- pulmonary carcinoma
- metastatic carcinoma
- haemangiosarcoma
- mesothelioma
- thymoma.

Neoplastic effusions may be transudates or exudates and are identified by the presence of neoplastic cells in the effusion and/or the identification of a mass by radiography or ultrasonography. Differentiation of reactive mesothelial cells from neoplastic cells may be difficult. Confirmation of the diagnosis by exploratory thoracoscopy and biopsy may be required.

Therapy is directed at the causative neoplasm. However, with the exception of lymphoma, the prognosis is poor. Intermittent pleural drainage or pleurodesis may be used as a palliative measure. Intracavitary chemotherapy has been attempted, e.g. with cisplatin. Systemic chemotherapy is indicated for lymphoma.

Pleural and mediastinal neoplasia   Mass lesions in the cranial mediastinum may be:

- thymic lymphosarcoma
- thymoma
- branchial cysts
- ectopic thyroid
- chemodectoma.

Thymoma   This uncommon tumour is derived from thymic epithelial cells. They may be non-invasive and well-encapsulated or locally invasive. A triad of clinical signs is associated with the presence of such a cranial mediastinal mass:

- respiratory distress
- precaval syndrome
- regurgitation.

Respiratory distress results from compression of the trachea, displacement of the lungs or pleural effusion. Precaval syndrome is swelling of the head secondary to obstruction of the venous return via the cranial vena cava. Regurgitation may occur because of extramural compression of the thoracic oesophagus or because of megaoesophagus secondary to acquired myasthenia gravis.

Radiography and ultrasonography will confirm the presence of a cranial mediastinal mass. Cytological examination of an ultrasound-guided fine needle aspirate will generally not reveal neoplastic epithelial cells, but allows differentiation from the more common cranial mediastinal lymphosarcoma, for which fine needle aspiration is generally diagnostic.

Surgical resection via a median sternotomy is the most appropriate treatment. Non-invasive thymomas are excised by ligating and dividing vessels supplying the tumour and carefully dissecting the tumour from surrounding structures such as the trachea, cranial vena cava and brachycephalic artery. Either one or both internal thoracic arteries may have to be ligated and divided. The most common complication is haemorrhage. Careful dissection is required, particularly at the craniodorsal margin of the thymus adjacent to the cranial vena cava. Iatrogenic trauma to the phrenic, vagus and recurrent laryngeal nerves and the terminal thoracic duct is also possible.

Approximately 50% of thymomas are locally invasive and not amenable to surgical resection. In these cases an incisional biopsy should be taken to confirm the diagnosis. Radiotherapy and chemotherapy have been attempted as palliative measures, but there is no proven benefit. If acquired myasthenia gravis is present, this requires therapy with immunosuppressive and anticholinesterase drugs. Postoperative morbidity and mortality is increased in animals with megaoesophagus.

Mesothelioma   This is a rare tumour which can occur in any body cavity lined by a serous membrane, including the pleural space, peritoneal cavity and pericardial sac. The most consistent finding is effusion into the cavity. Malignant cells are generally present in the effusion, but are difficult to differentiate from reactive mesothelial cells on cytological examination. The tumour may appear as a diffuse nodular thickening or uniform fibrous thickening of the serous lining. An incisional biopsy should be taken at the time of exploratory surgery, particularly if an obvious cause for the effusion is not identified. An effective treatment for mesothelioma has not been found. Intracavitary chemotherapy with cisplatin has been used as a palliative measure.

The thoracic wall

Anatomy

The thoracic wall is a strong and compliant structure which consists of 13 paired ribs, the intercostal muscles between them, and eight sternebrae (Fig 5.21). The first nine ribs articulate with the sternum. The costal cartilages of the next three ribs lie close to the sternum, but the 13th rib is a short, floating rib.

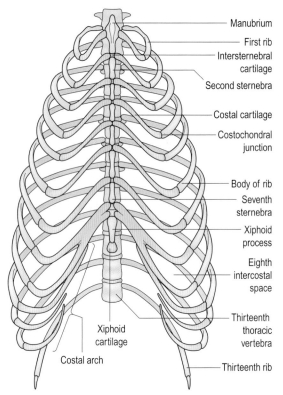

Figure 5.21   Anatomy of the thoracic wall.

Labels: Manubrium; First rib; Intersternebral cartilage; Second sternebra; Costal cartilage; Costochondral junction; Body of rib; Seventh sternebra; Xiphoid process; Eighth intercostal space; Thirteenth thoracic vertebra; Thirteenth rib; Xiphoid cartilage; Costal arch

Reconstruction of chest wall defects

Reconstruction of a defect in the chest wall may be required following trauma to the chest or surgical excision of one or more ribs. A defect involving five or six ribs is generally the upper limit that can be adequately reconstructed. Successful reconstruction of the chest wall must provide:

- an air-tight seal
- rigid stability
- protection for underlying organs
- an acceptable cosmetic appearance.

Primary closure   If the ribs cranial and caudal to the defect can be apposed without undue tension, then simple primary closure may be used. Encircling sutures are passed around the ribs cranial and caudal to the defect and tied to maintain approximation of the ribs. A rib approximator may be used to maintain the ribs in apposition during closure. The surrounding muscles (intercostal, latissimus dorsi, pectoral, external abdominal oblique) may be mobilised and sutured over the defect to provide additional protection. Primary closure is difficult to achieve if more than one rib has been removed.

Synthetic prosthetic material A variety of permanent or absorbable mesh materials, including polypropylene (Fig 5.22), carbon fibre and polyglactin, have been used to fill the defect. The materials should be durable enough to provide stability to prevent paradoxical chest wall movement, should be tolerated by the host, and should be easy to handle. Mesh will generally prevent paradoxical movement of the chest wall for defects of four ribs or less. The use of plastic spinal plates as prosthetic ribs is described, but is rarely necessary.

The prosthetic material is placed intrapleurally to bridge the defect, with the edges folded over against the parietal pleura to prevent trauma to intrathoracic structures from sharp edges. The material is secured to the surrounding ribs and intercostal muscles with mattress sutures. The material should then be covered with adjacent soft tissue, such as an omentum or a muscle flap. The skin may be closed directly, or may require an axial pattern flap (e.g. based on the thoracodorsal artery). The technique is relatively simple and the materials are readily available. However, implantation of a large piece of non-absorbable material predisposes to infection. If the implant becomes infected it must be removed.

Autogenous tissues The use of the animal's own tissues avoids the expense and risks associated with prosthetic materials. Muscle flaps or myocutaneous flaps, based on local muscles such as the latissimus dorsi or cutaneous trunci, may be used to close the defect.

For defects of the caudal chest wall, involving the last four or five ribs, the diaphragm may be advanced to close the defect. The attachments of the diaphragm to the costal arch are severed and the diaphragm is advanced cranially and sutured to the last rib cranial to the defect. Resection of the ipsilateral caudal lung lobe may facilitate advancement, but this is not usually required. This effectively converts the thoracic wall defect into abdominal wall defect. Closure of the defect is performed by apposing soft tissues, using a transposition flap from the transverse abdominal muscle if necessary.

The defect may also be closed with omentum. An omental pedicle, based on the left or right gastroepiploic artery and vein, may be harvested through a paracostal incision. It is then exteriorised and tunnelled subcutaneously to the defect. The omentum will contribute vascular supply to the area, but does relatively little to improve stability or durability.

Diseases of the thoracic wall

Chest wall trauma The chest wall is a compliant and resilient structure and any traumatic episode of sufficient magnitude to cause damage to the chest wall should alert the clinician to the possibility of damage to underlying structures. Chest wall trauma may be associated with the following conditions:

- severe compromise
  - airway obstruction
  - open pneumothorax
  - tension pneumothorax
  - flail chest
  - massive haemothorax
  - cardiac tamponade

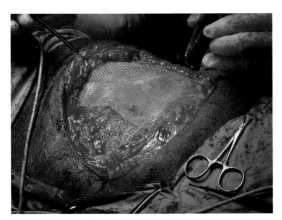

Figure 5.22 Repair of a chest wall defect with polypropylene mesh.

- moderate compromise
  - ruptured diaphragm
  - rupture of the tracheobronchial tree
  - pulmonary contusions
  - myocardial contusions
- mild compromise:
  - fractured ribs
  - mild pneumothorax.

It is vitally important to examine the animal carefully following such trauma and to stabilise the patient before attempting anaesthesia or surgery. Trauma to the chest wall is likely to result in a number of derangements in normal physiology:

- reduction in lung volume (pneumothorax, haemothorax, ruptured diaphragm)
- reduction in functional alveoli (lung lobe contusion, oedema or collapse)
- interference with chest wall (rib fracture, open chest wound)
- airway obstruction (haemorrhage, tracheal rupture)
- hypovolaemic shock (haemothorax).

Damage to the chest wall results in:

- reduced tidal volume
- increased work of breathing
- restriction of expansion of the thorax.

These result in hypoxaemia, hypercapnia and increased energy demand for breathing.

Initial management and stabilisation

- ensure a patent airway
- control any life-threatening haemorrhage
- administer supplementary oxygen
- stabilise the chest wall to improve the efficiency of breathing, or provide positive pressure ventilation
- treat hypovolaemia with appropriate fluids
- close any open chest wounds with sterile dressings
- remove any free air or blood from the pleural space.

The patient should be monitored closely, since changes in condition may occur rapidly. Once the patient is stabilised, then further diagnostic procedures, such as radiography, ultrasonography and electrocardiography, are indicated. Needle thoracocentesis or chest tube placement for pneumothorax or haemothorax and pericardiocentesis for cardiac tamponade may be performed. Indications for an early exploratory thoracotomy include:

- massive haemorrhage
- recurrent haemorrhage, exceeding 5% of the circulating blood volume
- open pneumothorax associated with a massive defect in the chest wall
- major air leak from a ruptured bronchus or traumatised lung lobe
- recurrent cardiac tamponade
- gross contamination of the pleural space with foreign bodies
- ruptured oesophagus.

Contusions   Contusions of the chest wall are common following blunt trauma. The resulting pain may prevent normal breathing – in the presence of associated pleural or pulmonary disease this may be significant. Adequate analgesia should be provided, using systemic (opioids and NSAIDs) and local anaesthetic techniques (e.g. intercostal nerve blocks, intrapleural local anaesthetic) and a search for other diseases induced by the trauma and their management should be instituted.

Fractured ribs and sternebrae   Rib fractures are relatively common following chest wall trauma. They may be single, but are more commonly multiple. The significance of rib fractures depends on:

- the number of ribs affected
- the number of fractures per rib
- the presence of displacement
- the presence of intrathoracic injury.

The animal may consciously limit respiratory excursions because of pain associated with fractured ribs. Non-displaced rib fractures are treated conservatively with adequate analgesia and cage rest. Bandaging the chest may provide support and reduce the pain associated with the fractures, but it may cause displacement of the fractures and further compromise ventilatory effort. An intercostal nerve block with bupivicaine is an effective method of achieving analgesia.

Rib fractures may be associated with laceration of the intercostal blood vessels and may lead to haematomas or haemothorax. Haemorrhage is usually self-limiting, although thoracic drainage may be required. Continuing accumulation of blood in the thoracic cavity necessitates exploration of the thorax and ligation of the vessels.

Rib fractures which are displaced into the pleural space may lacerate underlying lung lobes and should be reduced and stabilised surgically. Cross pinning with K-wires, cerclage wires and spinal plates are recommended. Occasionally, fractured ribs may have to be removed

Flail chest   A flail chest is created when more than one adjacent rib is fractured in two or more places. In immature animals, a flail segment may be produced with one fracture per rib dorsally, since the costal cartilage is very flexible. The flail segment lacks structural integrity with the rest of the chest wall and moves paradoxically during breathing, moving inwards during inspiration and outwards during expiration. This paradoxical movement compromises the efficiency of respiration and may cause contusion to the underlying pulmonary parenchyma. The flail segment may need to be stabilised, but the underlying pulmonary contusions are of more significance.

The animal should be placed in lateral recumbency, with the affected side down, and supplementary oxygen should be given. If stabilisation is indicated, external splinting techniques are preferred. The ribs of the affected segment are sutured to an external aluminium frame or splints made from aluminium rods or thermoplastic casting material. The sutures encircle the rib and incorporate the external splint. A sufficient number of sutures should be placed to incorporate the unstable segment and the normal chest wall. This may be performed under local anaesthesia in the severely compromised patient or under general anaesthesia after appropriate stabilisation. Internal fixation of the rib fractures is not commonly required.

Intercostal rupture   Tearing of the intercostal muscles breaches the integrity of the thoracic wall and may result in lung lobe herniation. The intercostal muscle is repaired as for closure of an intercostal thoracotomy. Multiple intercostal ruptures of consecutive intercostal spaces are repaired with a series of overlapping circumcostal sutures between adjacent ribs in a 'basket-weave' pattern.

Penetrating trauma and open chest wounds
Penetrating injuries may be caused by bite wounds or projectile injuries and result in open chest wounds. Treatment of other intrathoracic injuries sustained at the same time needs to be considered. Injury to the heart or great vessels is usually rapidly fatal. A minor cardiac puncture may result in haemopericardium and cardiac tamponade. Perforation of the lung will result in pneumothorax and moderate haemothorax. Perforation of the oesophagus and thoracic duct is rare. Bite wounds often look relatively innocuous, but the bruised skin may conceal gross damage to the intercostal muscles which will not be diagnosed unless surgical exploration is performed.

The open wound should be cleaned and closed to air penetration by application of petroleum jelly and a gauze bandage. The dressing must be large enough to cover the wound, extending 5cm in all directions, and must be impermeable to air. The edges should be secured with tape. The pleural space may then be evacuated of air. If there is continuing air accumulation in the pleural space, then the wounds may not have been closed adequately, or there may be damage to the pulmonary parenchyma or other intrathoracic structure. Whilst exploration of the abdomen is generally recommended following penetrating trauma, a more conservative approach may be taken with minor penetrating wounds of the thorax, as long as the patient remains stable. However, major wounds and all bite wounds should be explored surgically as soon as possible.

Surgery is indicated to remove foreign bodies in the lung or pleural space if they:

- are large (>2.5cm)
- have sharp edges
- are contaminated
- are in close proximity to the heart, great vessels, tracheobronchial tree or oesophagus.

Complications include wound infection and breakdown of any surgical repair, pyothorax, septicaemia and adhesions.

Sternal luxation Luxations of sternebrae are occasionally encountered. They may be treated conservatively or surgically, depending on the degree of instability.

Chest wall neoplasia Primary tumours of the chest wall are uncommon and are generally malignant sarcomas. Osteosarcoma and chondrosarcoma are the most common rib tumours, with fibrosarcoma and haemangiosarcoma being less common. Ribs are an occasional site for metastasis from other primary tumours, such as osseous neoplasia and carcinomas. Animals usually present with a palpable mass, although occasionally dyspnoea caused by a pleural effusion may be noted. Tumours are more common in large breed dogs, and there is a predilection for the costochondral junction.

Radiographs of the chest will document the site and extent of the lesion and the presence or absence of metastasis. A soft tissue mass protruding into the pleural space or externally, lysis of ribs and new bone production may be seen. A definitive diagnosis is achieved via incisional biopsy. The biological behaviour of chest wall osteosarcoma is similar to that of the appendicular form, with a median survival time of 5–12 weeks following surgery alone. Adjunctive chemotherapy with cisplatin increases the disease-free interval and survival up to approximately 9 months. Chondrosarcoma is associated with a more favourable prognosis, with median survival times of up to 3 years.

Surgery (Fig 5.23) involves *en bloc* excision (removal of the tumour and surrounding pleura, ribs, muscle, fascia, skin) involving the affected rib and at least one rib cranial and

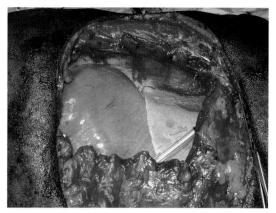

Figure 5.23 Chest wall resection for rib chondrosarcoma.

caudal to it. This may require excision of 3–6 ribs and creates a significant deficit.

Infection of the chest wall This may arise from penetrating foreign bodies, lacerations, bite wounds and surgical wound contamination. Pyothorax may co-exist. Treatment follows basic surgical principles and involves debridement and drainage. Osteomyelitis of the ribs and sternum may require resection of the affected ribs or sternebrae, which may create a defect requiring reconstruction.

Pectus excavatum This is an uncommon congenital deformity characterised by an inward concave deformation of the caudal sternum and costal cartilages. It is reported in dogs, particularly brachycephalic breeds, and cats. Clinical signs of exercise intolerance, dyspnoea and cyanosis reflect respiratory distress caused by restricted ventilation, paradoxical movement of the deformed segment and increased work of respiration. Cardiac murmurs, arrhythmias and mechanical tamponade may be caused by compression of the heart and great vessels, but concurrent congenital disease of the cardiovascular system may also co-exist. Chronic or recurrent respiratory infections and retarded growth may be seen.

Treatment is indicated in those animals with significant cardiopulmonary compromise. In immature animals, the most successful technique is the application of an external splint. Two or three large gauge monofilament sutures are placed percutaneously round the sternum and attached to an external frame which conforms to the ventral body wall. In the mature animal, no consistently successful technique is reported. A combination of several techniques may be required, such as multiple chondrotomy or excision of deformed costal cartilages, release of soft tissues contributing to sternal displacement, and internal fixation or external splinting to maintain the position of the sternum.

The diaphragm

Anatomy

The diaphragm is a musculotendinous structure (Fig 5.24) which separates the thoracic and abdominal cavities. Contraction of the diaphragm is a major force contributing to respiration. The diaphragm is composed of a U-shaped central tendon and a surrounding sheet of muscle arranged into four groups. The muscle attaches to the ribs on either side, the sternum and the lumbar vertebrae. Several structures traverse the diaphragm. The caval foramen allows the passage of the caudal vena cava and is located in the central tendon. The oesophageal hiatus is located in the dorsal muscular part of the diaphragm and allows the passage of the oesophagus and the phrenic nerves. The aortic hiatus is bordered by the paired crural tendons and permits passage of the aorta, azygos vein and thoracic duct.

Diaphragmatic reconstruction

The need to reconstruct a defect in the diaphragm too large to be closed by simple apposition is not commonly encountered. It may arise from congenital hernia; large,

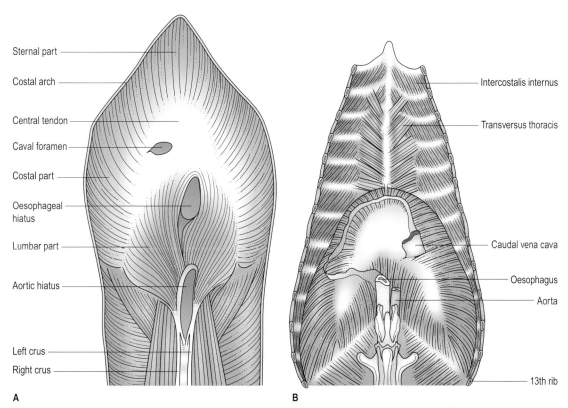

Figure 5.24   Anatomy of the diaphragm (a) abdominal surface from the ventral aspect, (b) thoracic surface from the dorsal aspect.

chronic diaphragmatic rupture; or resection of a tumour involving the diaphragm. The defect may be repaired using synthetic mesh repair, omental pedicle flap or transversus abdominis muscle flap.

Diseases of the diaphragm

Congenital diaphragmatic hernia The embryological development of the diaphragm is complex and involves several structures. Failure of development of any of these structures will result in a hernia, which may be of the following configurations:

- pleuroperitoneal hernia
- peritoneopericardial diaphragmatic hernia
- oesophageal hiatal hernia.

Traumatic diaphragmatic rupture This is a relatively common condition following trauma. Violent compression of the abdomen results in a rupture of the diaphragm and protrusion of the abdominal viscera into the thoracic cavity. Many pathophysiological derangements may ensue:

- loss of diaphragm contraction results in impaired ventilation
- pulmonary atelectasis and reduced resting lung volume causes impaired gas exchange
- the pressure of abdominal organs on major veins reduces venous return and cardiac output
- dilation of a herniated stomach may cause profound cardiopulmonary compromise
- ischaemia of herniated organs may occur.

Ruptured diaphragm is often missed at the initial clinical assessment following trauma. A high index of suspicion for this condition should be maintained in any patient that has suffered significant trauma until proven otherwise. Clinical findings include dyspnoea, tachypnoea and paradoxical respiration (the inward movement of the abdominal wall while the thoracic wall moves outward during inspiration). Palpation may reveal a relatively empty abdomen and a shift in the apex beat of the heart. Auscultation may reveal muffled heart and lung sounds and the presence of borborygmi within the chest. Percussion may reveal hyporesonance on one or both sides. Radiography (Fig 5.25) and ultrasonography will confirm the diagnosis.

Chronic diaphragmatic hernia occurs as a result of delayed presentation or failure of diagnosis after trauma. The animal may develop clinical signs months or years after the traumatic episode. The usual reason for presentation is the development of a progressive pleural effusion resulting from incarceration of one of the liver lobes in the thoracic cavity. Initial therapy consists of restoring and maintaining cardiopulmonary function and includes administering supplementary oxygen, treatment for shock and treatment of other injuries. The timing of the surgical intervention depends on:

- the extent of cardiopulmonary dysfunction
- the degree of pulmonary compromise and loss of pleural space
- organ entrapment.

There is a relatively high mortality rate in patients undergoing surgery within 24 hours of the trauma and in patients where surgery is performed more than one year following trauma. It is therefore important to stabilise the patient before attempting definitive repair. However, early surgical intervention may be required in cases where there is:

- massive organ displacement
- continuing haemorrhage

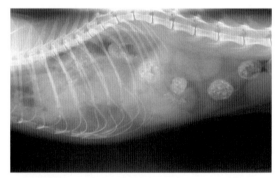

Figure 5.25 Lateral thoracic radiograph showing a ruptured diaphragm and abdominal viscera in the pleural space.

- an enlarging gas-filled viscus, particularly the stomach, in the thoracic cavity
- bowel rupture.

The surgeon should be scrubbed and all instruments prepared before anaesthesia is induced as rapid decompensation and emergency intervention may be required. Most ruptures can be repaired via a cranial midline laparotomy, although cranial extension of the incision via a caudal median sternotomy may be required. As soon as the abdominal cavity is opened, the thoracic cavity is exposed to the atmosphere and positive pressure ventilation is required.

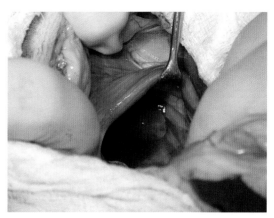

Figure 5.26   Radial tear in the diaphragm.

Surgery (Fig 5.26) consists of returning the abdominal contents to their normal position and repairing the diaphragm. It may be necessary to enlarge the tear in the diaphragm to enable the organs to be repositioned. Devitalised tissues, such as an incarcerated liver lobe, should be resected. In long-standing cases, adhesions may be present between the abdominal organs and intrathoracic structures.

A radial or circumferential tear or a combination may be present. The diaphragm is repaired with simple interrupted sutures. Cranial advancement of a circumferential avulsion from the costal arch may be used to reduce tension of the repair. Care is taken not to occlude structures which traverse the diaphragm, particularly the caudal vena cava.

Pulmonary oedema caused by re-expansion of previously collapsed lung lobes is a possible and sometimes fatal complication associated with ruptured diaphragm. This complication is more likely in long-standing hernias and where positive pressure is used to expand atelectic lobes. It may arise from inadequate surfactant production and increased capillary permeability. It is prevented by avoiding excessive positive pressure during ventilation and allowing the collapsed lobes to expand gradually postoperatively, while the pleural space is evacuated with a thoracostomy tube. If pulmonary oedema occurs, postoperative positive pressure ventilation with positive end-expiratory pressure (PEEP) may be necessary.

Chapter 6

The cardiovascular system

Stephen J Baines

CHAPTER OBJECTIVES

- Anatomy
  - Heart
  - Pericardium
  - Circulation
  - Conduction system

- Preoperative considerations
  - Patient preparation
  - Anaesthetic concerns
  - Surgical considerations
  - Postoperative care

- Techniques
  - Pericardiocentesis
  - Pericardectomy
  - Pacemaker implantation
  - Interventional cardiology
  - Cardiopulmonary bypass and total venous inflow occlusion
  - Intracardiac procedures

- Diseases of the pericardium
  - Pericardial effusion
  - Pericardial constriction
  - Peritoneopericardial diaphragmatic hernia
  - Intrapericardial cysts
  - Pericardial trauma

- Diseases of the great vessels
  - Patent ductus arteriosus
  - Vascular ring anomalies

- Diseases of the heart
  - Pulmonic stenosis
  - Aortic stenosis
  - Ventricular septal defect
  - Atrial septal defect
  - Atrioventricular valve disease
  - Tetralogy of Fallot
  - Cor triatrium
  - Cardiac neoplasia

ANATOMY

The heart is located within the mediastinum, which is the extrapleural space located between the medial reflections of the parietal (mediastinal) pleura (Fig 6.1). The mediastinum also encloses the oesophagus, trachea, vagus and phrenic nerves and the great vessels entering into or exiting from the heart. The vagus nerves (vagosympathetic trunks) pass across the base of the heart and the phrenic nerves pass across the heart more ventrally.

The great vessels in the mediastinum are:

- aorta
- cranial vena cava
- caudal vena cava
- azygos vein
- pulmonary artery
- pulmonary vein.

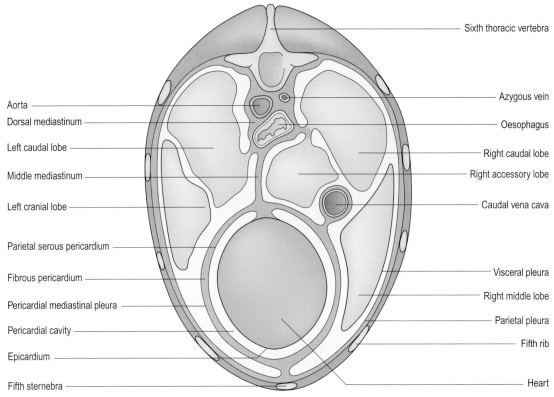

Aorta
Dorsal mediastinum
Left caudal lobe
Middle mediastinum
Left cranial lobe
Parietal serous pericardium
Fibrous pericardium
Pericardial mediastinal pleura
Pericardial cavity
Epicardium
Fifth sternebra

Sixth thoracic vertebra
Azygous vein
Oesophagus
Right caudal lobe
Right accessory lobe
Caudal vena cava
Visceral pleura
Right middle lobe
Parietal pleura
Fifth rib
Heart

Figure 6.1   Transverse section of the thorax at the level of the 5th rib.

Heart

The heart (Fig 6.2) is a muscular pump that is divided into four chambers. A muscular septum divides the heart into left and right sides and the atrioventricular valves divide each side into atria and ventricles. Valves between the atria and ventricles and between the ventricles and the corresponding outflow tract prevent regurgitation of blood. Each atrium has a small atrial appendage (auricle) attached to it.

The valves of the heart are:

- mitral valve: between the left atrium and ventricle
- aortic valve: between the left ventricle and aorta
- tricuspid valve: between the right atrium and ventricle

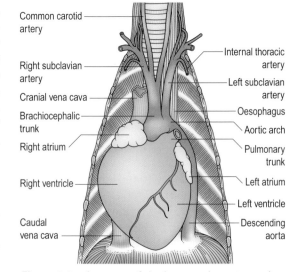

Common carotid artery
Right subclavian artery
Cranial vena cava
Brachiocephalic trunk
Right atrium
Right ventricle
Caudal vena cava

Internal thoracic artery
Left subclavian artery
Oesophagus
Aortic arch
Pulmonary trunk
Left atrium
Left ventricle
Descending aorta

Figure 6.2   Anatomy of the heart and great vessels from the ventral aspect.

- pulmonic valve: between the right ventricle and pulmonary artery.

The heart itself is composed of:

- epicardium: the outer surface
- myocardium: the muscular portion
- endocardium: the inner lining of the chambers.

The blood flow to the heart is via the coronary arteries, which leave the aortic bulb immediately distal to the aortic valve (Fig 6.3). The left and right coronary arteries, which subdivide into further branches, are usually present. Blood is returned from the heart via the coronary veins which drain either directly into the right atrium or into the coronary sinus, which then enters the right atrium.

Pericardium

The pericardium is a fibroserous envelope which covers the heart and great vessels. The parietal portion is composed of a thin, strong fibrous layer and a serous layer. The serous layer reflects over the heart to form the visceral pericardium. The pericardial sac formed between the two serous layers normally contains a small amount of clear fluid. Although the heart will function without the pericardium, the pericardium is thought to have several functions including:

- maintenance of the heart in an optimal position
- lubrication and protection of the heart
- influence on ventricular compliance and balance of left- and right-sided output.

Circulation

The right atrium receives unoxygenated blood from the systemic circulation via the cranial and caudal venae cavae and from the coronary circulation via the coronary sinus. Blood passes through the tricuspid valve into the right ventricle and then passes into the main pulmonary artery to be oxygenated in the

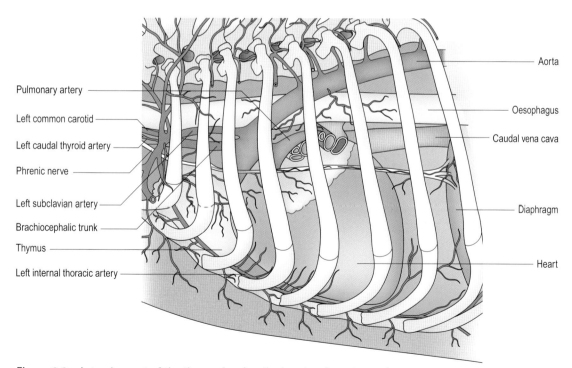

Pulmonary artery

Left common carotid

Left caudal thyroid artery

Phrenic nerve

Left subclavian artery

Brachiocephalic trunk

Thymus

Left internal thoracic artery

Aorta

Oesophagus

Caudal vena cava

Diaphragm

Heart

Figure 6.3   Lateral aspect of the thorax showing the heart and great vessels.

lungs. Oxygenated blood then returns via the pulmonary veins into the left atrium. Blood passes through the mitral valve into the left ventricle, from where it is ejected via the aorta to supply oxygenated blood to the body.

During relaxation of the heart (diastole), the pulmonic and aortic valves close to prevent regurgitation of blood into the ventricles, and the tricuspid and mitral valves open to allow blood to pass from the atria into the ventricles. During contraction of the heart (systole), the atrioventricular valves close, to prevent regurgitation of blood from the ventricles into the atria, and the pulmonary and aortic valves open to allow blood to be ejected into the pulmonary and systemic circulations respectively.

Conduction system

The electrical conduction system of the heart (Fig 6.4) is composed of three main parts:

- sinoatrial (SA) node
- atrioventricular (AV) node
- atrioventricular bundle and bundle branches.

The SA node is the principal pacemaker of the heart and is controlled by the parasympathetic and sympathetic nervous system. The AV node delays conduction of the electrical impulse between the atria and ventricles. The AV bundle divides into a left and right bundle

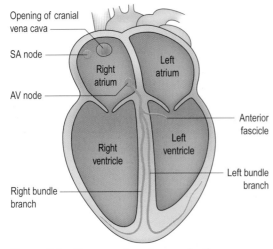

Opening of cranial vena cava

SA node

Right atrium

Left atrium

AV node

Right ventricle

Left ventricle

Anterior fascicle

Left bundle branch

Right bundle branch

Figure 6.4 The normal cardiac conduction pathways.

branch in the ventricular septum. These pathways conduct the electrical impulse down the interventricular septum and then up the ventricular free walls, allowing the heart to squeeze blood from the ventricles.

PREOPERATIVE CONSIDERATIONS

Patient preparation

Animals requiring cardiovascular surgery frequently have symptomatic cardiovascular disease that needs to be controlled prior to surgery.

Animals with congestive heart failure should be stabilised with diuretics (e.g. frusemide) and ACE inhibitors (e.g. enalapril) before surgery. Animals with supraventricular dysrhythmias may need treatment with digoxin, beta-blockers (e.g. propranolol, esmolol) or calcium-channel blockers (e.g. diltiazem). Those with ventricular dysrhythmias may require class I anti-arrhythmic drugs (e.g. lignocaine, procainamide). Animals with bradydysrhythmias may require atropine, isoproterenol or temporary transvenous or transthoracic pacing prior to surgery.

Animals with pre-existing pericardial or pleural effusion should have these effusions drained by pericardiocentesis or pleurocentesis prior to the induction of anaesthesia to improve cardiopulmonary function.

Animals in poor condition through cachexia or regurgitation (e.g. vascular ring anomaly) should have their nutritional needs assessed carefully and a plan should be prepared for their postoperative nutrition, which may include enteral tube feeding. Patients with congenital diseases may be young when surgery is performed. Hypothermia and hypoglycaemia are more common in these patients and care should be taken to prevent and treat these abnormalities.

Anaesthetic concerns

Careful consideration should be given to the choice of premedicant, induction and maintenance agents. Opioids have the potential to induce respiratory depression and brady-cardia, and anticholinergics may be required to prevent this bradycardia. Benzodiazepines have minimal depressant effects on the cardiovascular system and are often used synergistically with opioids.

Thiopentone and propofol can both cause cardiovascular depression, and the former is arrhythmogenic, although both provide a rapid induction. Etomidate is not arrhythmogenic, maintains cardiac output and allows a rapid induction and is therefore recommended in patients with cardiac disease. Ketamine may be used for induction of compromised patients, but should be avoided in patients with AV valve insufficiency, since it increases the regurgitant fraction. Ketamine may be used in conjunction with diazepam to offset some of its negative effects, e.g. muscle rigidity and potential seizure activity. Opioids, e.g. fentanyl, can also be used as induction agents in compromised animals, but they do not induce anaesthesia and intubation may be difficult in alert animals.

Isoflurane is the maintenance agent of choice in most cardiac patients. Its relative insolubility allows rapid induction, recovery and change in depth of anaesthesia. It is less arrhythmogenic than halothane and also has less depressant effect on the myocardium. A balanced anaesthetic technique should be employed, and the intraoperative use of opioids (e.g. fentanyl infusion) and muscle relaxants (e.g. atracurium) are considered.

Drugs, equipment and personnel required for cardiac resuscitation should be immediately available throughout the procedure and in the immediate perioperative period. Haemorrhage is one of the major complications of cardiovascular surgery and blood products and colloids should be available.

Surgical considerations

Instrumentation and sutures

Sutures   The more commonly used sutures are polypropylene (Prolene; Ethicon) and braided polyester (Ti-Cron; Davis and Geck). These sutures should be available in a range of sizes, from 3-0 (2 metric) to 6-0 (0.7 metric) with swaged-on, taper-point cardiovascular needles. Suturing may be facilitated by using double-armed (i.e. a needle at each end of the suture) sutures. Placement of pledgets (TFE polymer pledget; Ethicon) helps to buttress sutures in the heart and great vessels. Large gauge, 1-2 (4-5 metric), silk ligatures are useful for retraction or ligation of large cardiovascular structures, as tourniquets and for securing large cannulae (e.g. for cardiopulmonary bypass). Umbilical tape may also be used for vessel retraction. Silicone vessel loupes are useful to retract the phrenic nerves during pericardectomy. Vessels are temporarily occluded with a Rummel tourniquet (Fig 6.5), which may be made from a heavy gauge silk ligature and a piece of silicone chest drain. Cardiotomy incisions are usually closed with a continuous horizontal mattress pattern, oversewn with a simple continuous pattern. Stab incisions for access into vessels or heart chambers are closed with pledgeted horizontal mattress sutures. Larger incisions, e.g. for placement of bypass cannulae, are closed with a purse-string suture.

Instruments   A few specialised instruments will make cardiovascular surgery easier. Long-handled versions of standard dissecting instruments will make intrathoracic manipulations easier. DeBakey thumb forceps are generally used and at least one pair should have a tungsten-carbide insert for grasping sutures. Metzenbaum scissors are used as standard, but Potts scissors (45° and 90°) are useful. Mayo needle holders may be used in pairs with double-armed suture material and Castroviejo needle holders are used for fine sutures. Non-crushing tangential vascular occlusion clamps, such as Satinsky and Cooley, are used to temporarily close a cardiotomy or vascular incision so that it may be repaired while still maintaining luminal flow. Curved dissecting forceps, e.g. Mixter and Lahey, are used to dissect around vascular structures.

Surgical principles

The principles of good surgical technique apply to cardiac surgery. The presence of

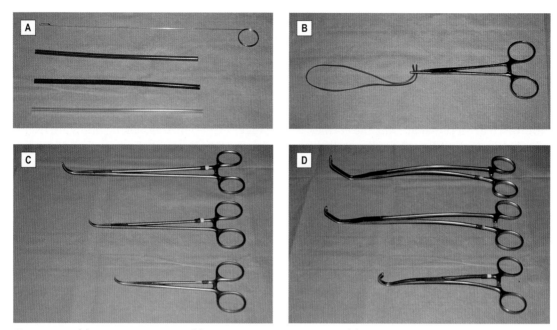

Figure 6.5   (a) Rummel tourniquet, (b) Silicone rubber vessel loops, (c) Mixter forceps, (d) Tangential vascular clamps.

motion at the surgical site makes surgery more demanding. Fine gauge suture with swaged-on atraumatic needles is generally used. Gentle placement of sutures to avoid bleeding from the needle tracks is important. Surgery of the cardiovascular system involves procedures performed on the atria, ventricles, pericardium, valves and great vessels. Some of these procedures are closed and do not require opening the heart or major vessels. Other procedures require an open-heart approach via venous inflow occlusion or cardiopulmonary bypass.

Surgical approaches   The surgical approaches to the heart and great vessels are described in Chapter 5 (Thoracic surgery). Most procedures may be performed via a left or right 4th–6th intercostal thoracotomy or a median sternotomy. Thoracoscopy may be appropriate for exploration and pericardectomy.

Postoperative care

Cardiovascular surgery is usually performed via thoracotomy and much of the postoperative care needed is detailed in Chapter 5.

For the patient undergoing cardiovascular surgery, particular care should be taken to monitor any abnormalities identified preoperatively, e.g. dysrhythmias, and to ensure that therapy for these disorders continues in the postoperative period. Continuous ECG monitoring, arterial blood pressure measurement, intermittent arterial blood gas analysis, pulse oximetry and palpation of the peripheral pulse are the main techniques used in the recovery period.

TECHNIQUES

Pericardiocentesis

This may be a diagnostic procedure, to remove a sample of the fluid in the pericardial sac, or a therapeutic procedure, to relieve the signs associated with a pericardial effusion. Sedation may be required for this procedure in some cases. The site for pericardiocentesis is immediately below the costochondral junction at the right 4th, 5th or 6th intercostal space. This site is chosen for several reasons:

there is no lung tissue between the chest wall and heart since this area overlies the cardiac notch (Fig 6.6)

the site is ventral to the thin-walled right atrium

there are no coronary arteries on the epicardium in this location

the right ventricle is at a lower pressure than the left and the risk of catastrophic haemorrhage is less.

The animal may be standing or in left lateral recumbency. The right thoracic wall from the sternum to above the costochondral junction, extending over the 3rd–7th intercostal spaces, is clipped and aseptically prepared. Local anaesthetic is introduced into the skin and intercostal muscles at the proposed site. A large (14–18 gauge), long (5–15cm) over-the-needle catheter is introduced through a stab incision in the skin. A syringe is attached to the needle and the catheter is advanced through the thoracic wall towards the heart. Slight negative pressure is applied to the syringe so that, once the pericardial sac is entered, fluid will be aspirated. Once the catheter is in the pericardial sac, the catheter is advanced and the needle withdrawn. A three-way tap and an extension set is connected to the syringe – as much pericardial fluid as possible is removed. A dedicated pericardiocentesis catheter, placed using the Seldinger guide wire technique (Fig 6.7) or a trochar, may also be used.

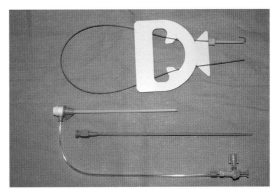

Figure 6.7 Catheter introducer, Seldinger wire and vessel dilator for angiography.

Continuous monitoring of the ECG allows dysrhythmias, induced by epicardial stimulation from the procedure, to be monitored. If the catheter or needle contacts the heart, then movement of the heart may be appreciated through the syringe and changes, such as ventricular premature complexes, may be seen on the ECG. The ECG changes generally resolve once the needle is retracted. The fluid is submitted for cytological and biochemical analysis and culture.

Pericardiocentesis causes an immediate clinical improvement, noted by slowing of the pulse rate and an increase in its volume.

Pericardectomy

Indications for pericardectomy include:

idiopathic pericardial effusion

constrictive pericarditis

heart base tumours

pericardial cysts

pericardial tumours.

Pericardectomy (Fig 6.8) involves removing all or part of the pericardium. It is indicated if pericardial effusion recurs after two or three episodes of therapeutic pericardiocentesis. In chronic cases, restrictive epicarditis may be present, for which pericardectomy may not be of benefit. Removal of a part or all of the pericardium may be achieved in a number of ways, as follows.

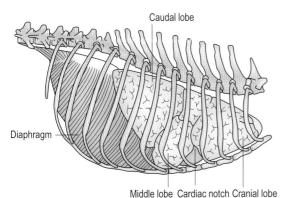

Caudal lobe

Diaphragm

Middle lobe Cardiac notch Cranial lobe

Figure 6.6 Thoracic wall and right lung, showing the cardiac notch.

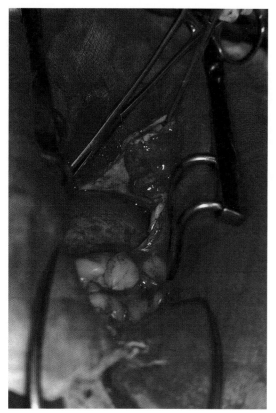

Figure 6.8   Pericardectomy via a median sternotomy approach.

Surgical pericardectomy

Pericardectomy may be performed via a left or right 4th or 5th intercostal thoracotomy or median sternotomy. Only a median sternotomy will expose the entire pericardium up to the heart base. Removal of the pericardium from the contralateral side is difficult from a lateral thoracotomy. This procedure allows removal of as much of the pericardium as possible.

The phrenic nerves, which run adjacent to the pericardium on either side of the thoracic cavity, should be identified, isolated and preserved. A subtotal pericardectomy may be performed, where the pericardium is removed ventral to the phrenic nerves. Alternatively, the phrenic nerves may be elevated from the pericardium and a complete pericardectomy performed.

Creation of a pericardial window may allow temporary resolution of clinical signs, but adhesions may close the aperture with time. If a palliative technique such as excision of a window of pericardium is chosen, consideration should be given to performing this via thoracoscopy or via percutaneous pericardiotomy.

The diseased pericardium is increased in thickness and vascularity and great care should be taken to ensure adequate haemostasis. A portion of the pericardium should be submitted for histological examination and, where appropriate, culture.

Thoracoscopic pericardectomy

A thoracoscope is placed via a subxiphoid portal and used to allow placement of additional instrument ports at the 4th–7th intercostal spaces, either on the same side or opposite sides. The mediastinum is opened to allow exploration of the thoracic cavity. The pericardium is grasped and a small incision made at the apex of the heart. This incision is continued in a cranial to caudal and lateral direction to allow either a subtotal pericardectomy or pericardial window to be performed.

Percutaneous balloon pericardiotomy

Percutaneous balloon pericardiotomy allows the creation of a pericardial window without a thoracotomy. Under general anaesthesia and image intensification, a guide wire is introduced into the pericardium with a catheter and, using the guide wire, a balloon catheter placed across the pericardium. The balloon is inflated, which tears a hole in the pericardium. This technique is of use for patients for whom a thoracotomy is not an option, or for those patients with a poor prognosis (e.g. neoplastic effusion).

Pacemaker implantation

The implantation of an artificial pacemaker (Fig 6.9) to regulate the heart rate is indicated in the following disorders:

- high grade second degree AV block
- third degree (complete) AV block

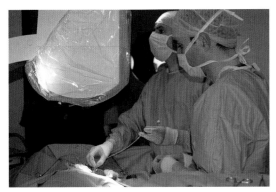

Figure 6.9   Transvenous pacemaker placement under fluoroscopic guidance.

- persistent atrial standstill
- sinus bradycardia
- sinus arrest
- sinoatrial (SA) block
- bradycardia-tachycardia syndrome
- sick sinus syndrome.

The pacemaker consists of the pulse generator and a lead which delivers the impulse to the heart. The leads may be implanted transvenously into the endocardial surface or via thoracotomy into the epicardial surface of the heart. The former is the most common approach.

Animals with symptomatic bradydysrhythmias are at risk of poor cardiac output during anaesthesia. The heart rate may be controlled preoperatively by placement of a temporary transvenous pacemaker in the conscious animal prior to anaesthesia, or by the use of temporary transthoracic electrodes which are stuck onto each side of the chest wall.

Endocardial lead placement

Endocardial lead placement involves implantation of the lead in the right ventricle via the right jugular vein. The lead is introduced into the vein and placed under fluoroscopic guidance such that the tip of the lead contacts the endocardium of the right ventricle. A subcutaneous pocket is created for the pulse generator, dorsal to the jugular vein. The right jugular vein is chosen because placement via the left jugular vein would be difficult in patients with a persistent left cranial vena cava, although this is an uncommon abnormality. Postoperatively, the animal is kept quiet, and sedated if necessary, for 2–3 days until the lead has become more firmly attached. Manipulation of the head and neck is avoided during this time, to prevent dislodgement or detachment of the lead.

Epicardial lead placement

Epicardial lead placement may be placed using the following approaches:

- left or right 5th intercostal thoracotomy
- cranial midline laparotomy and partial caudal midline sternotomy
- cranial midline laparotomy and transdiaphragmatic approach.

The latter approach is preferred. The left ventricle is exposed and an avascular area at the apex is identified. The corkscrew tip of the lead is introduced through the epicardium into the myocardium. The pulse generator is placed in a superficial site, where it may be accessed in cases of malfunction.

Interventional cardiology

Interventional cardiac catheterisation is performed for diagnosis (e.g. of congenital heart disease), to gain additional information (e.g. measurement of pressure gradients) and therapy (e.g. balloon valvuloplasty for pulmonic stenosis). In veterinary medicine, a diagnosis of cardiovascular disease is normally achieved via radiography and echocardiography.

Placement of a vascular access sheath

Access to the vessel is usually performed by percutaneous placement of a vascular access sheath. These comprise:

- a straight cannula through which catheters and wires may be placed
- a one-way valve to prevent blood leakage and air embolism
- a side arm to measure pressure or infuse agents.

The vascular access sheath usually measures 5–12 French and 20–35cm in length. For arterial access, the femoral or carotid arteries are chosen and for venous access the jugular or femoral veins are chosen. The entire procedure may be performed percutaneously, or a cutdown may be performed to isolate the vessel. The general procedure for gaining vascular access is as follows:

● introduce a catheter into the vessel
● introduce a guide wire
● remove the catheter
● introduce a vessel dilator over the wire
● remove the vessel dilator
● introduce a vascular access sheath over the wire
● remove the wire, secure the vascular access sheath to the vessel.

Once the procedure has been completed, the sheath is removed and haemostasis is achieved. If a surgical approach was made, the vessel may be ligated, or repaired with fine gauge polypropylene. If percutaneous placement of the sheath was performed, pressure is used to achieve haemostasis. Venous sites usually require 5–10 minutes of firm digital pressure, whereas arterial sites require 15–20 minutes of firm pressure, followed by 10 minutes of gentle pressure.

Interventional cardiac catheterisation procedures

Balloon valvuloplasty This technique has been used in human and canine medicine for over 20 years. It is a safe, effective and non-invasive technique and is generally the treatment of choice for valvular pulmonic stenosis. The procedure for pulmonic valvuloplasty is described.

A vascular access sheath is placed and a long end-hole catheter is placed through the sheath under fluoroscopic guidance from the femoral vein, into the caudal vena cava and the right side of the heart. The catheter is manipulated through the right atrium, tricuspid valve, right ventricle and into the main pulmonary artery. Pressure measurements across the pulmonary valve are made. Angio-cardiography, with direct injection of contrast medium under fluoroscopic guidance into the right ventricle, allows the site and size of the pulmonic stenosis to be identified.

A balloon catheter with an inflated balloon diameter of approximately 1.5 times the diameter of the pulmonic valve annulus is selected. A guide wire is placed through the end-hole catheter, which is then removed and replaced with the balloon catheter. The valvuloplasty catheter is placed so that the balloon lies across the stenotic region. The balloon is rapidly filled to its maximum pressure with contrast medium using a syringe with a pressure gauge, held at that pressure for 10 seconds, and then deflated. The procedure is repeated three or four times, repositioning the catheter as required.

During the first inflation of the balloon, indentation of the balloon at the level of the stenosis (a 'waist') is seen. Loss of this waist with subsequent inflations provides some visual evidence of success. Replacement of the balloon catheter with an end-hole catheter and measurement of the residual pressure gradient across the valve allows an objective measurement of success.

Transcatheter occlusion of vessels Transcatheter closure of patent ductus arteriosus (PDA) is the preferred technique for isolated PDA in children. This technique has been used in small animals and is safe and effective. The vessel is occluded with a vascular occlusion coil (e.g. Gianturco), which are spring coils made of stainless steel enclosing a mesh of Dacron strands. The strands promote the formation of an occlusive thrombus.

The advantages of transcatheter occlusion are:

● reduced morbidity from thoracotomy
● reduced risk of ductal rupture.

The disadvantages of transcatheter occlusion are:

● longer procedure time than surgery
● lower success rate of complete occlusion.

Other procedures A number of other interventional catheterisation procedures are performed in human cardiology, but have yet to gain widespread use in small animals. These include:

- closure of atrial septal defects
- closure of ventricular septal defects
- stent placement to prevent recurrence of stenosis.

Closure of septal defects is performed with a self-expanding device (Amplatz occluder) which consists of two discs, which sit either side of the defect.

Cardiopulmonary bypass and total venous inflow occlusion

Both of these procedures allow intracardiac procedures to be carried out without the loss of blood that would otherwise follow. A detailed description of these procedures is beyond the scope of this chapter, but an overview of the procedures will be given.

Inflow occlusion

This procedure involves occlusion of the veins supplying systemic blood to the right side of the heart. It is indicated for open heart surgery of short duration and may be performed from a left or right thoracotomy or a median sternotomy, although access from the left side is more difficult in the presence of cardiomegaly.

The main advantages of this procedure over cardiopulmonary bypass are:

- simplicity
- lack of need for specialised equipment or techniques
- minimal cardiopulmonary, metabolic or haematological derangement postoperatively.

The disadvantages of this procedure are:

- limited time available
- motion of the surgical field
- unavailability of another strategy if the procedure cannot be performed in the time.

The duration of inflow occlusion should be less than 2 minutes in the normothermic animal, extending to 4 minutes with mild hypothermia (32–34°C). Animals are hyper-ventilated for 5 minutes prior to inflow occlusion and then ventilation ceases for the period of inflow occlusion. Resuscitation is performed on re-establishment of venous inflow to the heart.

Cardiopulmonary bypass

This procedure involves removing venous blood from the systemic circulation as it returns to the heart and returning it via a systemic artery. While outside the body, the blood is oxygenated and thus the machine (Fig 6.10) replaces the function of both the heart and the lungs. During the procedure, the heart is stopped by infusing cardioplegia solution (containing potassium chloride) and the patient is cooled. The venous blood is removed via cannulation of the cranial and caudal vena cava or the right atrium and the caudal vena cava and the arterial blood is returned via the femoral or carotid artery. This procedure provides a bloodless, motion-free surgical site and allows the time to perform a complex surgical repair.

At the end of the procedure, the patient is warmed and resuscitated and the normal circulation is established while still maintaining the cannulae in place, should the patient need to go back on bypass. Before recovery, a tracheostomy tube may be placed to allow efficient ventilation in the postoperative period. Cardiopulmonary bypass requires a great deal of specialised equipment, and a competent team consisting of surgeons, anaesthetists, perfusionist and critical care specialists.

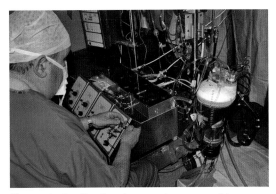

Figure 6.10 Cardiopulmonary bypass machine.

Intracardiac procedures

Intracardiac procedures which may be performed under venous inflow occlusion or cardiopulmonary bypass include:

- patch graft valvuloplasty
- atrioventricular valve repair
- atrioventricular valve replacement
- atrioventricular valve annuloplasty.

DISEASES OF THE PERICARDIUM

Pericardial effusion

Pericardial effusion is the collection of fluid within the pericardial sac. This fluid may be a transudate, an exudate or sanguinous. Possible causes are:

- right-sided congestive heart failure, e.g. feline cardiomyopathy
- hypoproteinaemia
- infectious pericarditis (bacteria, fungi, FIP, toxoplasma)
- neoplasia (haemangiosarcoma, mesothelioma, chemodectoma, lymphoma)
- acute haemorrhage (left atrial rupture, coagulopathy, trauma)
- idiopathic.

Neoplastic and idiopathic effusions are the most common. The pathophysiological changes depend on the rate and amount of fluid accumulation. Slow accumulation of fluid allows compensatory mechanisms to occur, such as the stretching of the fibrous pericardium and retention of intravascular volume to increase diastolic filling pressures. However, progressive right-sided congestive heart failure will occur, resulting in weakness, exercise intolerance, collapse and abdominal distension, caused by hepatomegaly and ascites. Cardiac tamponade occurs when the intrapericardial pressure approaches diastolic filling pressure, resulting in a profound drop in cardiac output and circulatory collapse. It may result from the rapid accumulation of fluid, or as the end stage of slow accumulation of fluid.

A rapid and weak arterial pulse, distended systemic veins and diminished heart sounds will be present. ECG analysis may reveal small complexes, ST segment deviation and electrical alternans (alternating large and small QRS complexes). Thoracic radiographs (Fig 6.11) will reveal globular cardiomegaly. Ultrasonography will confirm the presence of pericardial effusion and may identify a tumour.

Pericardiocentesis is performed to obtain a sample for analysis and to relieve the signs associated with the effusion. As much fluid as

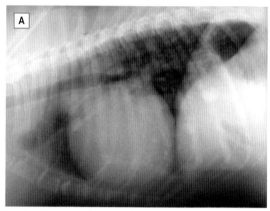

Figure 6.11 (a) Lateral thoracic radiograph showing pericardial effusion due to a heart base tumour. Pulmonary metastases are present.

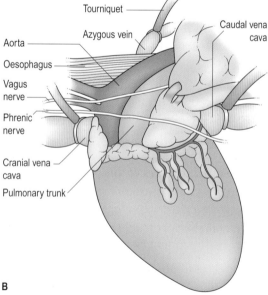

B
Figure 6.11 (b) Venous inflow occlusion from the left side.

possible should be removed. Urgent peri-cardiocentesis is required for animals showing signs of cardiac tamponade. If the effusion recurs after two or three episodes of drainage, then pericardectomy is required. This is cura-tive for idiopathic effusion and palliative for neoplastic effusion. Long-term palliation is possible for animals with mesothelioma or chemodectoma. Some animals with idiopathic effusion may be managed by periodic peri-cardiocentesis and corticosteroid therapy.

Pericardial constriction

This is a rare condition, which is suspected to be a late complication of chronic pericarditis. Fibrosis of the parietal or visceral pericardium, or both, leads to a reduction in ventricular compliance and restricted ventricular filling. The signs are similar to pericardial effusion. Establishing a definitive diagnosis may be difficult and this condition should be sus-pected in animals with right-sided heart fail-ure, with no evidence of pericardial effusion, congenital or acquired heart disease or pul-monary hypertension. Parietal pericardectomy will relieve the clinical signs in most cases. However, where there is extensive epicardial fibrosis, the restriction to diastolic filling will only be relieved by epicardial decortication. This involves peeling the fibrous layer from the surface of the heart and is associated with increased morbidity and mortality.

Peritoneopericardial diaphragmatic hernia (PPDH)

This is the most common congenital disease of the pericardium. It is uncommon and is seen in cats and dogs. It results from a failure of development of the transverse septum and is often associated with other midline defects, such as sternal dysraphism and abdominal hernias, and congenital cardiac anomalies, such as ventricular septal defects. The presence of a communication between the abdominal cavity and the pericardial sac allows the abdominal contents to migrate cranially and impinge on the heart.

Animals may be asymptomatic or may exhibit varying degrees of dyspnoea and exercise intolerance, depending on the struc-tures present in the pericardial sac. Auscul-tation may reveal diminished heart sounds. Thoracic radiographs reveal gross cardio-megaly, with a sharply defined but globular border and gas-filled loops of intestine over-lying the cardiac shadow. Echocardiography or a barium series (Fig 6.12a) will differentiate this disorder from pericardial effusion.

Surgical repair is indicated for any animals showing signs of cardiopulmonary distress. The approach is via a cranial midline laparo-tomy, which may be extended into a caudal midline sternotomy if further access is required

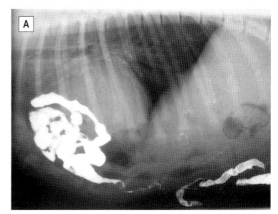

Figure 6.12 (a) Lateral thoracic radiograph following administration of liquid barium. Loops of small intestine can be seen in the pericardial sac and in an umbilical hernia.

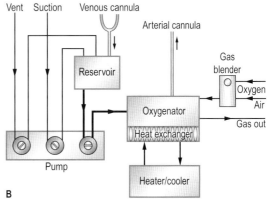

Figure 6.12 (b) Cardiopulmonary bypass circuit.

to relieve adhesions of abdominal organs. Unlike diaphragmatic rupture, the pleural space is not breached and the thoracic cavity remains closed to the atmosphere. Hence, positive pressure ventilation is not required. Repair is accomplished by closing the diaphragm and parietal pericardium with sutures. The presence of adhesions between the abdominal viscera and the pericardial sac is uncommon, but may necessitate resection of tissue, e.g. liver lobectomy.

Intrapericardial cysts

These are an uncommon finding in young dogs. The findings on physical examination, ECG analysis and radiography are similar to pericardial effusion and PPDH. Ultrasonography will delineate the presence of a unilocular or multilocular cystic structure within the pericardial sac. Surgical excision and subtotal pericardectomy via median sternotomy is curative. These cysts may derive from entrapment of omentum, falciform ligament or liver in the pericardial sac during development and may be seen in animals with PPDH.

Pericardial trauma

Pericardial trauma is not commonly identified, but may be more common than is diagnosed. Since the pericardium does not appear to be a vital structure, traumatic tears of the pericardium may cause no clinical signs. However, if the heart herniates out of the pericardium and the pericardium contracts around the heart base, obstruction of the venae cavae may occur. Obstruction of the caudal vena cava may result in ascites and hepatomegaly (Budd-Chiari syndrome) and obstruction of the cranial vena cava may result in swelling of the head and neck (caval syndrome).

DISEASES OF THE GREAT VESSELS

Patent ductus arteriosus

Patent ductus arteriosus (PDA) is a failure of the ductus arteriosus to close after birth, and results in left-to-right shunting of blood

through the ductus from the aorta to the pulmonary artery. The increased venous return to the left ventricle from the pulmonary circulation results in left ventricle volume overload. This may result in stretching of the mitral valve annulus with development of mitral regurgitation which worsens the volume overload. The increased pulmonary blood flow and pressure results in acquired pulmonary hypertension and pressure overload of the right ventricle. The development of pulmonary hypertension will increase the pressure of the pulmonary circulation, and may result in reversal of blood flow in the ductus, resulting in right-to-left shunting of blood. However, many dogs with a right-to-left shunt have had blood flowing this way since birth. Dogs with untreated PDA usually develop progressive left-sided heart failure and pulmonary oedema in the first year of life and die within a few years. Early surgical ligation of the ductus is recommended. Ligation of the ductus is contraindicated for right-to-left shunting PDA.

Most cases are diagnosed on physical examination at the time of first vaccination. Those that are not will present with a history of lethargy, exercise intolerance and poor growth. On auscultation, a characteristic continuous systolic-diastolic machinery-type murmur is audible over the left third intercostal space and a bounding pulse with a rapid fall-off (waterhammer pulse) may be palpated. In cases in which there has been time for the changes to develop, thoracic radiographs may reveal:

- biventricular enlargement
- enlargement of the aortic root, pulmonary artery and left auricular appendage (bulges seen at 1, 2 and 3 o'clock on a dorsoventral projection)
- pulmonary hypervascular pattern.

Surgical technique
The ductus arteriosus is approached via a left fourth intercostal thoracotomy. The cranial and caudal parts of the left cranial lung lobe are reflected and retained with a saline-soaked

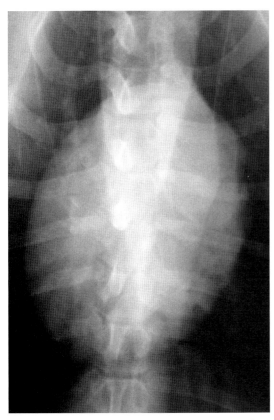

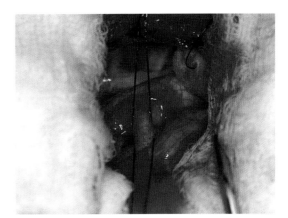

Figure 6.14   Isolation and ligation of a patent ductus arteriosus.

Figure 6.13   Dorsoventral radiograph in a dog with patent ductus arteriosus. Bulges in the cardiac silhouette at 1 o'clock (aorta), 2 o'clock (pulmonary artery) and 3 o'clock (left atrium) are visible.

swab. The ductus may be seen as a bulge between the aorta dorsally and the pulmonary artery ventrally and palpated as the site of fremitus during systole and diastole.

The ductus is approached by opening the pericardium immediately ventral to the vagus nerve and dorsal to the phrenic nerve and reflecting the vagus nerve dorsally, or by opening the pleura adjacent to the ductus and reflecting the vagus nerve ventrally. Ligation of the ductus (Fig 6.14) is then performed, with 3 metric silk, using the direct or indirect technique. The ductus is ligated twice, once on the aortic side and once on the pulmonary artery side. It may also be transfixed with 1–2 metric polypropylene between these ligatures.

For direct ligation, the fascia between the aorta and pulmonary artery is bluntly dis-

sected proximal and distal to the ductus. Care is taken to avoid the recurrent laryngeal nerve as it passes around the caudal aspect of the ductus. Right-angled forceps are passed around the ductus from distal to proximal. This manoeuvre is undertaken with great care to avoid rupture of the pulmonary artery or medial wall of the ductus. A loop of silk is then placed in the jaws of the forceps and the forceps withdrawn. The suture loop is divided, leaving two strands passing round the ductus. The aortic (high pressure side) is ligated first followed by the pulmonary side. Closure of this shunt will direct more of the left ventricular output into the systemic circulation and increase systemic blood pressure. Vagally-mediated reflex bradycardia (Branham's sign) may be seen and may be severe enough to result in asystole. An anticholinergic drug, such as atropine, should be available at the time of closure.

For indirect ligation (Jackson/Henderson technique), the mediastinum dorsal to the descending aorta is incised and further blunt dissection medial to the aorta is performed. This continues until the aorta is completely mobilised on its medial aspect, from the left subclavian artery cranially to a region caudal to the ductus caudally – often to the first intercostal arteries. Forceps are passed around the aorta cranial to the ductus in a ventral to dorsal direction. A loop of silk is placed in the jaws of the forceps and passed around the medial wall of the aorta. This manoeuvre is repeated around the aorta caudal to the ductus and the two ends of the silk ligature passed around this part of the aorta. Dividing the loop of silk results in two ligatures which pass around the ductus. The two sutures are positioned and tied as above.

Indirect ligation avoids dissection of the friable medial wall of the ductus and the pulmonary artery. However, the procedure takes longer, there is a risk of iatrogenic damage to the thoracic duct, which lies medial to the aorta, and the incorporation of mediastinal connective tissue in the ligature may lead to incomplete closure of the ductus.

If the ductus is very wide and/or very short, or if iatrogenic trauma has resulted in a tear, then the ductus must be divided and over-sewn with a double layer of 1 metric polypropylene. This is a technically difficult procedure and requires vascular occlusion clamps. In the event of rupture of the ductus, pressure is immediately placed over the site of haemorrhage and the blood removed with suction. The aorta is cross-clamped cranial to the ductus but caudal to the brachycephalic and left subclavian arteries, which reduces normograde haemorrhage but still allows perfusion of the head and heart. A second vascular occlusion clamp is placed across the aorta caudal to the ductus to prevent retrograde aortic haemorrhage. Bleeding will only now be coming from the low pressure pulmonary artery, which is controlled with digital pressure until the ductus is divided and ligated. The tear in the pulmonary artery or ductus is then repaired and the occlusion clamps removed.

The success rate is greater than 95% in experienced hands. Approximately 1.5–2% of ligated PDAs will recanalise, necessitating division and ligation.

Vascular ring anomalies

These are congenital malformations of the great vessels and associated structures which may lead to extramural compression of the thoracic oesophagus. The aorta, ligamentum arteriosum, and left subclavian artery all derive from left aortic arches. These disorders are caused by abnormal development of one or more, but not all, of these structures from the right aortic arches. A number of anomalies are reported:

- persistent right aortic arch and left ligamentum arteriosum
- persistent right aortic arch and aberrant left subclavian artery
- double aortic arch
- left aortic arch and persistent right ligamentum arteriosum
- left aortic arch and aberrant right subclavian artery.

Clinical findings are referable to extramural compression of the thoracic oesophagus and consist of regurgitation with a ravenous appetite and poor growth. Bulging of the dilated cervical oesophagus may be seen. Concurrent aspiration pneumonia will result in respiratory distress and signs of airway obstruction will be present if the trachea is compressed by a double aortic arch. Signs of cardiac disease are generally absent, unless a patent ductus arteriosus is present.

Radiographs (Fig 6.15) may reveal dilation of the thoracic oesophagus cranial to the heart and deviation of the trachea to the left.

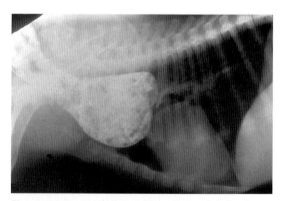

Figure 6.15   Lateral thoracic radiograph following a barium meal. Gross dilation of the oesophagus proximal to the heart base suggests a vascular ring anomaly.

Angiocardiography will allow the precise anatomic abnormality to be identified prior to surgery.

The earlier surgical correction is performed, the better the prognosis for return of normal oesophageal function. Many of these patients are small and underweight and anaesthesia is associated with greater risk because of this. Placement of a gastrostomy tube at the time of surgery may be considered if postoperative oral feeding is likely to be compromised by regurgitation. The surgery should be delayed until concurrent aspiration pneumonia is treated and nutritional support established by feeding liquid diets or placement of a gastrostomy tube.

It is unusual for the oesophagus to return to normal function postoperatively and persistent dilation of the cranial thoracic oesophagus is likely. Severe dilation of the cranial thoracic oesophagus is a poor prognostic sign. Continued dietary management, such as the feeding of a food of appropriate consistency, from a height, may be necessary. Some animals have a good clinical outcome in spite of the presence of radiographic evidence of mega-oesophagus.

Persistent right aortic arch (PRAA)

A left fourth intercostal thoracotomy is performed and the left cranial lung lobe reflected caudally with a moist swab. Additional anomalous vessels may be present, such as a persistent left cranial vena cava and a right hemiazygos vein. The latter vein often runs directly over the surgical field and may be ligated and divided. The former vein may be divided if a normal right-sided cranial vena cava exists. In PRAA, the ligamentum arteriosum is located as a fibrous ring between the proximal descending aorta and the pulmonary artery just cranial to the recurrent laryngeal nerve at the level of the oesophageal stricture. This ligament is dissected from the wall of the oesophagus, ligated and divided. Occasionally, the ligamentum arteriosum is patent and for this reason it is important to ligate this structure close to the aorta and close to the pulmonary artery.

The oesophagus is then dissected free from the aorta and pulmonary artery and any remaining constricting fibrous bands are freed from the oesophagus. A large bore stomach tube or oesophageal probe is passed across the site of stricture to ensure that all the fibrous bands have been removed and that no stricture remains.

Anomalous retro–oesophageal left or right subclavian artery

The anomalous vessel is elevated from the oesophagus, ligated and divided (Fig 6.16). There is sufficient collateral circulation to compensate for ligation.

Double aortic arch

This anomaly is rare. Surgery is technically difficult and involves ligation and division of the smaller of the two arches at its distal end, proximal to its junction with the other aortic arch. The ligamentum arteriosum is also ligated and divided.

DISEASES OF THE HEART

Pulmonic stenosis

This is obstruction of blood flow from the right ventricle to the pulmonary artery (Fig 6.17), and may occur at the valvular, subvalvular,

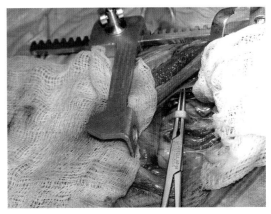

Figure 6.16 Isolation and division of a retro-oesophageal subclavian artery causing oesophageal compression.

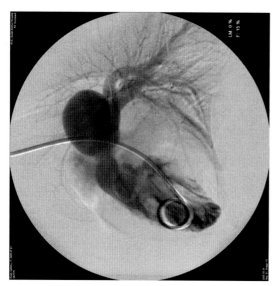

Figure 6.17 Selective right ventricular angiogram showing pulmonic stenosis and poststenotic dilation.

infundibular or supravalvular location. Valvular stenosis is the most common and results from thickening or fusion of the valve leaflets, with or without stenosis of the valve annulus. Subvalvular stenosis is caused by a fibrous membrane just proximal to the pulmonic valve, and differentiation from valvular stenosis may be difficult. Supravalvular stenosis is rare and presents as a stricture of the main pulmonary artery. Infundibular muscular hypertrophy of the right ventricular outflow tract is generally caused by concentric muscle hypertrophy of the right ventricle, often secondary to pulmonic valvular stenosis.

The severity of the lesion is quantified by measuring pressure gradients from the right ventricle to the pulmonary artery, either indirectly using Doppler ultrasound or directly during cardiac catheterisation. These gradients are classified as mild (<50mmHg), moderate (50–100mmHg) or severe (>100mmHg). Dogs with mild to moderate stenosis are asymptomatic, whereas dogs with severe stenosis show exercise intolerance, syncope, progressive right heart failure or sudden death. Echocardiography will confirm the diagnosis.

Surgical correction is indicated for moderate and severe stenosis, with a pressure gradient of >50mmHg and significant right ventricular hypertrophy. Several options are available:

- balloon valvuloplasty
- transventricular dilation valvuloplasty
- pulmonary valvotomy via inflow occlusion
- patch graft.

Balloon valvuloplasty

This is the simplest and safest technique for the initial treatment of pulmonic stenosis. It is most effective for treatment of valvular stenosis caused by fusion of the valve leaflet commissures. It is less effective for cases with marked muscular infundibular stenosis.

Transventricular dilation valvuloplasty

A pledgeted mattress suture is placed in the right ventricular outflow tract. A stab incision is made through the ventricle and a surgical valve dilator is introduced into the right ventricular outflow tract and across the pulmonic valve. The valve is dilated several times. The dilator is removed and the ventriculotomy incision closed with the mattress suture.

Pulmonary valvotomy

An incision is made in the pulmonary artery and right ventricular outflow tract and the valve is inspected. Fused valve leaflets may be incised or thickened leaflets may be excised. This procedure offers little advantage over balloon valvuloplasty in animals with valvular stenosis and is not likely to be sufficient in animals with infundibular hypertrophy or annular hypoplasia. One indication is in English bulldogs with anomalous left coronary artery, in which balloon valvuloplasty and patch graft valvuloplasty are contraindicated.

Patch graft

This technique (Fig 6.18) is used to treat all animals with severe stenosis caused by valvular dysplasia or hypertrophy of the outflow tract, or animals who have failed to respond to balloon valvuloplasty. This procedure opens

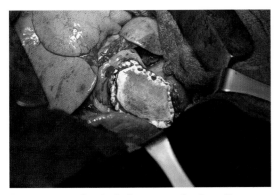

Figure 6.18 Surgical placement of a Gore-Tex patch graft for pulmonic stenosis.

up the obstructed portion of the right ventricular outflow tract and effectively turns the stenosis into an incompetence. The pulmonic valve is approached via a left fourth or fifth intercostal thoracotomy. The graft is either autogenous pericardium or a synthetic material, such as polytetrafluoroethylene (PTFE). A large rectangle of pericardium is harvested and cleaned of pericardial fat, taking care not to puncture it in the process. The coronary vasculature should be assessed carefully. In rare cases, an anomalous left coronary artery passes across the right ventricular outflow tract, prohibiting this surgical technique.

The procedure may be performed via venous inflow occlusion or cardiopulmonary bypass. An incision is made in the right ventricular outflow tract over the pulmonic valve and an incision is made in the valve (valvotomy) or a portion of the valve may be excised. If performed via venous inflow occlusion, the patch is sutured over the right ventricular outflow tract and then an incision is made through the patch and through the ventricular wall. Once the valve has been inspected and incision or excision performed, the incision in the patch is closed temporarily with a vascular clamp and the circulation is re-established. The incision in the patch is then repaired.

Aortic stenosis

Obstruction of blood flow from the left ventricle to the aorta may occur at the valvular, subvalvular or supravalvular levels. The subvalvular form is the most common in the dog and accounts for more than 90% of cases. Subvalvular stenosis can be subdivided into fixed and dynamic forms. The severity of the lesion is quantified by measuring pressure gradients across the region of stenosis. Clinical findings range from asymptomatic to exercise intolerance, collapse and syncope. Sudden death may be the first indication of stenosis in some animals.

Surgical intervention should be considered for animals with a systolic gradient of >75mmHg and substantial ventricular hypertrophy. However, the long-term improvement in survival is not as clear as it is for pulmonic stenosis. Surgical intervention includes:

- balloon valvuloplasty
- closed transventricular dilation
- open surgical dilation.

Balloon valvuloplasty
Balloon valvuloplasty is performed after catheterisation of one of the carotid arteries and requires image intensification.

Closed transventricular dilation
Transventricular dilation of the aortic valve may be accomplished via a median sternotomy or a left fifth intercostal thoracotomy. A valve dilator is introduced into the left ventricle through a stab incision, positioned across the stenosis and opened to dilate the subvalvular ring or split the fused commissures of the valve leaflets. There is little evidence that this procedure results in a long-term reduction in the systolic pressure gradient.

Open surgical dilation
Open membranectomy with or without septal myectomy is performed via cardiopulmonary bypass. Although this procedure will result in a sustained reduction in the systolic pressure

gradient and improved exercise tolerance, there is little evidence that it improves long-term survival.

Ventricular septal defect

Ventricular septal defect (VSD) is an important congenital defect in dogs and cats. It typically causes a left-to-right shunt, resulting in volume overload of the left side of the heart and, depending on its size and location, the right side as well. Chronic pulmonary over-circulation may lead to pulmonary hypertension and reversal of the direction of the shunt. Small defects are generally associated with a high-velocity shunt which is haemodynamically insignificant. Large defects are associated with lower shunt velocities and clinical signs of heart failure or pulmonary hypertension. Surgical therapy for this abnormality consists of palliation by pulmonary artery banding, or closure of the defect during an open heart procedure.

Pulmonary artery banding is achieved via a left fourth intercostal approach. The pericardium is incised and a plane of dissection between the aorta and pulmonary artery is created. Right-angled forceps are passed between the aorta and pulmonary artery, umbilical tape is grasped in the jaws and the forceps withdrawn. The forceps are then placed caudal to the pulmonary artery to grasp the other end of the tape. This results in a loop of umbilical tape around the pulmonary artery. The band is then tightened with the aim of increasing the pressure in the pulmonary artery to approximately half that of the systemic pressure, so that a balance is achieved between pulmonary and aortic blood flow.

Open repair consists of closure of the defect with a PTFE graft sutured over the defect during cardiopulmonary bypass.

Atrial septal defect

Atrial septal defect (ASD) is an uncommon defect which results in a left-to-right shunt and volume overload of the right ventricle. Bidirectional or right-to-left shunting may occur with large defects, or if right atrial pressure is increased by congestive heart failure, pulmonary hypertension or concurrent pulmonary stenosis. A small defect may be asymptomatic. A large defect will result in congestive right-sided heart failure.

Surgical repair is indicated for large haemodynamically significant ASD. This requires direct closure of the ASD or an autogenous pericardial patch graft via a right atriotomy approach under cardiopulmonary bypass. Palliation by pulmonary artery banding is not recommended because of the risk of reversing the shunt.

Atrioventricular valve disease

Atrioventricular valve disease and regurgitation is well recognised in the dog and is generally managed medically. It may be congenital (e.g. dysplasia) or acquired (e.g. endocardiosis). With the advent of cardiopulmonary bypass techniques, surgical therapy is a possibility. Therapeutic options include:

- valvuloplasty, to reconstruct a damaged valve
- annuloplasty, to narrow the valve ring and allow the cusps to meet
- prosthetic valve replacement.

Tetralogy of Fallot

This is a combination of congenital abnormalities, comprising:

- pulmonary outflow tract obstruction
- ventricular septal defect
- overriding of the aorta
- right ventricular hypertrophy.

This can be simplified into two haemodynamically significant defects – pulmonic stenosis (with resulting right ventricular hypertrophy) and the VSD (with overriding aorta as a consequence). The pathophysiological changes seen depend on the magnitude of these defects. In animals with a large VSD but insignificant pulmonic stenosis, the result is a left-to-right shunt and volume overload of the left heart, similar to an isolated VSD. In animals with severe pulmonic stenosis, a right-to-left shunt through the VSD exists. In some animals, both these defects are significant, similar to a VSD following pulmonary artery banding.

Animals with a left-to-right shunt are not cyanotic and may cope if the shunt volume is not sufficiently large to cause left heart failure. Animals with a right-to-left shunt are cyanotic and exhibit exercise intolerance and syncope. Progression of the pulmonic stenosis may result in reversal of the shunt from left-to-right to right-to-left.

Asymptomatic acyanotic animals do not need surgical intervention, but should be monitored closely. Surgical intervention is indicated for symptomatic animals and involves definitive repair or a palliative procedure. Surgical repair requires cardiopulmonary bypass and involves:

- closure of the VSD
- resection of excessive infundibular muscle in the right ventricular outflow tract
- enlargement of the pulmonary valve annulus by arteriotomy/ventriculotomy and patch-grafting.

Palliative surgical procedures attempt to increase pulmonary blood flow. Isolated correction of the pulmonic stenosis may be performed as described above. However, over-correction will result in a massive left-to-right shunt, and therefore the more conservative procedure of balloon dilation is preferred over patch grafting. The Blalock Taussig procedure involves creating a left-to-right vascular shunt between a systemic artery (the left subclavian) and the pulmonary artery by direct anastomosis. A modified procedure uses a PTFE graft between these two vessels.

Cor triatrium

This is subdivision of the atrium into two chambers by an anomalous embryonic membrane, such as persistence of the right sinus venosus valve. This may occur in the right (dexter) or left (sinister) atrium. Surgical therapy entails splitting or cutting the membrane via a right atriotomy under inflow occlusion.

Cardiac neoplasia

Heart base tumours

These tumours arise from the region of the ascending aorta and the most common type is the chemodectoma. These tumours are locally invasive, but do not tend to metastasise. The heart base is approached via a left or right fourth intercostal thoracotomy. Non-invasive tumours may be carefully dissected off the aorta, but most tumours are invasive or large tumours and are not candidates for surgical removal. Pericardectomy may be performed as a palliative procedure. The median survival time following pericardectomy is approximately 2 years, but this falls to 1–2 months if a pericardectomy is not performed.

Haemangiosarcoma

In the heart this tumour usually involves the right atrium or right atrial appendage. The tumour causes cardiac tamponade from pericardial effusion. Surgical excision of the mass may be performed via a right lateral thoracotomy or a median sternotomy, and should be combined with a pericardectomy. Surgical excision of the mass alone is associated with a relatively short median survival time of approximately 2–4 months. The addition of chemotherapy, e.g. a doxorubicin-based protocol, may increase this to 5–6 months. However, metastasis is the inevitable long-term result. Unlike heart base tumours, pericardectomy without excision of the primary mass does not prolong survival.

Other tumours

Other primary tumours such as fibrosarcoma, chondrosarcoma, rhabdomyosarcoma, fibroma, myxoma and ectopic thyroid carcinoma have been described in dogs. In cats, lymphoma and metastatic neoplasia are the most common.

Chapter 7

ENT surgery

Stephen J Baines

THE EAR

The ear (Fig 7.1) is composed of the pinna, the external ear canal, the middle ear and the inner ear.

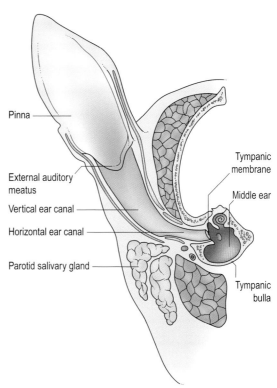

Figure 7.1   Anatomy of the pinna, external ear canal, middle ear and inner ear.

Pinna

Anatomy

The pinna is a cartilaginous sheet which extends dorsally from the external auditory meatus. Its lateral surface is concave and hairless.

Diseases of the pinna

Aural haematoma This is the most common physical injury of the pinna (Fig 7.2). It is usually self-inflicted by scratching and head-shaking, secondary to otitis externa. However, the presence of haematomas in some patients with no appreciable signs of otitis has lead to the suggestion that this condition may arise as a result of increased capillary fragility, e.g. associated with Cushing's syndrome, or may have an autoimmune basis.

The haematoma is a fluctuant, fluid-filled swelling on the concave surface of the pinna, which may involve the entire pinna or only a portion. The haematoma originates from branches of the great auricular artery within the auricular cartilage, rather than between the skin and cartilage. In time, the lesion undergoes fibrosis and may result in a scarred, shrunken 'cauliflower ear'. Therapeutic objectives are:

1. Identify and treat the underlying cause
2. Remove the haematoma
3. Maintain normal tissue apposition

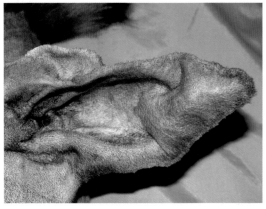

Figure 7.2 Aural haematoma.

4. Prevent recurrence
5. Maintain the normal appearance and function of the pinna.

Treatment
- *Needle aspiration.* A large gauge needle is inserted into the haematoma and the contents aspirated. The cavity may be instilled with a corticosteroid preparation. The aim is to reduce the inflammation, but this therapy may retard healing and prevents normal anatomic alignment of the tissues. Nevertheless, this therapy may be highly effective in early cases which are completely evacuated.
- *Incision and sutures.* A linear or curved incision is made on the concave aspect of the pinna and the haematoma evacuated. Longitudinal contracture is less likely to cause deformity with a curved S-shaped incision. The haematoma cavity is curetted and lavaged. Parallel, staggered rows of sutures are then placed to obliterate the haematoma cavity. These may be full-thickness through the entire pinna, or may pass from the concave surface, through the cartilage, without penetrating the skin on the convex aspect. These sutures should be placed parallel to the edges of the pinna to avoid incorporating the great auricular vessels. The augmentation of the sutures with a stent of radiographic film or individual buttons placed on one aspect of the pinna is generally not required.
- *Drain implantation.* In cases where there is little fibrin, a Penrose drain or teat cannula may be placed through stab incisions into the haematoma cavity.

Wounds of the pinna Traumatic lacerations of the pinna may be superficial, involving the skin on only one side of the ear; deep, involving one skin surface and the cartilage; or may perforate the entire pinna and involve both ear surfaces. Occasionally, a portion of the pinna may be avulsed. Depending on the severity, some wounds may be left to heal by second intention while others have a more cosmetic appearance and better function if sutures are placed. Second intention healing proceeds best if the underlying rigid cartilage template is intact.

Skin wound A simple linear laceration involving one skin surface may be left to heal by second intention or may be sutured. In general, suturing will result in an improved cosmetic appearance. The laceration should be cleaned and the edges debrided. The skin margins are apposed with simple interrupted sutures. Suturing is mandatory if a two- or three-sided flap is formed to prevent contracture and poor epithelialisation. Sutures should be placed to obliterate any dead space between the cartilage and skin.

Skin and cartilage wound The skin and cartilage should be sutured. Simple interrupted sutures in the skin may be sufficient if the wound is small. However, if the cartilage laceration is long, the edges of the cartilage should be approximated to avoid losing support. This may be achieved with a vertical mattress suture. The superficial portion of the suture approximates the skin and the deeper bite apposes the cartilage.

Full-thickness wound Full-thickness lacerations should be sutured, particularly those involving an ear margin. This may be achieved by placing simple interrupted sutures between the skin edges on either side of the ear or the skin and cartilage may be approximated with vertical mattress sutures on one side of the pinna.

Avulsions Small avulsions of the ear margin are treated by resection of surrounding tissue to achieve a normal contour. The skin edges are then apposed as before. Larger avulsions are repaired using a distant direct flap from adjacent tissue. This requires raising a flap from the skin of the head and neck adjacent to the pinna. The margin of the pinna is then sutured to the donor site and immobilised for approximately 2 weeks. The flap may then be removed from the donor bed and sutured to the remainder of the recipient bed.

Neoplasia of the pinna Any tumour which affects the skin may also affect the pinna. The most frequent tumour is squamous cell carcinoma (Fig 7.3), which commonly affects older cats – particularly white cats. Although these

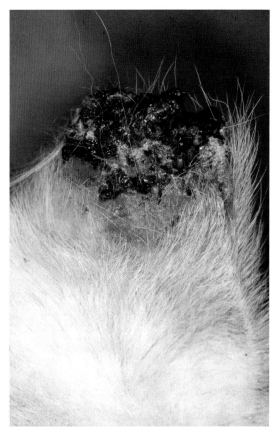

Figure 7.3 Squamous cell carcinoma of the pinna.

tumours are invasive, metastasis is uncommon. Similar lesions may also be present on the external nares and eyelids. Other tumours of the pinna in dogs and cats include fibrosarcoma, fibroma, basal cell tumour, melanoma, lymphoma, histiocytoma, papilloma and mast cell tumour. Tumours of the pinna may be removed by local excision or via a partial or total pinnectomy. Although this may result in a change in the cosmetic appearance, the functional result is good.

External ear canal

Anatomy

The external ear canal is a funnel-shaped cartilaginous tube which extends from the external auditory meatus to the tympanic membrane. It comprises a vertical canal and a horizontal canal. The terminal portion of the horizontal canal is formed by a bony projection of the petrous temporal bone.

Diseases of the external ear canal

Otitis externa   Otitis is defined as inflammation of the external ear canal (Fig 7.4) and is a common problem in small animals. The causes of otitis externa are numerous and in many cases more than one cause is present. The causes of otitis (Table 7.1) may be divided into predisposing factors, primary causes and perpetuating factors:

- Predisposing factors alone may not cause otitis externa, but increase the risk and act in conjunction with primary causes and perpetuating factors. It is vital that these factors are identified and dealt with during management of the otitis. For instance, the patient with a polyp in the external ear canal will continue to develop otitis externa until that lesion is removed.
- Primary factors are the inciting agents or diseases that directly result in otitis. These factors can induce otitis without predisposing or perpetuating factors. A thorough search must be made for the primary cause if therapy is to be successful. For instance, if the underlying cause is atopy and this is not recognised, then recurrent dermatitis and otitis is likely.

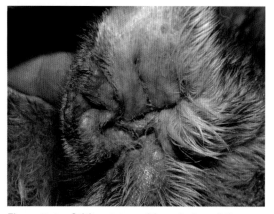

Figure 7.4   Otitis externa with occlusion of the external auditory meatus.

- Perpetuating factors prevent the resolution of otitis, even following what appears to be appropriate therapy. In early cases, treatment of the primary cause may be sufficient. In chronic cases, care must be taken to identify perpetuating factors and to include them in the treatment plan. For instance, treatment of otitis externa alone when otitis media is present will not resolve the condition.

The clinical signs of pruritus, headshaking and erythema are easily recognised. As the disease progresses, pain and aural discharge are noted and, with time, the external ear canal may become attenuated with granulation tissue and hyperplasia of the integument. Fibrosis and eventual calcification of the ear canal and ulceration of the integument may be present. Infection within the ear canal may erode through the wall of the canal to form a para-aural abscess or fistula. Neurological signs such as facial nerve paralysis, Horner's syndrome and vestibular signs may be found with severe disease.

Diagnosis of otitis externa is relatively simple; identifying the predisposing factors, primary cause and perpetuating factors is more difficult. Definitive diagnosis requires a thorough otoscopic examination, which will usually require sedation or general anaesthesia. Cytological examination of the aural exudate may be performed. Culture of the aural discharge is often performed, but is not always useful. Bacteria are often present but are considered perpetuating factors rather than a primary cause. Therapy will involve antibiotic therapy, but elimination of bacteria is not the end point of therapy. A thorough dermatological examination should be carried out to investigate the presence of an underlying dermatological disease.

Radiography is of limited use. Radiographs may reveal stenosis of the external ear canals and calcification of the cartilage. The tympanic bulla may have a soft-tissue opacity, indicating the presence of fluid or soft tissue. Bony proliferation or erosion of the bulla may be present later in otitis or if a tumour is present.

Table 7.1   Causes of otitis

Predisposing causes	Primary causes	Perpetuating factors
Conformation: – stenotic canals – hair in external canal – pendulous pinna – hairy concave pinna	Parasites: – *Otodectes cynotis* – Demodecosis – Sarcoptic mange – Ticks	Bacterial infection: – *Staphylococcus intermedius* – Proteus spp. – Pseudomonas spp. – *E. coli* – Klebsiella spp.
Excessive moisture: – humid climate – frequent swimming	Micro-organisms: – Dermatophytosis – bacteria (normally a perpetuating factor)	Yeast: – *Malassezia canis* – *Candida albicans*

Effects of treatment:
– trauma from cleaning
– irritation from topical
  medication
– superinfections (change
  in normal flora)
	Hypersensitivity:
	– atopy
	– food allergy
	– contact dermatitis
	– drug reactions
		Otitis media

Obstruction of the ear canal: – polyps – tumours – traumatic stenosis or scarring	Keratinisation disorder: – primary idiopathic seborrhoea – hypothyroidism – sex hormone imbalance – lipid-related	Progressive changes: – hyperkeratosis – acanthosis – oedema – apocrine gland Hyperplasia/hypertrophy – hidradenitis – fibrosis – calcification
Systemic disease: – pyrexia – immune suppression – debilitation – catabolic states	Foreign bodies: – grass seeds – hair	
	Glandular disorders: – ceruminous hyperplasia – altered secretion rate Autoimmune disease: – systemic lupus erythematosus – pemphigus foliaceous – pemphigus erythematosus Viral infection	

However, the changes seen in the external canal may all be appreciated clinically – apart from documenting bony lysis or proliferation radiographs are insensitive in identifying the presence of otitis media.

Cleaning the external ear canal   The first step in the diagnosis and management of otitis externa is careful examination of the external ear canal and tympanic membrane. If samples for cytology and culture are required, these should be collected first. A ceruminolytic agent may be instilled into the ear canal several hours before examination to soften and loosen the wax, debris and exudate. The ear canal is then lavaged under gentle pressure with sterile saline using a soft catheter and syringe. Residual debris and foreign bodies are then removed with alligator forceps. Neoplastic lesions may be examined and biopsy taken with small biopsy forceps. The external ear canal and tympanic membrane may then be examined with a hand-held otoscope or a small diameter rigid endoscope.

Medical therapy is aimed at treating the primary causes along with a consideration of, and therapy for, any predisposing or perpetuating factors. Surgical therapy is indicated when persistent or recurrent otitis fails to respond to medical therapy, when anatomic deformities exist, such as canal stenosis, and when obstructive lesions are present, such as tumours.

Tumours of the external ear canal Tumours of the external ear canal are relatively uncommon, and occur more frequently in cats. The most common tumours arise from the ceruminous glands (adenomas or adenocarcinomas). Other tumours found include squamous cell carcinoma, basal cell carcinoma and mast cell tumours. Benign tumours such as inflammatory polyps and papillomas are occasionally found. However, almost every type of cutaneous tumour has been reported at some time in the external ear canal.

Inflammation may be observed secondary to tumour growth, and chronic otitis externa may be a predisposing factor for the development of tumours. Clinical signs reflect the presence of a mass lesion and resulting otitis externa. Involvement of the middle ear and inner ear occurs in a proportion of cases and may be associated with neurological signs. Tumours of the ear canal are generally invasive, but with a relatively low potential for metastasis. Approximately 10% of animals will have regional lymph node or thoracic metastasis at presentation. Radiographs of the tympanic bulla may reveal a soft-tissue opacity in the bulla and bony proliferation or lysis. Diagnosis is by otoscopy and biopsy.

Most benign tumours can be readily managed with conservative surgical resection. For malignant tumours, aggressive excision, consisting of a vertical canal ablation, or more commonly, a total ear canal ablation (TECA), is indicated.

Malignant ear tumours are less aggressive in dogs than in cats. A fair to good prognosis is achieved in the dog, with the cat warranting a fair prognosis for ceruminous gland adenocarcinoma and a poor prognosis for squamous cell carcinoma or undifferentiated carcinoma. The median survival time following surgical management of all malignant ear tumour in dogs is more than 2 years compared with 1 year in the cat. However, ceruminous gland adenocarcinoma in the cat is associated with a median disease-free interval of 42 months following TECA and lateral bulla osteotomy (LBO). The presence of neurological signs, a diagnosis of carcinoma, and conservative rather than radical surgery are negative prognostic indicators. Radiotherapy is a possible adjunctive therapy for surgery. There is no objective information on the usefulness of chemotherapy.

Surgical management of otitis externa and otitis media

Surgery is indicated to:

- improve drainage and ventilation of the external ear canal.
- remove chronically diseased tissue
- gain access to the external ear canal or tympanic bulla.

Lateral wall resection Lateral wall resection (LWR) increases drainage and improves ventilation of the ear canal (Fig 7.5). It also facilitates placement of topical medications in the external ear canal. It is indicated:

- for patients with otitis externa where there is minimal hyperplasia of the epithelium of the external auditory meatus
- for removal of small mass lesions of the lateral aspect of the vertical canal
- to gain access to the lower portions of the canal.

It should not be performed on patients with obstruction or stenosis of the horizontal canal, concurrent otitis media or severe epithelial

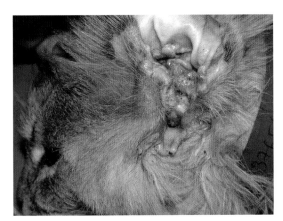

Figure 7.5 Lateral wall resection showing ventral drainage board.

hyperplasia. Dogs with an underlying disease, e.g. hypothyroidism, or primary seborrhoea, may respond poorly. This procedure is not curative, and long-term medical management of the underlying otitis externa may be required.

Surgery The patient is placed in lateral recumbency and two parallel incisions are made over the vertical canal, from the ventral aspect of the opening of the external ear canal. These extend for one and a half times the depth of the vertical canal. The incisions are joined ventrally and the skin flap thus created is dissected free of the underlying tissue and reflected dorsally.

The exposed vertical canal is dissected free of the overlying muscle tissue and the parotid gland is reflected ventrally. Two parallel incisions are made in the vertical canal and the cartilage flap is reflected ventrally. The majority of the cartilage is resected, leaving the distal one-third. This is sutured to the skin edges below the opening to the horizontal canal to act as a drainage board to prevent the skin from becoming excoriated. The skin edges are then apposed to the remaining vertical canal to close the wound.

Complications Wound contamination is difficult to avoid and some degree of minor wound swelling, exudation or dehiscence is not uncommon, but rarely requires any further attention. Despite its widespread use, it is apparent that this technique does not provide

a solution to all cases of chronic ear disease. The reasons for failure of LWR include:

- poor surgical technique e.g. failure to drain the horizontal canal properly
- poor patient selection, i.e. chronic irreversible changes in the remaining ear canal
- failure to control the underlying ear disease
- unremitting otitis media.

Vertical canal ablation Vertical canal ablation (VCA) is indicated in the management of cases of otitis externa in patients where the disease is confined to the vertical canal and who have a normal horizontal canal. In fact, this is an uncommon situation, and most patients will have chronic changes throughout the external ear canal and a total ear canal ablation is a more suitable alternative. Neoplasia or trauma to the vertical canal may be amenable to management with this technique. Since the tympanic membrane and bulla are left intact, VCA will interfere less with hearing postoperatively than total ear canal ablation.

Surgical technique A vertical incision is made over the vertical canal, extending to below the junction of the horizontal and vertical canal as for the LWR. A circular incision is made around the opening to the external auditory meatus and the entire vertical canal is dissected free of surrounding tissue. The vertical canal is transected 1–2cm dorsal to the horizontal canal and two parallel incisions are made in the cranial and caudal aspects of the remaining vertical canal. These flaps are reflected dorsally and ventrally to create a dorsal and ventral drainage board as described for the LWR, and are sutured to the skin. The dead space is obliterated and the wound closed.

Alternatively, this technique may be performed using a pull-through technique. A circular incision is made around the opening to the external auditory meatus and an incision is made at the junction of the horizontal and vertical canals. The vertical canal is then dissected free of surrounding tissue and pulled through the lower incision. This technique is technically more demanding and, apart from a claim for improved cosmesis, there is little to recommend it.

Total ear canal ablation/lateral bulla osteotomy This is indicated in:

- chronic proliferative changes in the ear canal beyond the vertical canal
- complete ear canal stenosis
- continuing otitis externa following LWR or VCA
- unremitting middle ear disease
- neoplastic disease of the ear canal or tympanic bulla.
- severe trauma to the external ear canal
- para-aural abscessation.

Many animals requiring this surgery will have undergone prolonged treatment previously and many will have had unsuccessful surgical intervention.

Surgical technique A circular incision is made around the opening of the external ear canal and a vertical incision is made over the vertical canal. The entire ear canal is dissected free of surrounding tissue to the level of the osseous external auditory prominence (OEAP) at the lateral aspect of the tympanic bulla (Fig 7.6). The external ear canal is amputated at the level of the OEAP, taking care to avoid the facial nerve, which exits the skull via the stylomastoid foramen, caudoventral to the OEAP.

The integument which lines the OEAP and tympanic bulla is removed with a curette. In the vast majority of animals, this requires a lateral bulla osteotomy. Rongeurs are used to remove the lateral aspect of the tympanic bulla, ventral to the OEAP. The tympanic cavity is irrigated and curettage proceeds until there is no integument or debris in the middle ear. The soft tissues are closed over the bulla, taking care to obliterate the dead space. A Penrose drain may be placed, extending from the bulla to exit ventral to the skin wound. The skin is closed in a T or inverted L shape.

Complications These include:

- facial nerve injury – this may be temporary, due to stretching (neuropraxia) or permanent, due to transection (paralysis)
- wound dehiscence and infection
- haemorrhage from the retroglenoid vein
- vestibular signs (inner ear disease)
- hypoglossal nerve dysfunction
- chronic sinus tracts and para-aural abscessation
- deafness.

The prognosis is good if a meticulous surgical technique is employed with long-term success rates of 90–95% reported. However, the complication rate may be high with poor surgical technique or if integument is left behind in the middle ear.

Middle ear

Anatomy

The middle ear consists of the tympanic membrane, the tympanic bulla, the Eustachian tube leading to the pharynx, and the three auditory ossicles (malleus, incus and stapes). The tympanic bulla is an air-filled cavity interposed between the external ear canal and the inner ear. Two nerves of clinical significance pass through the middle ear. A branch of the facial nerve (chorda tympani) leaves the brainstem, travels in the facial canal of the petrous temporal bone and enters the middle ear cavity. The sympathetic nerve leaves the cranial cervical ganglion behind the tympanic bulla and enters the middle ear cavity.

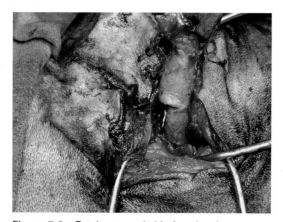

Figure 7.6 Total ear canal ablation showing mobilisation of the external ear canal.

Diseases of the middle ear

Otitis media   Otitis media is relatively common in dogs. The most common cause is otitis externa – middle ear disease should always be suspected in animals with chronic or recurrent otitis externa. One survey revealed that 16% of dogs with acute otitis externa and 50% of dogs with chronic otitis externa had concurrent otitis media. Other causes of otitis media include:

- foreign bodies
- trauma
- neoplasia
- haematogenous or ascending infection.

Patients with middle ear disease will generally also show the signs of otitis externa. Some animals may hold the head tilted because of pain, but this should be differentiated from the head tilt seen with vestibular dysfunction – the former patients can hold the head in a normal position if encouraged. Ipsilateral facial nerve paralysis and Horner's syndrome (Fig 7.7) may be apparent. Facial paralysis may be manifest by a drooping lip or ear, inability to move the ear, drooling of saliva, reduced or absent palpebral reflex and exposure keratitis. Horner's syndrome is characterised by ptosis, miosis, enophthalmos and protrusion of the third eyelid. If middle ear infection is severe or chronic enough to cause otitis interna, then signs of vestibular dysfunction may be seen. These include head tilt, nystagmus and ataxia.

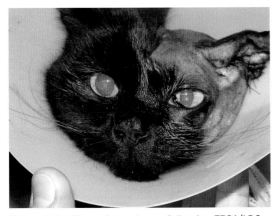

Figure 7.7   Horner's syndrome following TECA/LBO.

Diagnostic techniques include otoscopy and radiography. The normal tympanic membrane is slightly concave, translucent, pearly grey and glistening. Alteration in its colour, tension or integrity indicates pathologic changes in the middle ear.

Radiographs should include lateral and ventrodorsal projections of the skull, along with lateral oblique and rostrocaudal open-mouth projections centred on the tympanic bullae. A fluid opacity within the bulla may be caused by purulent exudates, granulation tissue, neoplasia or cellular debris. Bony proliferation or lysis of the bulla may be seen with neoplasia or osteomyelitis secondary to chronic otitis media. However, it is important to realise that many of these changes occur relatively late in the disease process and that radiography is insensitive, in that the bulla may contain appreciable quantities of fluid but have a normal radiographic appearance. Computed tomography is a more sensitive method of assessment.

Tumours of the middle ear   Neoplasia of the middle ear cavity is uncommon. Clinical signs are generally similar to otitis media, although invasion of the middle ear, inner ear and brain may cause severe central nervous system signs. A presumptive diagnosis may be made by clinical signs, otoscopy and radiography. Other imaging techniques, such as computed tomography or magnetic resonance imaging, may be required to define the extent of the lesion. A definitive diagnosis is made by biopsy.

Surgical treatment is often unrewarding because of the anatomic location, invasive nature and extent of the disease at the time of diagnosis.

Middle ear polyps   Middle ear polyps are pedunculated growths arising from the mucous membrane of the tympanic cavity, ear canal, nasopharynx and nasal passages. The cause of the polyp is unknown, but it is presumed to be due to inflammation, possibly arising from upper respiratory tract infection. A congenital predisposition has been suggested. The polyp generally arises from the tympanic bulla and may extend from the middle ear ventrally down the Eustachian tube into the naso-pharynx or dorsally into the external ear canal. Clinical signs include respiratory stridor, dyspnoea, dysphagia and signs of otitis externa or otitis media.

Treatment requires removal of the polyp. Nasopharyngeal polyps are removed by traction. This may require rostral retraction of the soft palate to identify the stalk of the polyp. Those polyps extending through the external ear canal are more difficult to remove by traction. A suitable approach is to remove as much of the polyp as possible by traction and then to treat the animal with anti-inflammatory doses of corticosteroids for a month. If clinical signs recur, then a ventral bulla osteotomy is indicated to remove the origin of the polyp.

Surgical techniques for middle ear disease

The aims of treatment are:

- to gain access to the tympanic cavity
- to remove inflamed or infected tissue and foreign debris
- to obtain material for biopsy or culture
- to provide an avenue for ventilation or drainage.

Myringotomy If the tympanic membrane is intact but discoloured or bulging outwards, a myringotomy or incision of the tympanic membrane is performed. The aims of myringotomy are:

- to obtain samples for culture
- to drain the middle ear
- to relieve pain and pressure associated with otitis media
- to allow lavage and instillation of medication.

After the external ear canal is cleaned, the otoscope is introduced and the tympanic membrane perforated caudal to the malleus. The contents of the middle ear may be sampled after introducing a 20 gauge spinal needle through the tympanic membrane and aspirating. The middle ear is then lavaged with sterile saline by repeatedly instilling and aspirating saline until the fluid recovered is clear. Long-term antibiotic therapy, for 3–6 weeks, is required – the choice of antibiotic being dependent on culture results. Common pathogens isolated from the middle ear include Staphylococcus spp., Streptococcus spp., Pseudomonas spp., *E. coli*, and *Proteus mirabilis*.

The disadvantages of myringotomy as the sole method of treatment include:

- poor exposure of the tympanic cavity
- poor postoperative drainage
- exposure of the middle ear to the external ear canal, which may itself be infected
- damage to the structures of the middle ear.

In addition, otitis media which is not secondary to otitis externa is relatively uncommon and this procedure is not commonly indicated. Surgical drainage is indicated if this therapy proves ineffective, or if a neoplastic lesion, inflammatory mass or foreign body is found.

Ventral bulla osteotomy Ventral bulla osteotomy (VBO) allows access to the tympanic cavity. It gives better access to the tympanic bulla than LBO, more consistent drainage and allows both bullae to be explored without repositioning the patient (Fig 7.8). In the patient with middle ear disease in conjunction with otitis externa, access to the tympanic bulla is best gained by a LBO following a TECA. Although this gives a more restricted

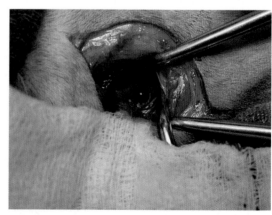

Figure 7.8 Ventral bulla osteotomy.

exposure, it avoids repositioning the patient. VBO is indicated in the management of middle ear neoplasia and nasopharyngeal polyps.

Surgical technique The patient is placed in dorsal recumbency. The bulla may be palpated immediately caudal and medial to the vertical ramus of the mandible. An 8–10cm paramedian incision is made just medial to the mandibular salivary gland and centred midway between the angular process of the mandible cranially and the wings of the atlas caudally. The incision is continued through the platysma muscle. The digastricus muscle and linguofacial vein are retracted medially and the styloglossus and hyoglossus muscles and the hypoglossal nerve are retracted laterally to expose the bulla.

A Steinman pin or small drill may be used to perform the osteotomy, which is then enlarged with small rongeurs. The contents of the bulla may then be examined. The feline bulla is divided by a thin bony septum into two compartments – a small craniolateral compartment and a larger caudomedial compartment. The bulla may be lavaged and, if necessary, a drain placed.

Lateral bulla osteotomy Lateral bulla osteotomy in conjunction with total ear canal ablation, which is the most appropriate technique for patients with concurrent otitis externa, is described above.

In rare circumstances, lateral bulla osteotomy may be performed without total ear canal ablation. The patient is placed in lateral recumbency and an incision is made over the vertical canal, extending 1–2cm ventral to the horizontal canal. The subcutaneous tissues are dissected to reveal the junction between the parotid salivary gland and the ventral aspect of the horizontal ear canal. Dissection continues ventrally along the caudolateral aspect of the ear canal to expose the lateral aspect of the tympanic bulla. The facial nerve is retracted ventrally. The bulla is then entered with a Steinmann pin or a drill, directed in a caudolateral direction to avoid the auditory ossicles. Rongeurs are then used to enlarge the osteotomy. The bulla is then curetted and lavaged.

General considerations for surgery of the ear canal

Surgical asepsis
It is difficult, if not impossible, to ensure that the surgical site is aseptically prepared. Rather than perform repeated lavage of the external ear canal, it is probably better to accept that aural surgery is a contaminated procedure. Hence, perioperative antibiotics are indicated. The requirement for postoperative therapy depends on the nature of the disease and the surgical procedure and may be determined once the degree of contamination has been assessed.

Analgesia
With the exception of minor surgery of the pinna, most aural surgery is extremely painful. Particular attention should be paid to achieving adequate analgesia, both from a humanitarian aspect and also to prevent self-trauma.

Wound management
Aural surgery is generally considered contaminated. Measures should be taken to prevent self-trauma. Bandaging the ears is difficult and incorporation of the ears into a bandage which passes round the neck may lead to asphyxiation. Prevention of self-trauma with an Elizabethan collar is recommended. The wound should be inspected frequently, and cleaned as required – particularly if a Penrose drain has been placed.

Nerve damage
Damage to the facial nerve may result in a loss of the blink response and a loss of parasympathetic innervation to the lacrimal glands. The eye should be kept lubricated with artificial tears or a suitable ophthalmic lubricant. Curettage of the tympanic bulla may result in Horner's syndrome, particularly in the cat. This is generally transient and may improve with a short course of corticosteroids. Vestibular signs, either as a result of extension of the disease from the middle ear or, rarely, from over zealous curettage of the bulla, may cause the patient to become disorientated.

THE UPPER RESPIRATORY TRACT

Indications for upper respiratory tract surgery

Anatomic divisions of the upper respiratory tract

Disorders of the following parts of the upper respiratory tract (Fig 7.9) may require surgical management:

- external nares
- nasal passages and paranasal sinuses
- hard and soft palate
- pharynx
- tonsils
- larynx
- trachea.

Common disorders of the upper respiratory tract include:

- brachycephalic airway obstruction syndrome (BAOS)
- nasal tumours
- nasal foreign bodies
- rhinitis
- laryngeal paralysis
- laryngeal masses
- tracheal collapse
- tracheal masses
- upper respiratory tract trauma.

Brachycephalic airway obstruction syndrome

Many disorders of the airway requiring diagnostic or surgical intervention are found in brachycephalic breeds. These include Bulldogs, Pekes and Pugs and, to a lesser extent, Mastiffs and Cavalier King Charles spaniels. The syndrome has many separate features which contribute to the overall problem of airway obstruction. Some of these are primary initiating factors, which may be heritable or congenital and arise because of conformational abnormalities, and some are secondary and are acquired later in life as a result of changes induced by the primary factors. The early diagnosis and management of the primary factors

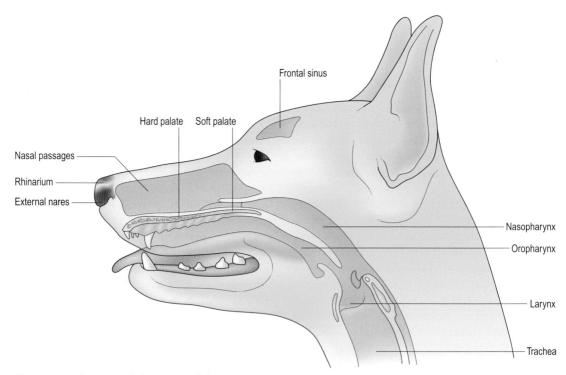

Figure 7.9 Anatomy of the nose and throat.

is important in order to limit the development of the more serious and potentially fatal secondary disorders.

The primary conformational changes include:

- stenotic nares
- overlong soft palate
- tracheal hypoplasia
- redundant pharyngeal mucosa.

The secondary changes include:

- tonsillar hypertrophy
- pharyngeal hypertrophy
- everted laryngeal ventricles
- laryngeal collapse.

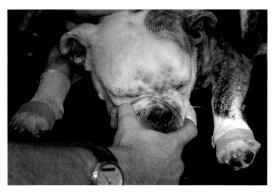

Figure 7.10   Administration of supplementary oxygen via face mask.

Preoperative assessment

General considerations

Surgical procedures of the upper airway are performed to remove, repair or bypass areas of obstruction, injury or disease. It is important to realise that many of the diseases cause airway obstruction and hence many of the patients will exhibit dyspnoea. Care should be taken to avoid exacerbating the respiratory distress on examination of these patients. Patients should initially be examined at a distance to avoid stress. Open-mouth breathing, abducted fore-limbs and restlessness indicate moderate to severe respiratory distress that may require emergency intervention. Minimal restraint should be used in severely dyspnoeic patients and they should be allowed to adopt the position they find the most comfortable.

Animals with marked dyspnoea will be distressed and may be hyperthermic. Supplementary oxygen may be given via face mask (Fig 7.10), nasal catheter, tracheostomy tube, endotracheal tube or oxygen cage. Sedation, with caution, may be beneficial for animals in distress. Cooling of the hyperthermic patient may be achieved by using a fan, applying ice packs or towels soaked in cold water to the head, axilla, inguinal area and extremities, and infusing cool fluids intravenously.

If it is possible that a temporary tracheostomy may be required, then the ventral neck should be clipped in readiness. If there is any doubt that the patient cannot maintain the airway, then intervention to achieve a patent airway should proceed. This may involve placing a tracheostomy tube in the conscious patient under local anaesthesia, inducing general anaesthesia and placing a tracheostomy tube or inducing general anaesthesia and performing definitive management of the condition. In many cases, an elective tracheostomy under general anaesthesia is easier and less stressful for the patient than performing it under local anaesthesia.

Diagnosis

A consideration of the patient's signalment should be made, since many of the disorders have strong breed predilections and many are congenital and will be noted in the young animal.

History and clinical signs will suggest the presence of upper respiratory tract disease and may allow assessment of the likely location. Inspiratory stridor (a whistling-type noise) is common in laryngeal disease, whereas stertor (a snoring-type noise) is found in patients with an overlong soft palate. Tachypnoea, dyspnoea and exercise intolerance may be found in more markedly affected individuals. Severely affected patients may exhibit marked dyspnoea, cyanosis and syncope. Gagging and regurgitation are common with nasopharyngeal, laryngeal and some tracheal diseases. Dysphonia (a change in the voice) may be noted with laryngeal disease and dysphagia may occur with obstructions rostral to the rima glot-tidis. Subcutaneous emphysema may accompany penetrating wounds of the larynx, trachea and nasal passages. Clinical signs may be exacerbated by excitement, exercise, stress, eating and drinking or high ambient temperatures.

Laboratory data is not commonly required for diagnosis of disorders of the upper respiratory tract. However, routine blood screens are of use to detect underlying diseases or diseases secondary to the primary disorder and to assess the general fitness for anaesthesia and postoperative therapy. Poor jugular venepuncture technique may result in iatrogenic damage to vital structures in the neck. In addition, the resulting haematoma may interfere with the surgical approach. In patients scheduled for unilateral procedures involving the neck, e.g. arytenoid lateralisation, it may be prudent to take blood from the contralateral jugular vein.

Direct inspection of the respiratory tract under general anaesthesia via rhinoscopy, laryngoscopy (Fig 7.11) or endoscopy, using a flexible or rigid endoscope, is the most common means of achieving a definitive diagnosis. Radiography and computed tomography are of use in assessing the nasal passages and trachea but are of less use for the pharynx and larynx. They are also indicated for evaluating the chest for secondary changes, e.g. aspiration pneumonia associated with laryngeal paralysis or metastases associated with tumours of the respiratory tract. Ultrasonographic examination may be employed as a non-invasive method to evaluate the larynx and trachea in the conscious animal.

The perioperative use of anti-inflammatory doses of corticosteroids (e.g. dexamethasone sodium phosphate 0.25–1mg/kg IV or methylprednisolone sodium succinate 0.5–2mg/kg IV) may help to reduce the oedema associated with diagnostic or therapeutic intervention, particularly intralaryngeal procedures.

Anaesthetic considerations

Preanaesthetic assessment

Patients with upper respiratory tract obstruction present an anaesthetic risk. The period of greatest danger is during induction and recovery. In addition, both the anaesthetist and surgeon often require access to the airway at the same time, so careful planning over the choice of anaesthetic regime and surgical procedure is necessary. The overall goal must be to maintain and support normal respiratory tract function.

The patient with upper respiratory tract disease must be treated in a calm and efficient manner until induction of anaesthesia and airway patency can be secured. Preoperative assessment is critical in evaluating the location, extent and severity of respiratory disease. Obvious injury to the chest wall, diaphragm, pulmonary parenchyma, trachea and bronchi or pleural space is managed before anaesthetic induction so that pulmonary gas exchange can occur in an unrestricted manner. This entails closing any open chest wounds, and draining the pleural space of air or fluid.

Whenever possible, potent respiratory depressants should be avoided in patients with respiratory tract disease in the perianaesthetic period. When sedatives or analgesics with this property are used (e.g. opiates), then the patient's breathing should be closely monitored. Mixed agonist-antagonist opioids (e.g. butorphanol, buprenorphine) minimise respiratory depression. Opiate antagonists (e.g. naloxone) may be used to reverse this respi-

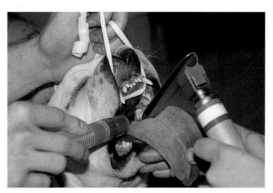

Figure 7.11 Laryngoscopy with supplementary oxygen administration.

ratory depression but will also reverse the analgesic effect. In patients undergoing anaesthesia for investigation and management of airway trauma, the possibility of cranial trauma should be investigated. Head trauma and secondary cerebral oedema will decrease ventilation independently of any obstruction. In these cases, additional respiratory depression must be avoided to prevent increases in intracranial pressure and neurological morbidity.

Vagal tone is often high in brachycephalic dogs. In addition, vagal stimulation associated with pharyngeal manipulation, from surgery or difficult intubation, and the use of vagotonic drugs may contribute to bradycardia. Consideration should be given to the use of anticholinergic agents preoperatively, or intraoperatively if bradycardia is a problem.

Presurgical preparation of the patient should be undertaken gently to avoid causing stress, and it may be preferable to delay it until the patient is anaesthetised. Emergency equipment and drugs should be available throughout the procedure – this includes suction to remove blood, secretions and debris from the airway.

Oxygen should be supplemented during airway examination and dyspnoeic patients should be pre-oxygenated before the procedure by supplying 100% oxygen for 5 minutes prior to the procedure via face mask or nasal catheter. Oxygen saturation should be monitored by pulse oximetry during the procedure.

Perioperative problems

Laryngospasm Laryngospasm in the perioperative period is a particular problem in cats, although it is recorded in dogs. It generally occurs following contact with the larynx under a light plane of anaesthesia, and may arise following irritation of the larynx by secretions or blood. Topical application of a local anaesthetic is therefore recommended prior to intubation to reduce the likelihood of this complication in cats.

Acute pulmonary oedema Acute pulmonary oedema may follow acute respiratory tract obstruction, e.g. acute exacerbation of laryngeal paralysis. A variety of factors may contribute to this:

- severe negative airway pressure
- reduced interstitial hydrostatic pressure
- release of catecholamines
- vasoconstriction
- increased vascular hydrostatic pressure
- hypoxia
- increased permeability of pulmonary vessels
- net accumulation of interstitial fluid
- inadequate removal of interstitial fluid.

The net result is acute pulmonary oedema and impairment to gas exchange. Because the cause is multifactorial, the therapy should be symptomatic initially, followed by management of any predisposing causes. Emergency therapy consists of oxygen supplementation, diuretics (e.g. frusemide) and corticosteroids. Endotracheal intubation and positive-pressure ventilation may be required in severe cases.

Induction of anaesthesia

Induction should be rapid, using an intravenous agent (e.g. propofol, thiopentone or ketamine) followed by immediate intubation and administration of oxygen. Mask or cage induction is likely to be too stressful and is not recommended. Anaesthesia is maintained with an inhalant agent. The presence of an indwelling intravenous catheter for prompt vascular access should be regarded as mandatory.

Whenever possible, a cuffed endotracheal tube should be placed and a known number of swabs or a taped sponge should be packed in the pharynx to absorb fluids. The endotracheal tube should ideally bypass the lesion and be present in the normal distal trachea (e.g. in the case of tracheal tumour or laceration). Pre-measurement of the lesion following endoscopy or from a radiograph will ensure that this is achieved. For lesions causing partial obstruction, e.g. tracheal neoplasia, a smaller endotracheal tube may be required. If an endotracheal tube cannot be placed, then consideration should be given to placing a tracheostomy tube to maintain a patent airway. Some procedures of the larynx and trachea may require temporary extubation. In these cases, consideration should be given to placing a cuffed tracheostomy tube and ventilating via the tube.

Anaesthesia for diagnostic procedures

For laryngoscopy, drugs which depress laryngeal function should be avoided. Propofol is a good choice for induction, since it is non-cumulative and may be given in small incremental doses to achieve a light plane of anaesthesia while still maintaining laryngeal function. Diazepam and ketamine also maintain laryngeal function, whereas thiopentone impairs laryngeal function.

The larynx is inspected with a laryngoscope as soon as a light plane of anaesthesia has been induced. Generally, this is just after jaw tone has been lost. It is important to inspect the larynx before an endotracheal tube is placed, to avoid compromising the diagnosis. However, it is important not to take too long in inspection. Once the examination is complete, the patient is intubated and is either allowed to recover or surgical correction of the disorder is performed.

Tracheoscopy and bronchoscopy places additional demands on the airway. Oxygen insufflation may be provided via the side port of an open bronchoscope. Flexible endoscopy is best performed via an endotracheal tube, with oxygen supplied via a side port on the endotracheal tube adapter. In small patients, it may not be possible to do this and endoscopy may have to be performed without an endotracheal tube in place. Oxygen may still be administered via a flexible catheter. In this case, the endoscopic examination should be brief and performed by someone with expertise.

Anaesthesia for surgical procedures

General anaesthesia is preferred for most upper respiratory tract procedures as it allows the establishment of a patent airway, allows controlled ventilation, facilitates asepsis and is less stressful for patients. Local anaesthesia may be used for tracheostomy tube placement when the patient is comatose or cannot tolerate general anaesthesia.

The presence of drapes around the surgical field obscures much of the patient's head and makes monitoring more difficult. The anaesthetist may have to rely on the character of the femoral pulse, the respiratory rate and blind palpation of jaw tone and lingual pulse to gauge the depth of anaesthesia. An oesophageal stethoscope is an invaluable aid. Attention should be paid to the re-breathing bag as well as the thoracic movements. A patient with respiratory tract obstruction is likely to show marked thoracic wall excursions but will only move small volumes of gas through the breathing system.

The breathing circuit and tube should be checked periodically to ensure no part is kinked or has become disconnected. Changes in the position of the endotracheal tube may occur during positioning of the patient. Flexion of the neck may result in caudal displacement of the tube, endobronchial placement or total occlusion of the tube. Extension of the neck or movement of the patient caudally may result in extubation.

Surgical considerations

Timing of surgery

Surgical procedures of the upper respiratory tract are best conducted at the beginning of the day's operating list. Careful observation is then possible throughout the remainder of the day for complications associated with the procedure, such as haemorrhage or oedema which may cause airway obstruction. Similarly, many of the procedures are not suitable to be performed on an outpatient basis or where adequate 24-hour intensive care facilities are not available.

Surgical intervention for patients which have suffered from marked haemorrhage, who are severely dyspnoiec or who cannot eat and drink voluntarily should be performed as soon as the patient has been stabilised. For those patients who are less severely affected, delaying the procedure until the weather is cooler may be of benefit. However, since the majority of these disorders are exacerbated by high ambient temperatures, many animals will present with acute exacerbations of their disease necessitating intervention when the weather is warm.

Surgical asepsis

Strict asepsis is not possible for many procedures within the mouth, nasal chambers and upper airway. Hence many of the procedures are regarded as clean-contaminated or contaminated and perioperative antibiotics are indicated. This should consist of a single intravenous bolus, 30–60 minutes before the start of surgery. Further doses may be given depending on the duration of the procedure and the nature of the surgery, but many patients will not require further prophylaxis. However, some patients will present with evidence of infection of a part of the airway, and in these cases antibiotic therapy is warranted on a therapeutic basis.

Streptococcus spp., *E. coli,* Pseudomonas spp., Klebsiella spp. and *Bordetella bronchiseptica* are commonly isolated from the respiratory tract of normal dogs. Ampicillin or clavulanate-potentiated amoxicillin are suitable choices for prophylaxis. Most canine respiratory tract infections are due to Gram-negative organisms and many are resistant to commonly-used antibiotics. The choice of a therapeutic antibiotic should be determined by cytological examination and culture of tracheobronchial or pulmonary secretions or discharges. Suitable empiric choices while waiting for these results are ampicillin, clavulanate-potentiated amoxicillin, trimethoprim-sulphadiazine and fluoroquinolones.

Instrumentation and technique

Most procedures may be performed with a standard surgical pack. Self-retaining retractors are of use for external approaches to the respiratory tract. Long-handled instruments facilitate procedures within the airway carried out from an oral approach. Right-angled tonsillectomy clamps are used for tonsillectomy (Fig 7.12) and soft palate resection. Diathermy should be used to ensure adequate haemostasis in the tissues outside the airway. Haemorrhage within the airway should be controlled with pressure using swabs, since diathermy used in this location may result in excessive tissue swelling and oedema. Suction is used to keep the surgical field free of haemorrhage intraoperatively and to remove blood and debris from the airway postoperatively. A drill is used to perform the initial rhinotomy or sinusotomy approach, which is then enlarged with rongeurs or an oscillating saw.

Meticulous, atraumatic surgical technique is important if good results are to be achieved. Postoperative swelling and oedema resulting from traumatic surgical technique may result in airway obstruction. A surgical assistant is of great benefit for most of the procedures involving the airway.

For each surgical procedure there is an optimal position for the patient to allow the best access to and visibility of the surgical site, to create tension on the tissues to be incised, thus allowing safer blunt dissection, and to allow safe anaesthesia and monitoring. Positioning the patient for some of the procedures, particularly those requiring access *per os*, may be awkward, but it is critical that the best access is gained and that the patient stays in this position. A little extra time spent ensuring proper patient positioning will pay dividends.

Aftercare

The results obtained by the surgeon are directly related to the quality of the after care

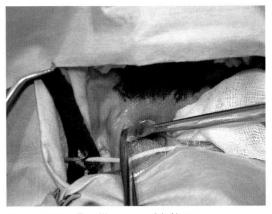

Figure 7.12 Tonsillectomy with Negus tonsillectomy forceps.

provided. The placement of the last suture does not signify the conclusion of the procedure. Postoperative care ranges from intensive care following recovery to long-term advice on diet and exercise – all of which are designed to return the patient to normal activity.

Recovery and intensive care postoperatively

The animal should be closely monitored at the end of the surgical procedure and the endotracheal tube should be left in place as long as possible. Recovery is generally accepted to be adequate when the dog strongly objects to the presence of the endotracheal tube. The airway should be inspected at the end of anaesthesia and suction used to remove any blood, secretions or debris from the airway or pharynx. The tube should be removed with the cuff still partly inflated, to reduce the risk of aspiration of blood or secretions. Because of the presence of redundant tissue in the pharynx, most brachycephalic breeds benefit from having the anaesthetist hold the tongue and extend the neck following extubation.

Supplementary oxygen should be available if required, especially if there is a risk of postoperative airway obstruction. Supplementary oxygen administration will increase the time available for institution of means of airway control if obstruction arises. Face mask and nasal catheter are the most practical means of providing this.

Intensive monitoring is particularly important once the tube has been removed. Ventilatory function should be monitored very closely for at least one hour after recovery. Postsurgical haemorrhage or oedema may develop later and can cause severe obstruction of the airway. All personnel concerned with nursing the patient should be aware of the signs of respiratory distress and should be competent in performing a temporary tracheostomy if required.

Postoperative medication

Careful attention should be paid to postoperative analgesia and a balanced regime, tailored to the individual patient and nature of the procedure be provided. An opiate is usually provided in the premedication and further doses may be given postoperatively. A balanced regime consisting of the addition of a non-steroidal anti-inflammatory drug (NSAID), such as carprofen, is likely to be successful. The first dose of this drug may be given perioperatively.

Corticosteroids have a role to play to reduce the inflammatory swelling which may accompany diseases of the upper respiratory tract and which will itself compromise the airway. In addition, they also have been recommended to reduce the oedema and swelling that may follow surgery. Generally, for most procedures, particularly those which do not encroach on the lumen of the airway (e.g. arytenoid lateralisation) or elective surgery, where gross oedema may not be present (e.g. tonsillectomy) they are not required as routine. Care should be taken not to administer NSAIDs postoperatively if corticosteroids have been given perioperatively.

Wounds of the head and neck are particularly vulnerable to self-trauma from rubbing and scratching, particularly during recovery. Many wounds of the head and neck cannot be bandaged satisfactorily and some device to limit self-trauma e.g. an Elizabethan collar, may be required. Adequate analgesia should be ensured in any animal showing self-trauma.

Sedation or tranquillisation may be required during recovery to minimise struggling and excitement, both of which will increase oxygen demand at a time when the patient is less able to provide this. Sedation may be required for agitated patients postoperatively. It is often preferable to discharge some patients (e.g. following arytenoid lateralisation for laryngeal paralysis) into their normal home environment as soon as possible.

Nutrition

Surgery of the upper respiratory tract and the original disease process may interfere with the animal's ability or inclination to eat and drink. Feeding should ideally be re-introduced as soon as possible. Patients with wounds in the oropharynx should not be given harsh or abrasive food. Surgical intervention in the larynx may interfere with normal swallowing and aspiration of fluid is a possibility. Such patients are better fed from a low position and sloppy or liquid food should be avoided. Animals fed canned food generally swallow discrete boluses of food, which reduces the likelihood of aspiration. Diseases affecting the nasal passages may impair the animal's ability to smell, which may result in reluctance to feed. Hand-feeding of palatable, warmed, strong-smelling food may be required to ensure adequate consumption.

Exercise

Postsurgical oedema will result in temporary partial obstruction of the respiratory tract. Vigorous exercise and excitement should be avoided for approximately 10–14 days while this resolves. A longer period of convalescence of 6 weeks is indicated for patients who have undergone arytenoid lateralisation, to allow ankylosis of the cartilages in their new position. Following laryngeal surgery, barking should be discouraged for 6 weeks.

DISORDERS OF THE AIRWAY

External nares

Anatomy

The rhinarium is the soft, hairless part of the nose, which is usually pigmented. The nostrils, or nares, are comma-shaped openings which allow air into the nasal passages. Dorsal and ventral lateral cartilages unite to form the tube of the nostril. Medial and ventral support is given by the nasal septum and lateral accessory cartilage. Dorsal support is provided by the dorsal lateral cartilage.

Diseases of the external nares

Stenotic nares Stenotic nares are often found in brachycephalic dogs (Fig 7.13) and it is one part of the brachycephalic airway obstruction syndrome (BAOS). The cartilaginous tissue of the lateral cartilages is broader and less rigid than is found in other breeds. The cartilages lack normal rigidity and col-

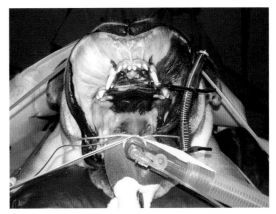

Figure 7.13 Positioning for an oral approach to the airway in a Bulldog.

lapse medially, causing partial occlusion of the external nares. The obstruction is worse during inspiration, when the cartilage may be drawn into the nasal passages because of its lack of rigidity. The reduced airflow necessitates a greater inspiratory effort.

In the normal animal, the external nares and nasal passages represent approximately one-third of the total resistance to the flow of air into the respiratory tract. Hence, obstruction at this level is likely to be significant. Stenotic nares (Fig 7.14) contribute both to obstruction of the airway and also increase the turbulence of air in the nasopharynx, which may exacerbate nasopharyngeal problems.

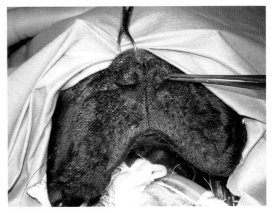

Figure 7.14 Stenotic nares: the left alar wing is moved to show a more normal patent nareis.

Diagnosis is by physical examination. The wing of the nostril occludes the external nares, and is sucked medially on inspiration. The degree of stenosis may vary between individuals. Signs of dyspnoea may be present.

Surgical technique Surgical treatment is directed towards resecting a portion of the wing of the nostril to increase the airflow. The wing of the nostril is examined to determine the amount of tissue to be removed. This tissue is highly vascular and bleeds profusely when incised. Pressure and the use of suction are indicated to control the haemorrhage, which generally stops once the sutures are placed. The wound is apposed with simple interrupted sutures of 3-0 to 5-0 suture material. The use of a soft braided material in this location, such as polyglactin 910 (Vicryl; Ethicon) or silk, is less irritating than monofilament material.

- Vertical wedge. A triangular wedge, with the base ventrally, is removed from the wing of the nostril and part of the alar cartilage.
- Horizontal wedge. A horizontal wedge, with its base directed dorsolaterally, is removed from the wing of the nostril.
- Lateral wedge resection. A portion of the caudolateral border of the wing of the nostril and a triangle of skin adjacent to it is removed.

Postoperative care The surgical site should be kept clean and an Elizabethan collar should be used to prevent self-trauma.

Prognosis In young dogs (less than 2 years old), the prognosis following surgery is favourable, as long as any other conditions causing airway obstruction, e.g. overlong soft palate, are corrected at the same time. However, in the older animal, when additional secondary changes such as everted laryngeal saccules or laryngeal collapse may contribute to airway obstruction, the prognosis is more guarded.

Neoplasia of the external nares Squamous cell carcinoma is the most common tumour of the nares and nasal planum in the dog and cat. The tumour is invasive but has a low metastatic potential in the cat. In the dog, the disease tends to be much more aggressive, infiltrating the nasal cartilages and rapidly metastasising via the regional lymph nodes. Other tumour types include lymphoma, fibrosarcoma, haemangioma, melanoma, mast cell tumour and fibroma.

Squamous cell carcinoma is often slow-growing and the tumour may progress from an early premalignant lesion (carcinoma-in-situ), characterised by superficial crusting, to the malignant form, characterised by an erosive lesion which bleeds easily. Secondary infection may be found once ulceration is present. The tumour may be overlooked as a non-healing sore. Associated lesions may be present on the eyelids and pinna. Early incisional biopsy should be performed for any such lesion. Prognosis is determined by histological grade, degree of infiltration into the nasal cartilages and metastasis.

Treatment Effective treatment depends on the extent of the tumour. Superficial, minimally invasive lesions can be managed effectively by almost any method, including cryosurgery, phototherapy, hyperthermia, irradiation or surgery. Surgical excision has the advantage of being able to document cure by examination of the margins of excision. Deeply invasive tumours are resistant to most non-surgical methods.

Surgery Wide local excision is the treatment of choice for premalignant and early malignant lesions without metastasis. This involves resection of the nasal planum and underlying cartilage with margins of 1cm on all aspects. Closure requires local advancement or rotation flaps. The functional result is excellent and the cosmetic appearance is satisfactory. In the dog, the cosmetic change may be more radical.

Radiotherapy Radiotherapy may be used as an alternative or adjunctive therapy to surgery, particularly where the lesion is more deeply invasive or aggressive than usual. However, long-term damage to the nasal cartilages is a possibility, and the resulting distortion is a common complication.

Photodynamic therapy   This is applicable for early, superficial lesions. A photosensitising agent is applied to the affected area for several hours. The area is then irradiated with a laser, or a light-emitting diode, which causes free radicals to be generated which are toxic to the tumour. Long-term control of superficial lesions with an excellent cosmetic result is possible.

Prognosis   The prognosis following excision of early premalignant lesions in the cat is good, with a good chance of achieving local cure. However, new lesions may develop at other sites. In the dog, the prognosis is poorer, with local recurrence and metastasis being more common. Radiotherapy as the sole therapeutic modality is generally reserved for more deeply invasive lesions – the prognosis for these tumours is poorer.

Rhinarial wounds   These will often heal rapidly by second intention because of the excellent blood supply. Primary surgical closure is indicated if there is damage to the dorsolateral nasal cartilages, since stenosis and collapse of the cartilage may occur.

Cleft of the primary palate (harelip)   The primary palate consists of the lip and premaxilla. Unilateral or bilateral clefts are occasionally seen in the dog, but rarely in the cat. Clefts are a congenital problem which may be attributed to inherited, nutritional, hormonal, mechanical and toxic factors. Concurrent clefts of the hard and soft palates (secondary palate) may be present.

Suckling is not possible since the cleft interferes with the generation of negative pressure in the oral cavity and animals may have a poor nutritional status. Such patients must be hand-reared until surgical correction can be performed at 2–3 months old. Surgical correction is aimed at closure of the nasal floor. The natural adjoining edges of the cleft are approximated. This technique requires mobilisation of sufficient tissue to avoid tension on the suture lines and is not a simple technique. Dehiscence and incomplete healing of the defects are common complications. Multiple surgeries may be required to achieve closure.

Nasal passages and paranasal sinuses

Anatomy
The two nasal passages extend from the external nares to the choanae, the junction with the nasopharynx, and are separated in the midline by the nasal septum. The passages are filled with scrolls of bone (conchae), which project medially into the passages from the lateral sides and the roof. A thin common passage, or meatus, is present immediately lateral to the nasal septum and leads from the nostril to the pharynx. This is connected to the three nasal meati (dorsal, middle and ventral) which fill the space between the conchae. The paranasal sinuses consist of the paired frontal sinuses and the maxillary recesses, which communicate with the nasal passages. The large frontal sinus occupies the brow ridge and supraorbital process of the frontal bone. The much smaller maxillary recess is present at the level of the carnassial tooth, between the orbit and the infraorbital canal.

Diagnosis of nasal passage disease
Diseases of the nasal passages and associated sinuses are common in the cat and dog. Many diseases will affect this area but may present with similar clinical signs, such as nasal discharge, epistaxis and sneezing. Establishing a definitive diagnosis requires a careful and systematic diagnostic plan:

- Presenting signs: sneezing, nasal discharge, epistaxis, dyspnoea
- History:
  - cute, chronic or intermittent signs
  - unilateral or bilateral discharge
  - nature of discharge: serous, mucoid, purulent, bloody
- Physical examination: facial deformity, pain, oculonasal discharge, dental disease, regional lymphadenopathy, obstruction of nasal passages
- Pattern of respiration: stertor, sneezing, cough, dyspnoea.

The most appropriate diagnostic plan is to anaesthetise the animal, make radiographs, perform endoscopy and then biopsy any lesions which are identified.

Radiographs   Radiographs are required to provide a presumptive diagnosis, to identify the extent of the disease and to identify that area of the nasal passage most likely to yield diagnostic material on biopsy. The dorsoventral projection of the nasal passages with the film placed intraorally is the most useful projection. The lateral projection of the skull and rostrocaudal skyline projection of the frontal sinus may also yield important information. Radiographs of the chest are indicated if neoplasia is suspected.

Endoscopy   Rhinoscopy may be performed with a small rigid endoscope (Fig 7.15) introduced via the external nares. The use of an external sheath, through which saline may be infused, aids visualisation by removing discharge and blood. The caudal nasal passages and choanae may be examined with a small diameter flexible endoscope introduced via the mouth and retroflexed 180° over the top of the soft palate. A cuffed endotracheal tube should be placed, the pharynx should be packed with a counted number of swabs and the patient should be positioned in sternal recumbency with the head tilted downwards.

Biopsy   Definitive diagnosis may require biopsy and should be performed following radiography. A biopsy is normally taken via the nostril using a blind grab technique with cup-action biting forceps or suction with a large-bore, end-opening catheter. The distance from the external nares to the medial canthus should be measured and marked on the biopsy instrument. The instrument should not be inserted further than the medial canthus to avoid penetrating the cribriform plate. A curette may be used to obtain material from rostral lesions if forceps are not available. Mild to moderate haemorrhage may accompany biopsy but will generally subside in a few minutes. A forceful, retrograde nasal flush, with collection of tissue debris in the nasopharynx has also been described as a way of collecting material. Cytological examination of nasal washings is largely unrewarding. Similarly, culture of discharge is largely unrewarding. Open surgical biopsy is occasionally required if diagnostic material cannot be obtained using the other methods outlined.

Serology   Antibodies to Aspergillus may be identified in a serum sample.

Disease of the nasal passages

Nasal aspergillosis   Clinical signs include the presence of a thick, green mucoid or mucopurulent nasal discharge, which may be accompanied by epistaxis. Depigmentation and ulceration of the external nares may be seen. Some patients show marked facial pain and resent handling of the head. Radiographs may show turbinate destruction (Fig 7.16), particularly rostrally. Destruction of the supporting bones of the nasal cavity is less common than with nasal tumours. Serology may reveal the presence of antibodies to Aspergillus and rhinoscopy may permit fungal plaques to be identified. Aspergillus is rarely cultured from samples of the nasal discharge.

Therapy for aspergillosis is directed at delivering a suitable antifungal agent to the site of infection for a sufficient period of time; many drugs have been proposed. The drug may be administered via:

- anterograde flushing via the external nares
- retrograde flushing via the frontal sinuses, which may be coupled with anterograde flushing via the external nares

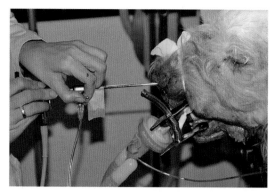

Figure 7.15   Rhinoscopy using a rigid scope with a sheath allowing irrigation.

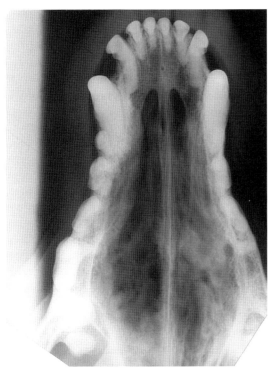

Figure 7.16 Dorsoventral intra-oral radiograph showing turbinate destruction indicative of Aspergillosis.

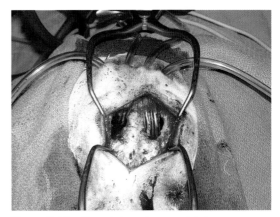

Figure 7.17 Dorsal sinusotomy and tube implantation for Aspergillosis.

- retrograde flushing via the frontal sinuses and nasal passages via tubes implanted for several days (Fig 7.17)
- oral therapy.

Flushing the nasal passages and sinuses with clotrimazole, and maintaining the drug in situ for one hour under anaesthesia is currently recommended. Refractory cases may be treated with implantation of tubes into the nasal passages and sinuses and flushing twice daily with enilconazole. This involves a longer treatment period but has a higher success rate. Open drainage of the nasal passages via a dorsal rhinotomy and topical instillation of an antifungal drug has been recommended for intractable cases. Oral therapy with ketoconazole, fluconazole or itraconazole does not have a high success rate, may be expensive, and has the potential risk of hepatotoxicity.

Neoplasia of the nasal passages and frontal sinuses Nasal tumours are uncommon – rep-resenting less than 2% of all canine tumours. Most tumours are malignant and of epithelial origin and include adenocarcinoma, squamous cell carcinoma and undifferentiated carcinoma. Mesenchymal tumours in the dog include chondrosarcoma, osteosarcoma and fibrosarcoma, whereas lymphoma is more common in the cat. Tumours may develop anywhere within the nasal passages and progressive local invasion is a common feature. Metastasis occurs in approximately 10–40% of tumours and may involve the regional lymph nodes or lungs. All breeds may be affected, although brachycephalics are somewhat under-represented.

The clinical signs may be insidious in onset or may begin acutely. Sneezing, a thin serosanguinous discharge (which may become purulent if secondary infection supervenes), and intermittent epistaxis are usual. These signs are usually unilateral at onset, but may become bilateral. With more advanced lesions, epiphora, facial distortion and exophthalmos may be seen. Neurological signs may be seen with invasion of the cranial vault.

Radiographs may show turbinate destruction and superimposition of a soft tissue opacity, particularly in the caudal half of the nasal passages (Fig 7.18). Destruction of the supporting bones of the nasal passages (nasal and frontal bones and hard palate) may also be seen. A soft tissue opacity in the sinuses may

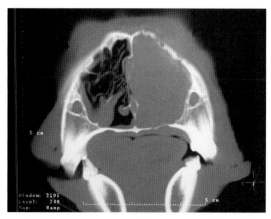

Figure 7.18   Transverse CT of the nasal passages showing a nasal tumour.

reflect retention of secretions secondary to obstruction of the outflow or neoplastic invasion of the sinus. Thoracic radiographs should be made, although they are usually unremarkable at presentation. Definitive diagnosis requires biopsy. The lymph nodes should be evaluated, e.g. by fine needle aspirate, if they are enlarged.

Treatment

- *Surgery*. Surgical excision of the tumour is not a curative process. At best, the procedure can only achieve cytoreduction, since a compartmental excision cannot be obtained within the confines of the nasal passages. Rapid local recurrence is therefore a consistent outcome unless the surgery is combined with an adjuvant therapeutic modality. Cryosurgery may provide short-term palliation but will not improve survival.
- *Radiotherapy*. External beam therapy, from either orthovoltage or megavoltage sources, is the main therapy for nasal tumours. This will treat the entire nasal cavity, including that tumour invading the nasal bones – which cannot be removed by surgery. The beam is directed via dorsal and lateral fields, to reduce damage to normal nasal tissue. Complications include the development of rhinitis, nasal fistulae and keratoconjunctivitis sicca. Brachytherapy, using iridium-192 isotopes after-loaded into catheters

placed into the nasal passages during cytoreduction of the tumour, has also been reported.

- *Chemotherapy*. Chemotherapy is restricted to the treatment of nasal lymphoma. There are no objective reports of response to cytotoxic therapy for other tumour types.

Prognosis   The prognosis for untreated nasal tumours is poor, with survival times averaging approximately 6 months or less. Surgical management may alleviate the signs of discharge and nasal obstruction, but does not improve the prognosis. The best results are achieved using radiotherapy, with or without cytoreductive surgery. Various studies report survival times ranging from 8 to 25 months. The prognosis for sarcomas is better than for carcinomas, and adenocarcinomas respond better than squamous cell carcinoma or undifferentiated carcinoma.

Nasal foreign bodies   Foreign bodies may either be inhaled directly via the external nares, or may be ingested and then gain access to the caudal passages and nasopharynx following retching or coughing. Occasionally, foreign bodies may penetrate the soft palate and enter the nasopharynx.

Rostrally located foreign bodies may be removed with forceps via the external nares. Foreign bodies in the caudal nasopharynx may be removed with forceps following rostral retraction of the soft palate. Flushing of the nasal passages with saline in a rostral to caudal direction may allow dislodgement of some foreign bodies. Inaccessible foreign bodies are removed via a dorsal or ventral rhinotomy. The foreign body is removed, along with any abnormal, inflamed tissue. The inflammation and infection caused by a foreign body may persist as chronic rhinitis.

Nasal trauma   Penetrating injuries to the nose and nasal passages will disrupt mucous membrane, cartilage and bone. Crush injuries are more likely to occlude the nasal passages. First aid measures such as the application of an ice-pack, topical adrenaline and cage rest are usually sufficient to control minor haemorrhage, but pressure-packing of the nasal passages under anaesthesia may be required if haemorrhage is severe.

Early exploration of the extent of damage should be performed either endoscopically or via open surgery. The aim is to re-establish an airway in the shortest period of time and to reduce the risk of chronic infection and airway stenosis. Blood clots, mucus and debris should be flushed away and the nasal passages examined. Depressed fractures of the nasal and maxillary bones should be elevated externally and alignment maintained with small pins and wires if required. Granulation tissue and bony proliferation may occlude the nasal passage if the mucosal discontinuity is large.

Surgery of the nasal passages
Indications:

- retrieval of foreign bodies
- removal of benign lesions
- management of neoplasia (in association with radiotherapy)
- management of chronic sinus disease
- management of fungal rhinitis.

Dorsal rhinotomy A dorsal midline skin incision is made from immediately caudal to the rhinarium to a point over the frontal area. The subcutaneous tissues and periosteum are reflected laterally and haemostasis achieved with diathermy. A unilateral or bilateral nasal flap is created using an oscillating saw or rongeurs, having established a rhinotomy opening with a drill. The upper limit of the flap is slightly above a line drawn between the medial canthi, while rostrally it hinges on the cartilaginous rhinarial attachment.

Access to the frontal sinus is achieved by increasing the length of a dorsal rhinotomy flap (Fig 7.19). Alternatively, the frontal sinuses may be trephined directly. A hole is made in the middle of the triangle of bone formed by the frontal process of the zygomatic bone and the zygomatic process of the frontal bone, immediately dorsal to the eye. The hole is then enlarged with rongeurs. The subcutaneous tissues and periosteum are closed with synthetic absorbable suture and the skin is closed routinely.

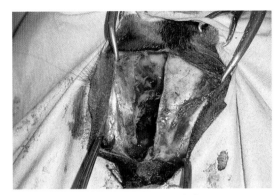

Figure 7.19   Dorsal rhinotomy and sinusotomy approach.

Ventral rhinotomy The ventral approach provides a more cosmetic approach and allows access to the ventral portion of the nasal passages, although access is more restricted. A ventral midline incision is made and the mucoperiosteum reflected laterally to expose the palatine bone. A section of the palatine bone is removed with a bone saw, cutting burr or osteotome. The palatine bone is not generally preserved. The incision may be closed in a one layer, or the periosteal/submucosal tissue and mucosal/submucosal tissue may be closed separately.

Palate

Anatomy
The soft palate forms the floor of the nasopharynx and the roof of the oropharynx. It is a mobile, muscular sheet, which has a valve-like action. It can be elevated to close the proximal airway during swallowing or depressed to close off the oral cavity during nose-breathing. It is continuous with the hard palate rostrally and its caudal free border curves laterally to form the palatopharyngeal arches, which merge with the walls of the pharynx. The hard palate forms a rigid bony partition between the oral and nasal cavities.

Diseases of the palate
Overlong soft palate An overlong soft palate is one of the major contributory features of the brachycephalic airway obstruction

syndrome. Its relative oversize in the compressed nasopharyngeal space of the brachycephalic dog causes obstruction of the nasopharynx and oropharynx.

Surgical management consists of resection of the caudal free border of the soft palate (Fig 7.20). The level of resection is important and should not generally be made cranial to the level of the caudal limit of the tonsils, to prevent nasopharyngeal reflux. The surgical technique consists of placing right-angled clamps across the palate at the appropriate level and resection of the palate, using the clamps as a guide. The free border is then oversewn with a synthetic absorbable suture material which is tightened as the clamps are removed. Haemostasis is of major importance, since even mild bleeding may compromise the already narrowed airway. Improvement is seen almost immediately postoperatively, although this may deteriorate temporarily with swelling of the tissues.

Cleft of the secondary palate The secondary palate consists of the hard and soft palates. Cleft hard palate may be present as a sole entity or as part of a cleft primary palate or cleft soft palate. Major clefts of the hard palate usually involve the soft palate (Fig 7.21). The criteria for successful closure of defects of the hard and soft palates are:

- closure in multiple layers

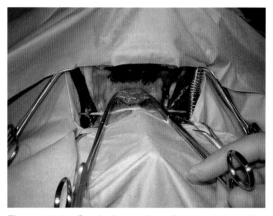

Figure 7.20   Surgical resection of an overlong soft palate.

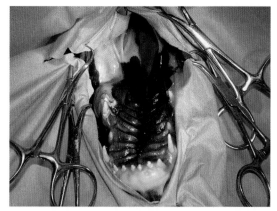

Figure 7.21   Cleft of the hard and soft palate (secondary palate).

- offsetting the suture lines from the midline and from each other
- tension-free apposition of the suture line
- support of suture lines by bone.

Dehiscence is a problem and may result from:

- sutures placed too tightly
- incomplete mobilisation of tissue
- growth of tissues
- lack of available tissue
- movement of tissues due to tongue movement and respiratory pressures
- poor blood supply.

Closure of hard palate defects These may be closed by sliding bipedicle flaps (Langenbeck technique) or by a single overlapping flap.

Bipedicle flaps are created by making releasing incisions in the mucosa and periosteum (mucoperiosteum) of the hard palate medial and parallel to the dental arcade. This creates a flap of tissue still attached rostrally and caudally. The mucoperiosteum is elevated and the flaps are moved towards the midline to cover the defect. This technique is relatively simple to perform. However, it places the suture line over the midline defect in the hard palate and it is difficult to close rostral defects with this technique.

An overlapping flap is created by making an incision as above along one side of the hard palate and elevating the mucoperiosteum to form a flap. On the other side of the defect, an incision is made in the hard palate at the border of the defect. The mucoperiosteal flap created first is flipped over and its free border tucked into the incision in the hard palate on the opposite side. This technique places the suture line away from the midline and is more successful for closing rostral defects.

Closure of soft palate defects   The margins of the cleft are incised to separate the oral and nasal mucosa. Three layers should be evident: the nasal mucosa, the palatal muscles and the oral mucosa. Each of these layers is closed separately with simple interrupted or continuous sutures.

Oronasal fistulae   Acquired oronasal fistulae are communications between the nasal and oral cavities. They may be caused by:

- trauma
- dental disease
- oronasal neoplasia
- radiotherapy
- iatrogenic factors following oral or nasal surgery.

Most oronasal fistulae require reconstruction, although small or traumatic fistulae may close spontaneously. They may be closed by:

- simple apposition of the wound edges
- mucosal flaps
- mucoperiosteal flaps.

Flap techniques are likely to be more successful because they result in less tension and more support of the repair. Flaps of adjacent mucosa or mucoperiosteum are prepared and advanced, transposed or flipped over to close the defect.

Pharynx

Anatomy

The pharynx may be divided into the oropharynx (caudal to the oral cavity), the nasopharynx (caudal to the nasal passages) and the laryngopharynx (immediately rostral to the larynx). The nasopharynx is a tubular space which extends from the caudal limits of the nasal passages (choanae) to the larynx.

Diseases of the pharynx

Pharyngeal hypertrophy   Chronic negative airway pressure and obesity may contribute to pharyngeal wall hypertrophy and weakening. The pharyngeal wall may become thrown up into redundant folds which, because of their inherent weakness, permit partial collapse of the pharyngeal diameter during respiration. Resection of mucosa may be performed, but it is difficult to improve pharyngeal rigidity.

Pharyngeal mucocoele   A salivary mucocoele is a collection of saliva in the tissues that has leaked from a gland or its duct. In the dog, this commonly affects the sublingual gland. This generally gives rise to a fluctuant ventral cervical swelling. Collection of the saliva in a sublingual position occurs in some cases and leads to a sublingual mucocoele or ranula. The least common manifestation of this disease is collection of the saliva in the tissues adjacent to the pharynx, as a pharyngeal mucocoele. In this location the accumulation of saliva causes the wall of the pharynx to bulge medially, producing progressive airway obstruction. Treatment is by surgical removal of the sublingual and mandibular salivary glands and drainage of the mucocoele.

Tonsils

Anatomy

The paired palatine tonsils are masses of lymphoid tissue in the lateral walls of the oropharynx caudal to the palatoglossal arch and ventral to the soft palate. The tonsils sit within and are generally covered by the tonsillar crypt.

Diseases of the tonsils

Tonsillar hypertrophy   Enlargement of the tonsils contributing to airway obstruction (Fig 7.22) is generally considered to be a secondary change. This may occur because of the conformation of the brachycephalic pharynx, which tends to result in tonsillar eversion and chronic inflammation of their exposed surfaces, or the increased negative airway pressure developed by animals with airway obstruction,

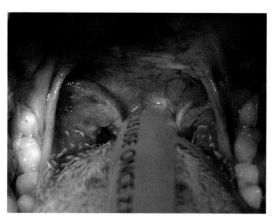

Figure 7.22   Tonsillar hypertrophy.

which leads to collapse of structures within the pharynx.

Their contribution to the syndrome of upper airway obstruction is not clear. However, it is generally considered that removal of enlarged tonsils will improve airway dynamics. Tonsillectomy is performed by resecting the tonsil distal to a right-angled clamp placed across the base of the tonsil. The pedicle is then over-sewn to control haemorrhage, and the clamp removed as the suture is tightened.

Tonsillar tumours   Tonsillar tumours are uncommon and most are squamous cell carcinomas. Melanomas and lymphoma have been reported. Metastasis to the cervical lymph nodes occurs very early in the disease and some patients present with marked lymphadenopathy in the absence of gross changes in the tonsil. Dysphagia may result from pain associated with the lesion and the physical size of the enlarged lymph nodes. Pulmonary metastases are present in 10–20% of cases at presentation. Systemic spread of the disease is considered to be present in more than 90% of patients at the time of diagnosis.

Fine needle aspirate of the tonsil or lymph nodes or tonsillectomy will confirm the diagnosis. Tonsillectomy is not likely to be curative, but it should be performed bilaterally, if at all, because of the high incidence of bilateral disease. Regional irradiation of the pharynx and cervical lymph nodes is a palliative measure, with only 10% of animals alive at

one year. No effective chemotherapeutic agents exist.

Larynx

Anatomy

The larynx (Fig 7.23) is a semi-rigid fibroelastic cylinder which joins the upper and lower respiratory tracts. Three major and two minor hyaline cartilages are embedded in this fibroelastic membrane to maintain a patent airway and to provide support for the moving parts. The larger cartilages comprise the flap-like epiglottis rostrally, the horseshoe-shaped thyroid cartilage in the middle and the ring-shaped cricoid cartilage, which attaches to the trachea, caudally. The cricoid and thyroid cartilages are joined by the firm cricothyroid articulation and provide the rigid chassis of the larynx. The paired arytenoid cartilages, which are joined dorsally in the midline by a sesamoidean band, protrude into the lumen of the larynx. The gap between their corniculate processes forms the dorsal part of the rima glottidis.

A vocal ligament arises from the most ventral part of each arytenoid (the vocal process) and these meet in the ventral midline. These form the core of the vocal folds and the ventral part of the rima glottidis. Similar, but smaller, vestibular folds lie parallel to and rostral to the vocal folds. The laryngeal ventricles consist of a ventricular depression lateral to the vocal fold and a ventricular saccule at its base.

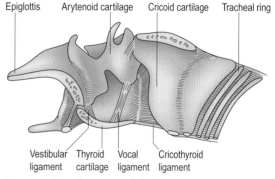

Figure 7.23   Anatomy of the larynx.

The extrinsic muscles of the larynx work with the muscles of the hyoid apparatus to elevate, depress, protract or retract the larynx. The intrinsic muscles of the larynx control the diameter of the rima glottidis. The only abductor of the rima glottidis is the cricoarytenoideus dorsalis. The caudal laryngeal nerve, which is the terminal branch of the recurrent laryngeal nerve, is the motor supply to all the intrinsic muscles apart from the thyroideus, which is supplied by the external branch of the cranial laryngeal nerve.

The larynx has a valve-like function and is concerned with:

- control of airway diameter during breathing
- vocalisation
- protection of the lower airway from inhalation of debris.

Diseases of the larynx

Laryngeal paralysis Laryngeal paralysis is the complete or partial failure of the arytenoid cartilages and vocal folds to abduct during inspiration. This usually results from an interruption of the innervation of the intrinsic muscles of the larynx, although dysfunction of the intrinsic muscles of the larynx and cricothyroid ankylosis will have a similar effect.

Interruption of the innervation of the intrinsic muscles of the larynx prevents normal function. Inadequate abduction of the arytenoids increases airway resistance and results in respiratory stridor and exercise intolerance. Inadequate laryngeal adduction during swallowing predisposes to aspiration of food and secretions, and may lead to coughing and aspiration pneumonia. Alteration in the control of the arytenoids will lead to a change in vocalisation.

Idiopathic laryngeal paralysis accounts for the majority of the cases and is particularly prevalent in the medium to large breeds, especially males. The defect is unknown, although paralysis may also arise in the context of a generalised polyneuropathy or myopathy syndrome. It has been suggested that animals with hypothyroidism may be predisposed. Congenital laryngeal paralysis is recorded in the Bouvier des Flandres and Siberian Husky. Acquired paralysis may also occur from trauma to the neck, space-occupying lesions of the neck and cranial mediastinum, and iatrogenic damage during head and neck surgery.

Clinical signs Generally, laryngeal paralysis has a slow and insidious onset. Inspiratory stridor is the main finding and may be associated with a variable degree of exercise intolerance. Severely affected animals may exhibit cyanosis and syncope. Signs are exacerbated by a warm environment and by exercise, excitement or stress. A change in the character of the bark (dysphonia) and dysphagia while eating or drinking may be noted.

Diagnosis The presenting signs and signalment will lead to a high index of suspicion. Auscultation of the airway may localise the stridor to the larynx. Radiography is of use to rule out other causes of abnormal respiratory noises and dyspnoea and to identify conditions which may be associated with laryngeal paralysis, e.g. a cranial mediastinal mass, megaoesophagus, and aspiration pneumonia. Ultrasonographic examination of the larynx may be performed and the lack of movement of the vocal folds and arytenoids may be appreciated.

Definitive diagnosis rests on observation of the larynx under a light plane of anaesthesia. Incremental doses of an intravenous induction agent should be given until jaw tone is just lost. Too deep a plane of anaesthesia will abolish laryngeal function in all patients and will result in a period of apnoea. Laryngoscopy will reveal that the arytenoid cartilages and vocal folds lie in a paramedian position and there is lack of abduction during inspiration. Movement of the arytenoids and vocal folds may be out of phase with respiration, and they may be drawn into the lumen of the larynx on inspiration or may oscillate. Inflammation of the tonsils, pharynx and larynx may be present. The majority of cases of idiopathic laryngeal paralysis are bilateral; unilateral paralysis suggests a unilateral lesion.

Treatment Animals with asymptomatic laryngeal paralysis may initially require no treatment, particularly if they maintain a sedentary lifestyle and avoid excessive weight gain and stress. However, clinical signs are likely to progress and surgery is recommended for animals which display respiratory distress. Medical therapy may be required to alleviate animals in an acute respiratory crisis and immediately postoperatively. If possible, aspiration pneumonia should be treated before surgery. The presence of concurrent mega-oesophagus is a poor prognostic sign.

Emergency medical therapy for animals in a cyanotic crisis

- Administer oxygen by mask, nasal catheter, or oxygen cage
- Cool if hyperthermic (>105°F/40.5°C) with an alcohol or ice water bath or shower
- Give corticosteroids (0.1–1mg/kg dexamethasone IV) to reduce laryngeal oedema and inflammation
- Sedate, with caution, if markedly distressed (e.g. acepromazine 0.01–0.03mg/kg IM, SC with an opiate)
- Additional therapy for pulmonary oedema if present (frusemide 2–4 mg/kg IV, IM, SC)
- Intravenous fluids may be indicated but should be instituted with caution in patients with pulmonary oedema
- Emergency tracheostomy
- General anaesthesia followed by gradual wakening or elective temporary tracheostomy.

In most cases, it may be better to perform definitive surgical correction than a tracheostomy.

Surgical management of laryngeal paralysis
The aim of surgical management of laryngeal paralysis is the permanent enlargement of the rima glottidis to improve the restricted airflow. A number of procedures have been suggested, and there is some controversy as to which is the most appropriate. Each technique has its advantages and disadvantages and ultimately the surgeon's choice may depend on familiarity with the technique and personal preference. The adoption of one surgical technique, which is associated with a high success rate and a low incidence of complications, in order

to gain familiarity and proficiency with it, is a suitable goal. To this end, unilateral arytenoid lateralisation has much to recommend it, and the other procedures are described solely for completeness.

The procedures may be divided into those which remain outside the lumen of the larynx and those which disrupt structures with in the laryngeal lumen:

Extralaryngeal procedures

- arytenoid lateralisation
- laryngeal re-innervation
  these procedures aim to dilate the rima without entering the laryngeal lumen and, in most cases, are preferred. They have the following advantages:
  - endotracheal intubation can be performed and routine inhalation anaesthesia used
  - the risk of aspiration during surgery and postoperatively is low
  - the postoperative care required, particularly temporary tracheostomy, is reduced
  - the incidence of intralaryngeal scarring is very low

Intra-laryngeal procedures

- partial laryngectomy (ventriculocordectomy, partial arytenoidectomy)
- castellated laryngofissure
  these procedures involve entering the lumen of the larynx and are associated with significant intraoperative and postoperative complications:
  - endotracheal intubation may be precluded during the procedure, necessitating either a temporary tracheostomy or total intravenous anaesthesia
  - blood, secretions or debris may be aspirated into the lower airway, particularly if an endotracheal tube is not in place
  - the tracheostomy tube may need to be maintained postoperatively until the surgically-induced laryngeal oedema has resolved
  - surgical disruption of the laryngeal mucosa or cartilages is associated with intralaryngeal scarring and webbing, which may lead to stenosis of the airway.

Laryngeal collapse and eversion of the ventricles Chronic obstructive airway disease results in increased negative pressure in the airway on inspiration and turbulent airflow, which leads to progressive, secondary changes in many structures in the airway. Initially, the mucosa of the larynx and pharynx becomes thickened and oedematous. This also involves the mucosa of the laryngeal ventricles, which may be forced to evert into the ventral rima glottidis. As the condition progresses, the laryngeal cartilages lose their structural rigidity and collapse toward the midline. The leading and lateral edges of the epiglottis roll inward and the cartilage folds dorsally towards the glottis. The weaker regions of the arytenoids, including the cuneiform processes, collapse medially, drawing the corniculate processes with them. The rima glottidis becomes progressively narrowed by these changes.

The condition generally arises secondary to another obstructive disease of the upper airway in brachycephalic dogs, such as stenotic nares and overlong soft palate. It may also be seen as a sequel to tracheal collapse and hypoplasia. Laryngeal collapse is occasionally seen in young Bull terriers during the first year. This may be due to an underlying cartilage abnormality, causing a weakened larynx. Laryngeal collapse will result in inspiratory stridor and exercise intolerance. Clinical signs associated with stenotic nares and overlong soft palate may also be present. The presence of continuing dyspnoea following management of these two conditions should raise the suspicion of laryngeal collapse.

Laryngoscopy will reveal glistening, pea-sized everted laryngeal saccules immediately rostral to the vocal folds in the initial stages. In more severely affected animals, the rima glottidis will be obscured by the inverting epiglottis and arytenoids. In many animals, this disease is progressive and secondary to an underlying problem. Hence, early detection and management of the underlying disease is necessary to limit the progression of the disease. Surgical management of primary lesions such as stenotic nares and overlong soft palate,

and resection of hyperplastic tonsils or hypertrophic pharyngeal mucosal folds may improve airway dynamics sufficiently to allow the resolution of mucosal oedema and eversion of the saccules.

Resection of the laryngeal saccules may be performed if the condition does not respond as above. Partial laryngectomy, consisting of ventriculocordectomy and partial arytenoidectomy, is of theoretical benefit to enlarge the diameter of the airway. However, the relatively high complication rate and the need for repeated surgery to maintain the airway means that long-term results are not good. Arytenoid lateralisation is not effective in this condition, since these animals lack the normal rigid laryngeal chassis essential for the success of the procedure. Permanent tracheostomy has a role to play in the management of this condition, since it not only bypasses the narrowed airway but also relieves the high negative airway pressures generated by these patients and may slow the progression of the laryngeal collapse.

Laryngeal trauma Trauma to the larynx is uncommon, due to the relatively protected position of the larynx and its mobility. Blunt trauma may be caused by bite wounds, choke chain injuries and crushing injuries from road traffic accidents. Penetrating trauma may occur from stick penetration injuries or bite wounds. Trauma may result in fracture or dislocation of the cartilages and associated hyoid apparatus, direct penetration of the lumen or nerve damage, which may result in laryngeal paralysis. Acutely, the laryngeal lumen may be obstructed by haemorrhage, oedema or prolapsed cartilages. In the long term, fibrosis of the normal cartilage articulations and glottic stenosis, resulting from intralaryngeal scarring, may cause obstruction.

Obstruction of the airway will generally cause obvious signs of respiratory distress. External wounds may be present, along with subcutaneous emphysema from air leaking out of the larynx into the perilaryngeal tissues. Laryngoscopy should be performed to assess the severity of the damage once the patient has been stabilised. Emergency measures may be required to ensure a patent airway, such as removing haemorrhage and debris from the airway by suction or performing a temporary tracheostomy to bypass the larynx.

Laryngeal stenosis   Any disease or trauma to the laryngeal cartilages or overlying mucosa may result in the development of scar tissue or proliferative granulation tissue which narrows the glottis. External trauma, intralaryngeal surgery, traumatic endotracheal intubation and proliferative laryngitis may be the cause of the original injury.

Laryngeal tumours   Tumours of the larynx are rare in the dog and cat. In the dog, squamous cell carcinoma, adenocarcinoma, chondrosarcoma, fibrosarcoma and osteosarcoma have been recorded, whereas in the cat, lymphoma, squamous cell carcinoma and adenocarcinoma may occur. The benign tumours chondroma and oncocytoma have also been recorded in the dog. The cell of origin of the oncocytoma is unclear, but it may be related to striated muscle cells, akin to rhabdomyoma. Oncocytomas may attain a large size, are minimally invasive and do not appear to metastasise. Most other laryngeal tumours are locally invasive and have a significant metastatic potential.

Clinical signs are those of a progressive obstructive disorder at the level of the larynx. Inspiratory stridor, exercise intolerance, dysphonia, dysphagia and cough may be seen. Laryngeal tumours are not generally palpable externally. Radiographs of the larynx may reveal the lesion, but are rarely required. Thoracic radiographs should be taken to rule out metastases. Definitive diagnosis is by laryngoscopy and biopsy. Care should be taken, since the airway may be compromised already by the space-occupying lesion and biopsy carries with it the risk of haemorrhage, which may further compromise the airway lumen, and the risk of post-biopsy scarring. An endotracheal tube should be placed, or tracheostomy performed.

Very few laryngeal tumours are candidates for definitive surgical excision. The single exception to this is the oncocytoma, which is usually found as a discrete mass underneath the laryngeal mucosa and which may be removed by careful submucosal dissection. Partial laryngectomy is a theoretical option, but is associated with all the risks of intralaryngeal surgery – postoperative function and survival times are not good. Total laryngectomy with permanent tracheostomy is another theoretical option, but is associated with a high rate of complications and a relatively short survival time. Permanent tracheostomy alone may be used as a palliative measure. There are few reports of the use of radiotherapy for laryngeal tumours, although this option is more likely to preserve laryngeal function. Chemotherapy has a role in the management of lymphoma of the larynx in the cat, but its role in the management of other tumour types is not clear.

The prognosis associated with malignant laryngeal tumours is poor. Radical excision is not possible and since the main concern is interference with airway function, many animals are euthanased at an early stage of the disease.

Granulomatous laryngitis   This is an uncommon, chronic proliferative inflammatory disease of the larynx of dogs. It must be differentiated from neoplasia by biopsy. The proliferating lesions are found around the arytenoid processes and cause airway obstruction. Treatment is with prednisolone, with or without surgical debulking of the lesions. Surgery may allow immediate increase in the diameter of the airway, but carries with it the risk of scarring and adhesions postoperatively.

Laryngeal surgery

Surgical management of laryngeal paralysis is the most common indication for laryngeal surgery in small animals, and most of the procedures discussed are involved with this. Apart from this, laryngotomy is occasionally performed to gain access to the lumen of the larynx for inspection, biopsy or removal of lesions. Total laryngectomy with permanent tracheostomy has been recommended for the management of gross laryngeal lesions (e.g. malignant tumours, severe trauma), but is not commonly performed.

Arytenoid lateralisation The aim of this technique is to mobilise the arytenoid and to fix it in abduction, thus mimicking the action of the dorsal cricoarytenoid muscle. Although idiopathic laryngeal paralysis is a bilateral condition, unilateral surgery is usually performed. This is because a small increase in the diameter of the larynx will result in a large increase in the airflow through it. In addition, bilateral surgery is associated with a high risk of aspiration pneumonia. For most right-handed surgeons, it is convenient to operate of the left side of the larynx.

Surgical technique The jugular vein is occluded and its course from the confluence of the linguofacial and external maxillary veins is identified. The hyoid apparatus, larynx and trachea may also be palpated directly and wing of the thyroid may be flexed laterally. These manoeuvres are difficult in obese animals. A skin incision is made immediately below the jugular vein extending from the caudal aspect of the vertical ramus of the mandible for 6–8cm. The subcutaneous fascia and fat is divided to reveal the panniculus muscle, which is divided along the same line.

The thyropharyngeus muscle, which wraps around the body of the larynx, is identified and incised. The junction between the cricoid and thyroid cartilages is identified and disarticulated with scissors and the wing of the thyroid cartilage reflected laterally with retractors. The muscular process of the arytenoid is identified by palpation. This is easier in long-standing cases where atrophy of cricoarytenoideus dorsalis is more marked. This muscle is isolated and incised mid-belly. The cricoarytenoid articulation is identified and disrupted with scissors.

The approximate position of the interarytenoid sesamoid band, which lies immediately rostral to the rostromedial limit of the cricoarytenoid articulation, is identified. This band lies between the two arytenoid cartilages in the midline and is approximately 1mm in diameter. This structure is difficult to see and must be sectioned blindly.

The arytenoid is now only attached to the laryngeal mucosa and the vocal fold. The muscular process is grasped and the mobility compared to that present before sectioning of the interarytenoid band. Successful cricoarytenoid disarticulation and sectioning of the interarytenoid band confers increased mobility such that the muscular process may easily be retracted caudally from its original position to lie adjacent to the caudal aspect of the wing of the thyroid.

A horizontal mattress suture of 3 metric polypropylene (Prolene; Ethicon) is placed from the caudal aspect of the wing of the thyroid through the muscular process of the arytenoid and then back through the arytenoid and thyroid. Gentle technique, a sharp atraumatic needle and relatively large bites of tissue are required to avoid fragmenting the arytenoid cartilage. The suture is tied with care, ensuring sufficient abduction of the arytenoid. Alternatively, cricoarytenoid laryngoplasty may be performed, which should theoretically give more anatomic abduction, but a thyroarytenoid suture is more easily and accurately placed.

The adequacy of arytenoid abduction may be ascertained by inspection of the airway. The patient is extubated, the airway cleaned of mucus with a swab in the jaws of long-handled forceps and the larynx examined.

Postoperative care The animal should be monitored very closely during recovery. The patient is maintained in sternal recumbency and restrained until extubation, which is delayed as long as possible. The animal should be allowed to recover in a cool, stress-free environment, and allowed to adopt a comfortable position.

With successful surgery, the respiratory distress is usually relieved immediately. However, supplemental oxygen should be available and an agitated patient may require sedation. If signs of upper respiratory tract obstruction persist, then inspection of the airway and re-intubation followed by an elective, temporary tracheostomy may be required.

An intravenous bolus of a broad-spectrum bactericidal antibiotic is given prior to surgery and further doses are given at intervals dictated by the half-life of the drug, but need not continue beyond 24 hours. In a debilitated patient, the implantation of a permanent suture material in a potentially clean-contaminated surgical site may prompt additional therapy. Aspiration pneumonia should be treated aggressively with antibiotics and coupage. Corticosteroids may be given in patients with marked laryngeal oedema. Adequate analgesia should be provided.

It is often recommended that feeding should begin 12–24 hours postoperatively, although many animals can tolerate food earlier. Dogs are better fed from a low position and abrasive or sloppy food should be avoided. Animals fed canned food generally swallow discrete boluses of food, which decreases the likelihood of aspiration. Many dogs will initially cough and gag somewhat when eating because of temporary glottic dysfunction.

Strenuous exercise and barking should be discouraged for 6 weeks postoperatively. Sedation may be required for agitated patients postoperatively. For these reasons it is often better to discharge these patients into the home environment as soon as possible.

Complications Unilateral arytenoid lateralisation is a technique with a relatively simple anatomical approach. However, it requires meticulous surgical technique and great familiarity with the regional anatomy of the larynx. It is recommended that the surgeon observes the technique before performing it. Attention to haemostasis is particularly important. Various studies have demonstrated an excellent clinical outcome in more than 90% of patients.

Many complications are common to other surgical techniques of the upper respiratory tract. The potential complications include:

- haemorrhage
- laryngeal oedema
- aspiration

- penetration of the laryngeal lumen
- oesophageal laceration
- inadequate dilation of the rima glottidis
- fragmentation of the arytenoids.

Haemorrhage is generally mild to moderate and relatively easily controlled with pressure and the judicious use of electrocautery. Meticulous haemostasis is important to prevent submucosal bleeding which may compromise the airway diameter, or may result in aspiration of blood if the laryngeal lumen is inadvertently entered. Postoperatively, laryngeal and perilaryngeal oedema, if it did not exist preoperatively, is rarely of clinical significance, and is reduced by gentle surgical technique, the appropriate use of corticosteroids and minimal electrocautery. Animals are predisposed to aspiration because arytenoid lateralisation interrupts normal glottic closure during swallowing and results in a permanently enlarged rima glottidis. However, aspiration pneumonia is uncommon after unilateral procedures.

Inadvertent penetration of the laryngeal lumen may occur, particularly when sectioning the interarytenoid sesamoid band. This will often cause no problems, although animals should be closely monitored for signs of upper respiratory obstruction. Oesophageal laceration is a potential complication which may be avoided by dorsal retraction of the oesophagus and a thorough knowledge of the regional anatomy. Treatment is with copious lavage and closure of the defect with sutures.

Inadequate dilation of the rima glottidis, resulting in continued clinical signs, may be caused by inadequate mobilisation of the arytenoid, incorrect suture placement, inadequate tension on the suture or suture pull-through. In addition, complete lateralisation is not possible if the arytenoids are chronically fixed in the midline. Success is also poor if the animal has concurrent laryngeal collapse. Fragmentation, fracture or laceration of the arytenoid during surgery is an occasional complication and may require that the contralateral arytenoid is abducted. Occasionally, poor results are obtained with unilateral lateralisation, particularly when generalised neuromuscular disease is present. In this case, bilateral procedure may be indicated, although this carries with it an increased risk of aspiration pneumonia.

Laryngeal re-innervation Re-innervation of the larynx by neuromuscular pedicle grafts or nerve anastomosis has been reported in dogs. Experimental studies have shown that the dorsal cricoarytenoid muscle can be re-innervated by transplanting a neuromuscular pedicle based on the first cervical nerve. Dogs gain abductor function over 9–11 months. The sternothyroid muscle is chosen since it is not innervated by the recurrent laryngeal nerve, it is an inspiratory muscle (and therefore provides synchronous abduction of the rima), and it has a nerve supply long enough to allow transplantation without undue tension on the graft.

However, there are a number of practical problems associated with this procedure. Firstly, it has only proved to be of use in acutely denervated muscle and its effectiveness in idiopathic laryngeal paralysis, where a chronic neuropathy is the underlying cause, is unknown. Secondly, re-innervation of the intrinsic muscles of the larynx may be indiscriminate, such that simultaneous contraction of the abductors and adductors may occur, resulting in inco-ordinated movements of the arytenoids. Finally, the long interval between surgery and an acceptable function is too long a delay for the animal with marked laryngeal obstruction.

Microsurgical repair of the caudal laryngeal nerve has been proposed for acute traumatic lesions.

Partial laryngectomy This technique aims to remove a portion of the vocal folds or arytenoids which are obstructing the airway. A temporary tracheostomy is performed, or alternatively the endotracheal tube may be placed and removed intermittently to allow access to the surgical site.

Ventriculocordectomy is performed by grasping the vocal fold with long dissecting forceps and tensing it rostrally. The vocal fold and adjacent vocalis muscle is then resected, beginning at its attachment to the vocal process. Leaving a small section of mucosa at the ventral commissure of the rima glottidis between the resected folds may reduce the risk of postoperative scarring. The procedure is performed bilaterally.

Partial arytenoidectomy is performed in conjunction with ventriculocordectomy. Crocodile-action cup biting forceps are used to resect a portion of the arytenoid cartilage. Removal of the corniculate, cuneiform and vocal processes may be performed, although removal of the corniculate process alone may reduce the incidence of postoperative complications.

Haemorrhage is controlled by applying pressure with a small dental sponge in the jaws of long-handled forceps. Blood clots and debris should be removed using suction.

Complications Aspiration pneumonia is a relatively frequent complication following ventriculocordectomy and partial arytenoidectomy. Performing ventriculocordectomy alone and the use of a tracheostomy tube with an inflatable cuff may reduce the incidence of this complication. Glottic stenosis may be seen as a long-term complication. Granulation tissue proliferation and intralaryngeal scarring and webbing are difficult to manage and may recur after resection. Postoperative oedema may cause laryngeal obstruction, necessitating temporary tracheostomy. The perioperative use of corticosteroids (dexamethasone sodium phosphate 0.25–1mg/kg IV) or methylprednisolone sodium succinate (0.5–2mg/kg IV) may reduce the incidence of this complication.

Castellated laryngofissure This technique involves making a step-like ventral laryngotomy incision in the thyroid cartilage. The two halves of the thyroid cartilage are then separated, thus dilating the rima glottidis. One half of the thyroid cartilage is then moved rostrally with respect to the other and the two halves of the thyroid cartilage are then anchored in this dilated position. This procedure is combined with ventriculocordectomy and is associated with many of the complications associated with intralaryngeal surgery.

A modification of this technique involves performing bilateral arytenoid lateralisation at the same time. However, it is well known that arytenoid lateralisation alone is successful in managing laryngeal paralysis, so the rationale for the combined procedure is not clear. There are few reports of the standard or modified procedure and it is not in common use.

Resection of laryngeal saccules This is indicated in the management of the eversion of the laryngeal saccules, before the condition has progressed to laryngeal collapse. The patient is positioned in sternal recumbency, and intubated. The laryngeal saccules are approached *per os*. They are identified as small, white or reddened pea-like protrusions immediately behind the vocal folds. The saccules are grasped with dissecting forceps, tensioned rostrally and amputated at their base with fine scissors. Haemorrhage is controlled with direct pressure at the site with a small dental sponge in the jaws of a long-handled forceps.

Laryngotomy This procedure is indicated to gain access to the lumen of the larynx to inspect, biopsy or remove lesions. If the lesion can be approached *per os* through the rima glottidis, then this should be performed. An incision is made through the cricothyroid ligament and continued rostrally through the keel of the thyroid cartilage. Retractors are used to separate the two halves of the cartilage.

Total laryngectomy This technique is suggested for the management of laryngeal tumours or gross laryngeal trauma, but is not commonly performed. The trachea is transected at its junction with the cricoid cartilage and the entire larynx, including the epiglottis, is removed. The pharyngeal mucosa is then closed. A permanent tracheostomy is then performed with the proximal end of the trachea. Care of the tracheostomy site is particularly important, since this is the only way the animal can breathe.

Trachea

During tracheal surgery it is imperative that a patent airway is maintained. The surgical procedure may be complicated by the presence of an endotracheal tube in the surgical field.

Postoperative complications, such as wound dehiscence, infection and contraction, resulting in stenosis (which may cause only minor effects in other locations), pose serious threats to the success of the surgery.

Anatomy

The trachea extends from the cricoid cartilage to the bifurcation dorsal to the heart base. It consists of 35–45 C-shaped cartilages united by fibroelastic annular ligaments. The tracheal membrane forms the dorsal aspect of the trachea and is composed of the trachealis muscle and connective tissue. The trachea is lined by a ciliated columnar epithelium rich in goblet cells, which secrete mucus. During inspiration the lumen widens slightly, as a result of the trachealis muscle widening and the natural tendency of the cartilages to open, and narrows on expiration.

The trachea has a segmental blood supply which originates from the cranial and caudal thyroid arteries and runs in the lateral pedicles. Disruption of both lateral pedicles will cause ischaemia and necrosis, although preservation of one pedicle will allow sufficient blood supply to the trachea. The recurrent laryngeal nerves lie in close apposition to the trachea and should be identified and preserved. Other structures in the region include the paired thyroid glands, the oesophagus, the carotid arteries and the vagosympathetic trunk.

Diagnostic techniques

Clinical signs associated with tracheal disease include coughing, stridor, retching and exercise intolerance. Palpation may reveal focal or generalised abnormalities, e.g. collapse, hypoplasia, focal masses or stenosis, and compression may exacerbate clinical signs. Auscultation may localise focal lesions.

A full radiographic study involves separate lateral views of the cervical and thoracic trachea, during inspiration and expiration. A skyline view of the trachea at the thoracic inlet provides a transverse view, but may be difficult to obtain. Fluoroscopy improves visualisation of the trachea throughout the respiratory cycle.

Tracheoscopy may be performed with a rigid or flexible endoscope. Open tracheoscopy with a rigid endoscope has the advantage of allowing ventilation during the procedure. Endoscopic evaluation should be combined with external compression to evaluate for the presence of tracheal collapse. A tracheal wash, to collect samples of mucosal debris, may be obtained via tracheoscopy or percutaneously with a catheter.

Surgical approaches

Cervical trachea The cervical trachea extends from the cricoid cartilage to the thoracic inlet. The animal is placed in dorsal recumbency with the forelimbs secured cranially and a sandbag or towel under the neck. A ventral midline skin incision is made directly over the trachea. This incision extends through the thin platysma muscle to reveal the paired sternohyoideus and sternothyroideus muscles, which extend from the larynx to the manubrium. These muscles are separated in the midline. Extension of the incision to the level of the manubrium requires sharp division of the sternocephalicus muscles. Retraction of these ventral muscles exposes the trachea, which is easily dissected from the surrounding loose connective tissue.

Thoracic trachea The thoracic trachea and carina are approached through a right third intercostal thoracotomy. On entry into the thorax, the right cranial lobe is retracted dorsocaudally to remove it from the surgical field. The trachea is associated with the longus colli muscle dorsally, the oesophagus medially and the cranial vena cava and vagosympathetic trunk ventrolaterally. The costocervical vein crosses the cranial thoracic trachea, while the azygos vein crosses the caudal thoracic trachea. Gentle retraction of these structures allows adequate visualisation of the trachea, although both these veins may be ligated and divided to achieve adequate exposure of the trachea. The left recurrent laryngeal nerve is closely associated with the trachea and should be preserved during medial dissection of the trachea.

Tracheal wound healing

The aims of tracheal wound healing are:

- re-establishment of normal mucociliary function
- retention of normal flexibility
- retention of inherent resistance to collapse
- avoidance of stenosis.

Superficial wounds which do not extend below the tracheal submucosa, such as caused by foreign bodies and endotracheal intubation, are rapidly healed by epithelialisation within one day and a fully differentiated epithelium is present at 4 days.

Deeper wounds which penetrate the submucosal layer heal by formation of granulation tissue, with subsequent coverage by epithelium. However, this epithelium may be poorly differentiated, which interrupts normal mucociliary function, and is associated with some degree of stenosis. Hence, healing of tracheal wounds by first intention healing of accurately apposed wound edges is preferred over second intention healing.

Excessive tension at the wound will cause wound disruption, scar formation and stenosis. Stenosis is more likely in immature than mature animals. Tension increases with the number of tracheal rings which are resected. The absolute maximum number of rings which may be safely removed varies with the age and conformation of the dog and the elasticity of the trachea. Whilst experimental studies have demonstrated that 60% of the trachea may be resected in mature dogs, resection of more than 25% should not be attempted in immature animals. Resection of up to five or six tracheal rings is a reasonable upper limit for resection. Techniques to relieve tension at the anastomotic site include the use of tension sutures, division of adjacent tracheal annular ligaments, and bandages to maintain the neck in flexion. Normal mucociliary clearance is impaired by resection and anastomosis, but should return to normal within one month.

General techniques in tracheal surgery

Tracheal resection and anastomosis This is indicated for the management of:

- tracheal stenosis
- trauma
- neoplasia.

During mobilisation of the trachea, the lateral pedicles should only be dissected over the area to be resected. This should be performed as close to the trachea as possible to avoid trauma to the recurrent laryngeal nerves. Stay sutures are placed around the first cartilage ring cranial and caudal to the proposed site of resection before resection of the affected segment. Following resection, these sutures are used to manipulate the ends of the trachea during anastomosis.

Approximately five to six rings may be removed with simple local dissection of the trachea from the surrounding connective tissue. Resection of more rings requires mobilisation of a larger segment of the trachea and other measures to decrease tension on the anastomosis. Resection and anastomosis may be performed in three ways:

1. Split cartilage The trachea is divided by incising through the tracheal cartilages. Simple interrupted sutures of a synthetic monofilament material, which pass around these split cartilages and penetrate the lumen, are used to appose the two segments. Three or four retention sutures are placed around the second ring cranial and caudal to the anastomosis to reduce tension. This technique results in less stenosis, but should not be performed in smaller animals where the tracheal rings are difficult to split without causing fragmentation.

2. Split annular ligament This technique is indicated for smaller patients. The trachea is incised through the annular ligament. Suture placement is as above. Apposition of the tracheal segments is less accurate and the cranial segment tends to override the caudal segment. The risk of stenosis may be increased.

3. Split annular ligament and annular ligament repair Resection is performed through the annular ligaments, preserving as much as possible of the ligament. Simple interrupted monofilament sutures are placed through the annular ligament cranial and caudal to the site of excision. Retention sutures are used as above. This technique has a number of problems and is not recommended. There is a relatively high risk of tracheal stenosis, tissue pull-out of sutures is more likely and the technique is technically demanding.

Following resection and anastomosis, the repair should be examined for leaks. The endotracheal tube is withdrawn into the cranial segment and the trachea covered with sterile saline. Ventilation with moderate inspiratory pressure will allow the presence of leaks to be identified. The application of a Martingale-type splint to restrain the animal's neck in flexion and prevent excessive tension on the anastomotic site has been described. This needs to be maintained for 2–3 weeks postoperatively.

Complications Complications include haemorrhage, a change in vocalisation, fistula formation and cartilage malacia. Dehiscence may occur if there is excessive tension or movement at the anastomotic site. Dehiscence may be manifested as subcutaneous emphysema, acute dyspnoea, haemoptysis and subcutaneous swelling. Tracheal stenosis is promoted by excessive tension, second intention healing following dehiscence and ischaemia following damage to the blood supply. Trauma to the recurrent laryngeal nerves may result in laryngeal paralysis.

Temporary tracheostomy A temporary tracheostomy is indicated for short-term maintenance of a patent airway (Fig 7.24), usually in animals with airway obstruction at the level of the larynx or pharynx. In an emergency, they may be placed under sedation and local anaesthesia, but general anaesthesia and elective tracheostomy is preferred if possible. Indications:

- bypass of upper airway obstruction
- ventilatory management
- access to the lower airway.

Several types of tubes are available (Fig 7.25). Most tubes can be re-used after ethylene

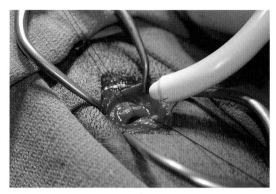

Figure 7.24 Placement of a tracheostomy tube.

oxide sterilisation. The tubes may be cuffed or non-cuffed. A cuffed tube is only essential if positive pressure ventilation is to be applied. The tubes should be flexible and minimally irritating to tissues. Tubes with an inner cannula allow the tube to remain in place while the cannula is removed and cleaned of secre-

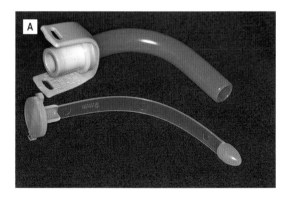

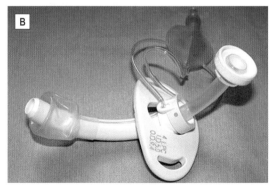

Figure 7.25 Tracheostomy tubes: (a) single piece, uncuffed, (b) two-piece, cuffed.

tions. Tracheostomy tubes may be placed in the region of the second to fifth tracheal ring. The tube may be introduced into the trachea via:

- transverse incision through the annular ligament
- longitudinal incision through tracheal rings and annular ligaments
- U-shaped flap incision
- excision of a portion of tracheal rings.

It is a matter of debate whether the precise technique influences the development of stenosis. Placement of the tube through a transverse incision between the third and fourth tracheal ring is a simple technique and is recommended. The incision should be less than 50% of the tracheal circumference to minimise stenosis. Placement of stay sutures of a synthetic monofilament suture material around the tracheal rings immediately above and below the tracheotomy incision aids manipulation of the trachea and introduction and replacement of the tube. The diameter of the tube should be approximately 50–70% of the diameter of the trachea. This avoids irritation to the trachea from a tightly-fitting tube and allows the animal to breathe around the tube if required. The tube is secured by tying loops around the animal's neck.

Postoperative management of the tube is of paramount importance. Obstruction of the tube with respiratory secretions may result in compromise and death of the patient and animals should be monitored closely and continuously if possible. Management and removal of secretions is important. A humidifier in the cage will reduce the viscosity of the secretions. If a tube with a cannula is used, the cannula should be removed and cleaned as often as required. This may be as often as every 15 minutes initially, and then every 1 hour or more as required. If a single lumen tube is used, this is removed and replaced as necessary. The use of two tubes, so that a clean tube can be immediately placed once the old one is removed is preferable.

Periodically, 2–10ml of sterile saline should be instilled into the trachea via the tube to loosen tracheal secretions. A few minutes later, the trachea should be suctioned with a long, flexible catheter to remove the secretions. The tube should be removed as soon as possible. It is difficult and detrimental to the animal to maintain the tube for longer than a few days. If maintenance of an airway is required for this period of time, a permanent tracheostomy should be performed.

Permanent tracheostomy A permanent tracheostomy (Fig 7.26) is indicated when prolonged bypass of the upper airway is required. Following exposure of the trachea, a rectangular segment is excised from the ventral trachea. This should be two to four tracheal rings in length, approximately one-third of the diameter of the trachea and centred at the third to fifth tracheal ring. The trachea may be brought into close apposition with the skin by suturing the sternohyoideus muscles dorsal to the trachea with one or more horizontal mattress sutures. A skin segment equivalent in size to the tracheal window is removed.

The subcutaneous tissues are sutured to the tracheal fascia with simple interrupted sutures. The tracheal mucosa is then incised and sutured to the skin edges with simple interrupted sutures. In animals with redundant cervical skin folds, occlusion of the stoma by these folds is occasionally encountered as a problem, and may necessitate excision of redundant tissue as a separate procedure. The stoma should be gently cleaned with warm water or saline to remove accumulated secretions, as often as required, depending on the quantity of secretions produced. Great care should be taken to avoid disrupting the suture line. After 2 weeks the stoma requires minimal care.

Animals with a permanent tracheal stoma are prone to aspiration of foreign bodies and water via the stoma. Animals should not be allowed to swim and appropriate care should be taken during bathing. Some animals may be prone to chronic respiratory tract infections and chronic mucus discharge from the airway.

Diseases of the trachea

Tracheal collapse This is a syndrome characterised by dorsoventral flattening of the tracheal rings with laxity of the dorsal tracheal membrane. It is most common in middle-aged to old toy and miniature dogs, particularly toy Poodles, Yorkshire terriers, Pomeranians and Chihuahuas, although approximately 25% of dogs are symptomatic by 6 months old. The major sign is a chronic persistent paroxysmal cough, exacerbated by exercise, excitement and pulling on the lead. The cough is typically harsh, dry and unproductive and easily elicited on tracheal palpation. A deep 'goose-honk' type cough may be present in some individuals. Gagging after coughing is often noted. Mildly affected animals may be otherwise asymptomatic, whereas more severely affected dogs may show tachypnoea, dyspnoea and, occasionally, cyanosis or syncope.

The aetiology is multifactorial. Development of the condition requires both the presence of an underlying congenital defect in the tracheal cartilage, resulting in a weakening of the rings, and the presence of secondary factors which may cause this weakness to progress to the symptomatic state. The secondary factors include:

- obesity
- recent endotracheal intubation
- respiratory tract infection
- cardiomegaly
- cervical trauma
- inhalation of irritants or allergens.

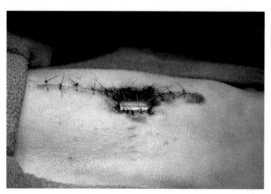

Figure 7.26   Permanent tracheostomy.

Tracheal collapse may be seen in association with other obstructive lesions of the airway, such as laryngeal collapse. Each of these diseases may exacerbate the other, and it may be difficult to know which the primary problem was.

The dynamic changes of tracheal collapse may involve the cervical or thoracic trachea, or both. The changes are often most pronounced at the thoracic inlet. Cervical tracheal collapse occurs on inspiration, because of the increased negative pressure within the trachea. Thoracic tracheal collapse occurs on expiration or coughing, because of the increased intrapleural pressure. In severely affected dogs, collapse may be observed in the bronchi. Concurrent laryngeal paralysis is reported, but is more likely to develop following surgery, with iatrogenic damage to the recurrent laryngeal nerve.

As the tracheal rings lose their normal C-shape and become flattened, the dorsal tracheal membrane becomes widened and flaccid and is drawn into the tracheal lumen, worsening the obstruction. Once clinical signs are apparent, the syndrome is perpetuated by the cycle of chronic inflammation which exacerbates the cough, which itself worsens the inflammation. Chronic inflammation results in increased viscosity of the tracheal mucus, which impairs the normal tracheal mucociliary clearance mechanism and contributes to tracheal obstruction and lower airway disease.

The presenting history is generally of a chronic, deep, 'goose-honk' type cough, which may be accompanied by intermittent bouts of acute dyspnoea. The dyspnoea may be associated with cyanosis and a variety of inspiratory and expiratory sounds. Excitement and pressure on the trachea may trigger bouts of coughing. Although the signs may wax and wane, it is a progressive condition.

Physical examination may reveal palpable collapse of the cervical trachea. Sinus arrhythmia may be marked. Auscultation of the cervical trachea may reveal turbulent airflow, and referred sounds or wheezing sounds may be heard on thoracic auscultation. Palpation may elicit a cough and may reveal some degree of collapse of the cervical trachea.

Definitive diagnosis is achieved via endoscopy and radiography. Inspiratory and expiratory radiographs (Fig 7.27) of the neck and chest may allow a diagnosis to be made in approximately 60% of patients with severe collapse. A tangential rostrocaudal view of the thoracic inlet has also been described. Fluoroscopy will demonstrate dynamic collapse in relation to the phases of respiration. Tracheoscopy will allow the degree of collapse and extent of the airway involved to be determined; laryngeal paralysis or collapse may also be noted. A grading system has been developed (Table 7.2).

Therapy   Many potential therapies exist for this multifactorial disease and a stepwise approach, tailored to the individual case, is the most appropriate. It must be remembered that anatomic collapse will not lead to clinical signs in all individuals and therefore any potentiating causes should be sought and treated. Long-term medical management is possible for many cases and this avenue should be exhausted before surgical therapy is considered.

Treatment of the potentiating causes

1. Weight reduction
2. Treatment for left-sided heart failure
3. Removal of inhaled irritants, including owner's cigarette smoke

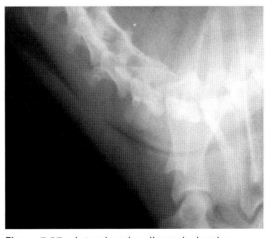

Figure 7.27   Lateral neck radiograph showing tracheal collapse.

Table 7.2   Grading system for tracheal collapse

Grade	Reduction in lumen (%)	Trachealis muscle	Cartilage shape
I	25	Slightly pendulous	Nearly circular
II	50	Pendulous, stretched	More flattened
III	75	More stretched	Nearly flat
IV	<100	Stretched, touches rings	Completely flat or inverted

4. Treatment of respiratory tract infections
5. Replacement of collar with a harness
6. Exercise restriction.

Treatment of the coughing patient

1. Antitussives. e.g. diphenoxylate/atropine (Lomotil; Searle), butorphanol
   - the aim is to reduce the chronic irritation caused by coughing
2. Glucocorticoids, e.g. prednisolone
   - a short course of these agents will also reduce the inflammation with this condition
3. Bronchodilators e.g. theophylline (Corvental; C-Vet), terbutaline
   - bronchodilation may reduce the high intrapleural pressure during expiration and reduce tracheal narrowing; however, evidence for their benefit is not clear cut.

Surgical management   The indications for surgery and appropriate technique remain controversial. Dogs which suffer significant and persistent clinical signs, despite conservative management, or which have life-threatening compromise of ventilatory function should be considered candidates for surgical management. Candidates should be free of congestive heart failure and collapse of the lower airway, since these animals are rarely improved by surgery. However, animals with advanced disease are often debilitated, with increased risk of anaesthetic and surgical complications. The aim of surgery is to support the tracheal cartilages and trachealis muscle, while preserving as much of the segmental blood and nerve supply to the trachea as possible. Many techniques have been proposed, but few are in routine use. Surgical techniques include:

tracheal ring chondrotomy, plication of the dorsal membrane, extraluminal prosthetic supports, intraluminal prosthetic supports.

1. Tracheal chondrotomy.   This involves division of alternate tracheal rings in the ventral midline. This results in the tracheal ring and the dorsal tracheal membrane adopting a triangular rather than a flattened configuration. However, the redundant tracheal membrane still falls into the trachea – this technique is associated with limited success.

2. Plication of the dorsal tracheal membrane.   This involves placing horizontal mattress sutures through the dorsal tracheal membrane to reduce its width. This has the effect of pulling the tracheal rings into a more normal C-shape. However, this technique reduces the diameter of the tracheal lumen and long-term improvement is not maintained.

3. Extraluminal prostheses.   Extraluminal prostheses, in the form of rings or spirals (Fig 7.28), may be used to support the trachea. The prostheses are made from 32ml syringe barrels or their rigid cases and have holes punched out to pass sutures through. The rings are 5mm wide and are placed at 5–10mm intervals along the trachea, with their open portion ventrally, and sutured to the trachea. Complications include some loss of tracheal flexibility, inability to support the trachea between the prostheses, and potential erosion of the ring through the trachea.

Spiral prostheses are rotated onto the trachea and fixed similarly. They have the theoretical advantage of supporting the trachea along the entire length of the prosthesis. However, the original technique involved dissection of both lateral pedicles, which is associated with a considerable risk of disrupt-

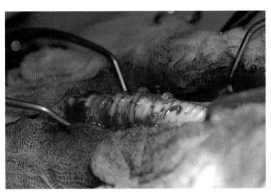

Figure 7.28   Surgical placement of external tracheal ring prostheses.

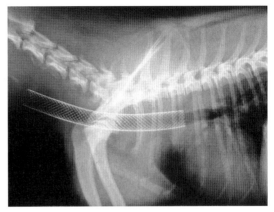

Figure 7.29   Lateral chest radiograph showing intra-luminal tracheal stent.

ing the blood supply and tracheal necrosis. A modification of this technique involves dissecting only one pedicle and making small fenestrations in the other pedicle to pass the prosthesis.

4. Intraluminal prostheses. Expandable wire cylinders have been used to provide an internal stent (Fig. 7.21).

External support with prosthetic rings is the most commonly used technique. Prosthetic rings or spirals made from polypropylene (e.g. 2-ml syringe barrels or cases) are used – rings are preferred since they interfere with the blood supply less. Rings 5–8mm wide should be created, with five or more staggered holes. Although it is recommended that the cervical and the thoracic segments should be supported if affected, application of prostheses to the thoracic trachea is associated with a high morbidity rate.

The peritracheal tissue is gently dissected only in the region of ring placement and the ring is guided around the trachea so that the gap in the ring is directed ventrally. Simple interrupted sutures are placed between the tracheal rings and holes made in the prosthetic rings. At least one suture should engage the trachealis muscle. Rings should be placed approximately 5–8 mm apart, such that approximately five or seven will be required to support the cervical trachea (Fig 7.29).

A number of complications are associated with implantation of prosthetic tracheal sup-

ports, including loosening or failure of the implant, infection, laryngeal paralysis and tracheal necrosis. Damage to the trachea results in significant impairment of the tracheal blood supply and the risk of necrosis. Arytenoid lateralisation, at the time of surgery, has been reported to improve the results. Permanent tracheostomy may be indicated for those patients with laryngeal collapse. The prognosis for older dogs (over 6 years old) is significantly worse than that for young dogs, independent of the severity of collapse on tracheoscopy.

Postoperative care Animals should be maintained in a quiet, stress-free environment. Cough suppressants should be used in the immediate postoperative period. Adequate analgesia and, in some cases, sedation may be required to reduce ventilatory stress. The presence of normal laryngeal function at the end of the procedure should be ensured. It should be emphasised that surgery for tracheal collapse may improve the condition, but will not cure it.

Tracheal hypoplasia In this condition, the tracheal rings are of normal rigidity but are reduced in diameter. The tracheal profile is normal but the reduced airway diameter results in dyspnoea. This may be exacerbated if other conditions causing airway obstruction are also present. The condition is found predominantly in English Bulldogs; pups generally show clinical signs during the first few weeks of life. In some cases, they may remain asymptomatic until the condition is exacerbated by other components of the brachycephalic airway obstruction syndrome.

Tracheo-oesophageal and broncho-oesophageal fistula   This is an abnormal communication between the lumen of the oesophagus and the trachea or a bronchus. Both are rare. Broncho-oesophageal fistulae may arise from trauma, e.g. penetrating trauma secondary to foreign bodies, or may be congenital, the majority of which are the result of a traction diverticulum.

Clinical signs are primarily referable to the respiratory system. Coughing after eating and drinking, anorexia and weight loss are seen. Regurgitation may be a problem. Diagnosis requires endoscopy or positive contrast oesophagraphy.

Surgical correction involves identification, dissection and resection of the fistula. The involved bronchus and oesophagus are then reconstructed. If significant secondary pathologic changes are present in the lungs, then lobectomy may be required. The prognosis for simple correction of the fistula is good. If secondary complications such as pneumonia and pulmonary abscesses are present, then the prognosis is more guarded.

Tracheal foreign bodies   Inhaled foreign bodies are occasionally found in the trachea (Fig 7.30), particularly at the carina, although most are relatively small and will migrate into the mainstem bronchi or lower. Grass seeds and heads of cereal crops are the most commonly encountered.

Animals present with coughing, halitosis and a variable degree of dyspnoea, depending on the degree of airway obstruction. Secondary infection within the trachea or pulmonary parenchyma is common and may progress to abscesses or pyothorax and fistulous tracts. The cough will remain until the foreign body is removed. Radiographic changes may be minimal if there is little involvement of the lung and if the foreign body is radiolucent. A definitive diagnosis is often only confirmed by endoscopy.

Many tracheal foreign bodies can be removed with forceps during tracheoscopy. Postopera-

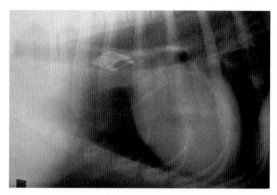

Figure 7.30   Lateral chest radiograph showing a tracheal foreign body (snail shell).

tive therapy with antibiotics is warranted, along with bronchodilators if bronchiole wall damage has occurred. More distal lesions may require a thoracic approach and either tracheotomy or bronchotomy for removal of an uncomplicated foreign body or lobectomy when significant pulmonary parenchymal inflammation is present. Following removal of the foreign body, the viability of the trachea is assessed. The presence of a devitalised portion may necessitate resection and anastomosis. The wound should be apposed with care and the incision checked for leaks under positive pressure ventilation. A pleural or pericardial patch may be placed over the incision to ensure an airtight closure.

Tracheal trauma   This may arise from:

- bite wounds
- penetrating injuries, e.g. gunshots
- blunt trauma
- iatrogenic trauma, e.g. during endotracheal intubation.

Penetrating injury to the cervical trachea will result in deep subcutaneous emphysema, which may dissect extensively along the head neck and trunk. Intrathoracic tracheal penetration will result in pneumomediastinum, which may progress to pneumothorax and pneumoretroperitoneum. Tracheal avulsion may result from violent trauma, particularly secondary to hyperextension of the head and neck. The site of the avulsion is generally between the thoracic inlet and the carina. This injury will compromise respiration, but may not be lethal if the peritracheal tissues maintain their continuity. In fact, many cats will present with clinical signs referable to tracheal avulsion several months after the original trauma. Physical examination, radiography and endoscopy are indicated to determine the site and extent of the injury.

Small defects in the trachea may heal with conservative management. Bandaging the neck may control leaks from the cervical trachea and placement of a chest tube and evacuation of the pleural space may reduce signs associated with thoracic tracheal penetration. Surgical management will result in a more rapid and predictable response, and is indicated for larger injuries. Small defects should be debrided and repaired primarily. Larger defects may require resection and anastomosis. Local muscle flaps may help to control air leak from a damaged segment.

Tracheal avulsion   This is generally caused by violent trauma, particularly secondary to hyperextension of the head and neck, e.g. following a bite from a larger dog or other external trauma. The site of the avulsion is generally between the thoracic inlet and the carina. This injury will compromise respiration, but may not be lethal if the peritracheal tissues maintain their continuity. In fact, many cats will present with clinical signs referable to tracheal avulsion several months after the original trauma. Radiographs may reveal a discontinuity in the tracheal lumen which may be associated with a dilated pseudotrachea at the site of avulsion.

The avulsion is repaired (Fig 7.31) via a right fourth intercostal thoracotomy. The right cranial lung lobe is packed off and the azygos vein ligated and transected. A stay suture is placed in the distal trachea at the carina. The peritracheal tissue overlying the avulsion is dissected to reveal the ends of the trachea. The endotracheal tube is inserted into the distal segment of the trachea from the proximal segment, or alternatively a sterile endotracheal tube may be inserted into the distal segment via the surgical site. Abnormal scar tissue at

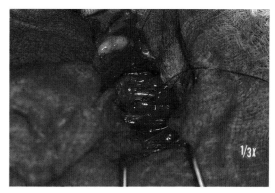

Figure 7.31   Surgical repair of a tracheal avulsion.

the avulsed ends of the trachea is removed and an end-to-end anastomosis is performed.

Tracheal stenosis   Stenotic lesions of the trachea usually arise from acquired injuries, such as laceration from intubation, pressure necrosis from prolonged use of an over-inflated endotracheal tube cuff, penetrating wounds and scarring after tracheotomy or other tracheal surgery. Ethylene-oxide sterilised tubes may cause local irritation and necrosis if not subject to adequate ventilation. Congenital stenosis is rare.

Animals may present with a history of coughing, dyspnoea, exercise intolerance and stridorous respiration. The severity of the signs will depend on the degree of stenosis and the activity level of the dog. Auscultation may localise the site of the lesion, and palpation may exacerbate the cough. Plain radiographs will often indicate the site and extent of the lesion. Tracheoscopy should be performed with care to avoid asphyxiation.

Conservative management of minor lesions by bougienage with open bronchoscopes may be attempted, but is often accompanied by recurrence. Concurrent treatment with corticosteroids may reduce the degree of scarring. Small, web-like stenoses may be ablated with the use of a surgical laser via tracheoscopy. More severe or recurrent lesions should be managed by resection and end-to-end anastomosis. Some degree of stenosis is inevitable following the repair.

Tracheal neoplasia Neoplastic lesions of the trachea are rare in the dog and cat. Benign tumours include osteochondroma, chondroma, leiomyoma, polyps and oncocytoma. Malignant tumours include osteosarcoma, chondrosarcoma, lymphoma, plasmacytoma, adenocarcinoma and squamous cell carcinoma. Local extension or metastasis from thyroid carcinoma and pharyngeal rhabdomyosarcoma may occur. Oncocytoma is a rare benign tumour peculiar to the larynx and trachea, which is associated with prolonged survival times following excision. Osteochondromas are generally found in young dogs, less than one year old. These lesions grow from the cartilage rings and are composed of cancellous bone capped by cartilage. They may reflect a malfunction of osteogenesis rather than a true tumour and are benign.

A biopsy is essential to differentiate tumours from granulomatous masses and lesions of *Filaroides osleri*. This may be made via tracheoscopy, or an open-surgical biopsy may be coupled with excision. Malignant lesions are often locally extensive with a high rate of metastasis. Small benign lesions are potential candidates for resection and anastomosis. Permanent tracheostomy may be used as a palliative measure for animals with a proximally-located lesion. Little objective information is available on the use of radiotherapy or chemotherapy.

Chapter 8

Orthopaedics

Nicholas J Bacon

CHAPTER OBJECTIVES

■ Preoperative considerations
   Protection and support of soft tissue
      injuries
   Protection and support of closed
      fractures
   Treatment and management of open
      fractures
   Antibiotics
   Fluid therapy
   Analgesia

■ Postoperative considerations
   Drug therapy
   Support dressings
   Management of surgical wounds
   Management of surgical drains
   The urinary/faecally incontinent
      patient
   Care of the incontinent patient
   Decubital ulcers

Fluid therapy
Physiotherapy
Special nutrition to meet increased
   needs

■ Surgical procedures and the role of the
   assistant

■ Special considerations perioperatively

■ Advanced orthopaedic surgical
   procedures and techniques
   Bone grafts
   Total hip replacement
   Tibial plateau levelling osteotomy
   External skeletal fixators
   Arthroscopy

■ Specialised surgical instrumentation
   General orthopaedic instruments
   Internal fixation
   External fixation

Many surgical orthopaedic patients are otherwise clinically healthy. Their procedures are termed elective and the scheduling of their surgery is not critical. The major considerations with elective surgery are sterility, analgesia, minimal complications and a rapid return to normal function.

The management of these cases differs significantly from the true orthopaedic emergency such as an open fracture patient, which may have extensive soft tissue injury and multiple organ damage. These are nursing challenges where preoperative triage and stabilisation are priorities, more complex anaesthesia is to be anticipated and a possible intensive period of care and recovery is to be expected after surgery. These cases cannot be conveniently labelled 'orthopaedic' or 'soft tissue' and the nursing they require reflects this.

PREOPERATIVE CONSIDERATIONS

Protection and support of soft tissue injuries

Acute soft tissue injuries are associated with swelling, erythema and pain, through a combination of local release of inflammatory mediators, vasodilation, haemorrhage, or lymphatic and venous congestion. Joint luxations have additional pain through synovial membrane and ligament damage; fractures combine soft tissue injury with often explosive bone injury.

Acute skin wounds should be protected from the environment as soon as possible. All open wounds should be considered contaminated even if they are caused by 'clean' sharp objects such as glass or metal. Contamination is initially from the patient's own skin flora and is typically coagulase-positive *Staphylococcus intermedius* but environmental organisms soon begin to colonise the wound. Once in the hospital setting nosocomial pathogens/flora can soon overtake a wound.

Initial treatment actions or inactions can have a profound effect on the subsequent healing of the injury – wound management at presentation is critical. All open wounds should be covered prior to transport to the clinic or immediately on presentation. A clean/aseptic technique should be followed during all wound manipulation and latex gloves should be worn throughout.

High volume lavage should be used to clean the wound, even using tap water through a shower head for vast contaminated wounds with extensive foreign material embedded in them. Precise lavage can then be applied through a 21G needle and 20ml syringe which achieves pressures of approximately 8 pounds per square inch (psi). Hartmann's is the lavage fluid of choice as this has less cytotoxic effect on tissue fibroblasts (Buffa et al 1997) compared with isotonic saline solutions. Wound dressings should then be applied which will prevent further contamination, provide analgesia and can further clean the wound. One of the most effective wound coverings in the acute phase is a wet-to-dry dressing (Table 8.1). This creates a primary layer of moist sterile swabs on the wound which adhere to the superficial tissue as they dry. Removal of the adherent layer strips off dead tissue (Fig 8.1) back to a bleeding capillary surface.

Human wound management has moved away from wet-to-dry dressings and more towards hydrogels. These are insoluble polymers that absorb and retain water. When placed in contact with wounds they absorb exudate, rehydrate dead tissue and promote debridement through hydrolysis. They are particularly useful in large defects or cavities where there is extensive tissue loss. The gels need to be applied generously and need a suitable secondary layer to hold them in place, e.g. Allevyn, Opsite (Smith & Nephew)

Table 8.1 Features of wet-to-dry debriding dressings

Advantages	Disadvantages
Sterile swabs are a cheap and widely available dressing material	Need to be changed every 24 hours; every 12 hours in very exudative wounds
Effective and rapid debriding action	Painful to remove as adherent to wound surface; most patients will require pre-analgesia or sedation
Even severely contaminated wounds can be clean within 2–4 days	Can macerate surrounding skin if wet swabs overlap wound edges
Can freshen indolent pale chronic granulation tissue	Can debride epithelialisation at wound edges

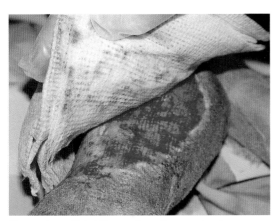

Figure 8.1 Debriding action of a wet-to-dry dressing is evident once removed.

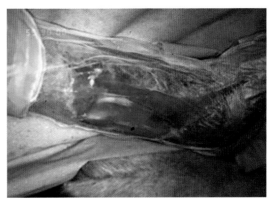

Figure 8.3 Adhesive dressing keeps hydrogel in close contact with wound.

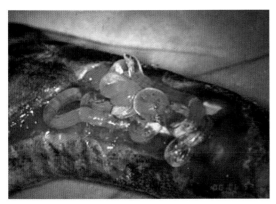

Figure 8.2 Hydrogel applied generously to wound surface.

(Figs 8.2, 8.3). They can be left in situ for 48 hours and when hydrated the gels assume a sticky brown appearance commonly mistaken for purulent exudate. Although much more expensive than wet-to-dry dressings they are more comfortable for the patient when in position and are less painful to remove.

Protection and support of closed fractures

A closed fracture is when the fracture site does not communicate with the skin. Its support varies depending on the fracture type and location. Some fractures (e.g. the femur) are often best left unsupported preoperatively

to avoid heavy dressings acting as pendulums should they slip distally down the limb. In other sites, immobilisation and support can provide significant analgesia by minimising repetitive trauma between bone ends, or between bone and soft tissue and is very useful in the short-term prior to definitive fracture repair. Some minimally displaced closed fractures (especially involving the carpi, hocks and feet), greenstick fractures and non-displaced stable fractures in immature patients can be treated by external co-aptation alone and satisfactory healing should be expected. A simple and versatile short-term solution is a mouldable splint (e.g. Orthoboard, Millpledge) or a preformed plastic splint (Mason Metasplint) (Fig 8.4). These are incorporated into the secondary or intermediate layer of the dressing. The rigid preformed splints are not suitable long-term as they do not adequately immobilise the limb and loosen easily when the patient starts to weight-bear.

The main role of the secondary layer is absorption and trapping exudate away from the primary layer. This layer can be highly padded (e.g. a Robert Jones bandage) which will achieve additional support, minimise dead space, reduce swelling and oedema and protect the wound (Figs 8.5, 8.6). A number of bandage techniques to specifically immobilise certain joints or limbs have been described (Table 8.2).

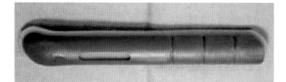

Figure 8.4 Mason meta splinting suitable for short-term support of closed fractures.

Treatment and management of open fractures

Key points:

- assess whole patient
- provide analgesia and broad-spectrum intravenous antibiotic
- clip and clean surrounding area
- cover wound with sterile dressing
- support fracture site.

Classification

A fracture is described as open when the bone ends are in communication with the air through the skin. There is a greater potential for bacterial infection and osteomyelitis in open rather than closed fractures, largely due to the loss of the skin's protective barrier but also through often large areas of traumatised

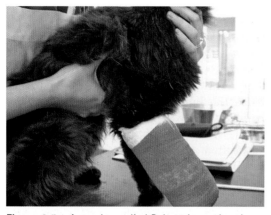

Figure 8.5 A poorly-applied Robert Jones dressing used to support a mid-radial fracture in a cat. The top of the dressing is level with the fracture line and the weight of the dressing encourages instability at the fracture site.

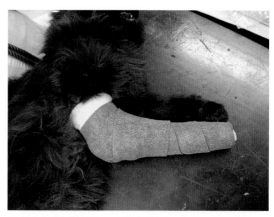

Figure 8.6 The heavy dressing is replaced with a lighter but more effective one including the elbow, providing much greater comfort prior to surgery.

or devitalised tissue which has lost its blood supply and so cannot be reached by the body's immune system or antibiotics.

Open fractures are classified according to the amount of soft tissue damage and the mechanism by which the bone ends become contaminated:

- Grade I: There is generally only a small puncture wound, caused by a sharp bone end puncturing the skin from the inside, either at or following the time of fracture (e.g. during transport to the clinic) (Fig 8.7).
- Grade II: The external force creating the fracture has also created moderate skin and tissue damage or loss, exposing the bone ends to the environment. Although some are comminuted, most fractures tend to be simple.
- Grade III: Severe skin and soft tissue damage or loss typifies this most severe form of open fracture. An example is of a distal limb shearing injury caused by the animal being dragged along the road (Fig 8.8). Significant bone loss and contamination may also occur with ballistic injuries, e.g. bullet or air gun wounds (Fig 8.9).

Presentation

If offering telephone advice prior to the patient arriving, you should recommend the fracture

Table 8.2 Co-aptation techniques used to immobilise limbs or joints

Affected area	Type of external co-aptation	Notes
Scapula/shoulder	Velpeau sling Carpal flexion bandage	To discourage weight-bearing
Shoulder	Spica splint	Moulded splint to length of lateral limb with figure-of-eight bandage over the body wall
Humerus	Spica splint	
Elbow	Full limb cast (toes to axilla) Spica splint Lateral splint (no body wrap) Robert Jones	Lateral splint applied toe to proximal humerus ± body bandage Robert Jones to include upper limb
Radius and/or ulna	Full limb cast (toes to axilla) Lateral splint Robert Jones	Robert Jones to above elbow
Carpus, metacarpals	Short cast (toes to proximal antebrachium) Caudal splint Robert-Jones	
Hip	Ehmer sling (to prevent weight-bearing)	
Stifle	Full limb cast (toes to groin) Robert Jones	Robert Jones to include as much thigh as possible
Tibia and/or fibula	Full limb cast (toes to groin) Robert Jones	
Tarsus, metatarsals	Short cast (toes to proximal crus/tibia) Lateral splint Robert Jones	

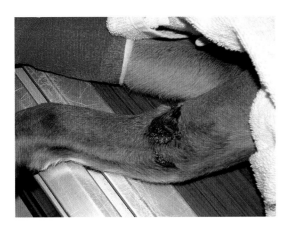

Figure 8.7   Grade 1 open radius and ulna fracture in a Lurcher 30 minutes after being involved in a road traffic accident.

is covered with a clean cloth or bandage. *No attempt should be made to push exposed bone back beneath the skin*. Instruct the owner to try to support the limb during transport to minimise further damage.

Trauma sufficient to cause an open fracture may also have caused other injuries, particularly to the chest and abdomen, which may not be immediately apparent on initial examination. Lung tissue bruising, pneumothorax, haemothorax, rib fractures and diaphragmatic tearing are frequently seen in association with such patients, and these should be identified prior to sedation or anaesthesia. Concurrent abdominal trauma to the larger organs such as the liver, spleen or kidneys may cause sig-

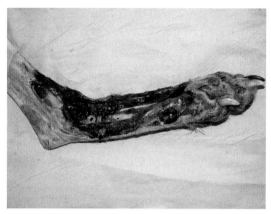

Figure 8.8   Grade III open fracture of the distal medial malleolus of the tibia/shearing injury leading to loss of medial collateral ligament support.

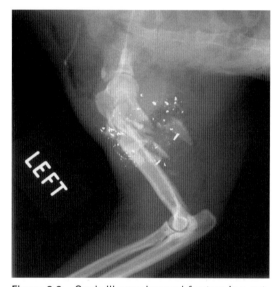

Figure 8.9   Grade III open humeral fracture in a cat caused by an air gun pellet. Gas opacities indicative of an open fracture can be seen in the soft tissue.

nificant blood loss. Urinary, biliary or intestinal leakage will cause varying degrees of peritoneal contamination which, if ignored, may not cause clinical signs for several days. Blood tests and imaging should therefore be prioritised without being distracted by the more obvious external injuries.

The open wound and fracture site will be contaminated and this can rapidly progress to infection due to the local avascular bone and soft tissue, combined with the pathogenicity of the organisms and the time since the injury. Following presentation, open fractures must be treated early and aggressively with broad-spectrum intravenous antibiotics, ideally within 3 hours of injury.

After stabilisation, including analgesia and haemostasis, the patient should be sedated or anaesthetised and radiographs of the fracture taken. Open fractures are characterised by gas opacities near the fracture site within the soft tissue; many also have mineral densities present such as embedded grit off the road. Orthogonal views (two projections at right angles to each other) should be taken of the fracture site, including the joints proximally and distally. Similar views of the opposite limb should be taken for comparison and use in planning fracture repair.

The wound should be protected with water-soluble gel, the surrounding fur clipped and the skin cleaned with 0.1–1% povidone iodine. The wound should then undergo copious lavage followed by sharp debridement. This should be performed in a sterile fashion with the area draped and all personnel in theatre-wear including masks, caps, gowns and gloves.

Grade I open fractures

Wounds typically have little dead tissue and this can be debrided at the time of definitive repair. If this is to be delayed then the wound should be covered with a sterile non-adherent dressing (e.g. Allevyn, Smith & Nephew) and the limb supported with a splint and bandage to prevent further contamination and provide soft tissue protection and analgesia. Larger compressive dressings such as a Robert Jones can reduce the amount of swelling preoperatively which will make it simpler to identify bony landmarks and orientation at surgery.

Grade II open fractures

Debridement is dictated by the amount of soft tissue loss. Some simple cases can be closed primarily and can be treated the same as grade I, but many require early debriding dressings (e.g. wet-to-dry), followed by fracture stabilisation, and finally allowing the defect to heal by delayed primary or second intention healing, or through reconstructive techniques such as skin flaps or free skin grafts.

Grade III open fractures

These are the most challenging, time-consuming and ultimately costly cases. The wounds are heavily traumatised and require initial sharp debridement in theatre, often repeated for 2–3 days as more devitalised tissue dies and becomes obvious. This is followed by several days of sterile debriding dressings until healthy granulation tissue begins to cover the wound (Fig 8.10) thereby protecting the underlying bone. Non-adherent dressings can be used once granulation tissue is present. Orthopaedic repair, especially of shearing injuries, can be performed during this phase. External skeletal fixators provide rigid immobilisation but still allow access to the wound for daily care (Fig 8.11). This is not possible with techniques such as casting or splinting without repeatedly destabilising the limb at every dressing change.

Antibiotics

Antibiotics are not a substitute for a poor sterile or surgical technique but are part of a balanced approach to minimise the bacterial load in the surgical site. The implication of a

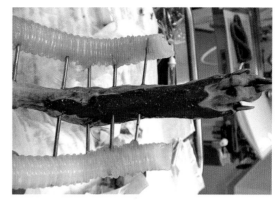

Figure 8.11   Use of an external fixator allows the joint to be immobilised yet still allow active wound management.

postoperative infection involving only the skin is minor. Postoperative infection involving a joint or fracture site can be catastrophic.

Elective surgery

Many orthopaedic surgeries are elective and are 'clean' procedures performed in a sterile fashion. Perioperative broad-spectrum antibiotic cover (e.g. cefuroxime) should be given intravenously 30 minutes before the first incision to ensure an adequate concentration is present in the tissues at surgery. The dose should be repeated every 90–120 minutes following the start of surgery for as long as the patient is anaesthetised. With no break in sterile technique and with no introduction of permanent materials (e.g. metal, nylon, bone cement) there is no indication to continue antibiotics after surgery. The exception to this is if the patient has decreased wound defences, e.g. through senility, malnutrition, immuno-suppressive drug therapy, endocrine disease or metabolic disease.

When permanent material has been used it may act as a focus for infection and continuing the antibiotic cover postoperatively would be prudent. A bacteriological swab of any implants should be taken prior to wound closure if concerns exist over sterility of the surgery or if infection in that site would be disastrous (e.g. hip replacement).

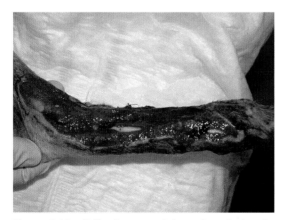

Figure 8.10   Following several days of surgical and dressing debridement, granulation tissue is beginning to cover and protect the exposed bone.

Closed fractures

Although closed fractures have no immediate contamination, damaged tissue and haematomas at the fracture site create a suitable environment into which bacteria from other sites in the body can settle and multiply and so antibiotic treatment is indicated once the fracture is diagnosed. The use of traditional implants in the repair means postoperative antibiotics are also required due to a possible interaction between bacteria and the surface of the implant.

Infective bacteria can produce a coating called a biofilm or glycocalyx which covers the stainless steel implants. This layer promotes both bacterial growth and adherence to the implant which seemingly 'protects' the bacteria and allows them to avoid detection and clearance by the body's immune system. This establishes low grade infections which can present with persistent pyrexia, non-healing sinus tracts or with vague non-specific systemic or orthopaedic signs.

Bacteriological swabs should be taken from the surface of implants following long or contaminated surgeries.

Open fractures/osteomyelitis

Aggressive antibiotic therapy should be started as soon as the wound has been lavaged, debrided and a bacteriological swab taken. The agent chosen should be bactericidal, have activity against Gram-negative and Gram-positive bacteria (especially staphylococci) and be able to be given intravenously. Amoxicillin + clavulanic acid and cefuroxime are both sensible first choices pending bacteriology culture and sensitivity results.

Antibiotic cover should be continued postoperatively as infection from soft tissue wounds communicating with fracture sites can become established in the bone in the presence of dead tissue or an unstable fracture repair. However, a fracture will heal in the presence of infection as long as the repair is stable. The infection may not be completely eliminated, though, until the implants are removed due to the persistence of infective organisms in the implant biofilm layer.

Animals with established bone infection (osteomyelitis), either as a consequence of an open fracture or through introduced infection at time of surgery (Fig 8.12), require prolonged courses of antibiotics of at least 2 months. Prior to stopping treatment there should be radiographic evidence of bone healing, and/or implant removal and culture.

Fluid therapy

Elective procedures in healthy patients do not require preoperative fluids. Intraoperative fluid support is sufficient and an intravenous infusion of 10ml/kg/h of an isotonic crystalloid should replace anticipated surgical and anaesthetic losses. Unexpected fluid loss may mean fluids are continued postoperatively until the calculated deficit (e.g. as determined by counting blood soaked swabs, volumes lost through drains, abnormal gastrointestinal losses etc) is replenished.

Patients who have suffered trauma with resulting orthopaedic injury may require supportive fluids prior to anaesthesia and fracture repair. The type, volume and rate of fluid administration are dictated by the perceived losses and condition of the patient. It is important not to underestimate the 'hidden' volume of blood which can be lost at a frac-

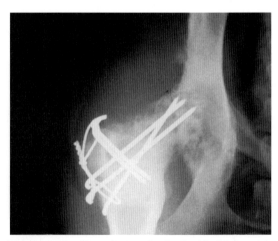

Figure 8.12 Bone destruction in the hip joint following introduction of infection at time of surgery.

ture site to form a haematoma. This can be large with fractures of the femur or pelvis – clinical signs and laboratory findings associated with hypovolaemia or anaemia are often noted.

Occasionally patients are reluctant to eat or drink after injury, e.g. through pain or nervousness, or it may be undesirable for the patient to eat by mouth, e.g. open facial fractures, and they may require additional fluid support prior to surgery.

Analgesia

Patients exhibiting orthopaedic pain may be suffering acutely following trauma and/or surgery, or chronically associated with long-standing joint or bone disease. Growing evidence suggests that wherever possible, pain should be prevented rather than treated and every attempt should be made to reduce the amount of pain induced at surgery. This not only relies on drug therapy, but also nursing and surgical considerations that will make the patient's recovery and rehabilitation more comfortable.

At presentation, initial management of cold-lavaging open wounds or contused swollen tissue will provide immediate relief, followed by supportive dressings or splints for unstable fractures. Provision of a warm quiet environment with soft bedding will further reduce preoperative stress and discomfort. A combination of analgesic drugs is usually then employed preoperatively, intraoperatively and during recovery but these cannot compensate for poor surgical technique, patient care or nursing. Drugs that can be employed to prevent surgical pain include opioids, local anaesthetics and non-steroidal anti-inflammatories (NSAIDs).

Opioids
These provide analgesia by binding to receptors in the brain, spinal cord and peripheral tissue. Opioids are used for both their analgesic and sedative effects, and are commonly included in the premedication in combination with a sedative (e.g. acepromazine maleate).

Care should be taken when head trauma is suspected as some degree of respiratory depression might be seen following opioid administration. Pure agonists like morphine and methadone have the advantage that repeated doses at fairly short intervals can be given in severe pain. Partial agonists, however, such as buprenorphine and butorphanol have a ceiling effect whereby pain is only controlled up to a certain maximal dose, beyond which higher doses may in fact become less effective and start blocking pain-relief (Tables 8.3, 8.4).

Opiates are usually given following triage and are repeated as necessary. Intraoperatively during painful fracture or tissue manipulation boluses of fentanyl can be used to provide fast-onset short-acting analgesia. Excessive use or high doses, however, can result in intraoperative bradypnoea or apnoea from reduced respiratory drive.

Excellent sensory analgesia can be provided by injecting preservative-free morphine into the epidural space at L7–S1. This is normally done immediately following induction of anaesthesia prior to surgery. It can provide pain relief for up to 24 hours and is most useful for hind limb procedures. The morphine can be combined with local anaesthetics for additional motor nerve blockade, although this may lead to temporary pelvic limb paresis or faecal incontinence on recovery.

Long-term opioid analgesia is possible with the use of adhesive dressings containing fentanyl. The drug is absorbed from the patch across the skin at a constant rate and so the patch is cut to the correct size to provide the correct dose for the dog's weight. The patches are typically applied at least 24 hours before surgery to ensure sufficient preoperative drug uptake, and can be left in situ for up to 3 days to provide continuous pain relief. Precautions need to be taken to ensure they are not eaten by the patient and being a controlled drug (CD), patients cannot be discharged to the owner with patches in place.

Local anaesthetics
These provide analgesia by completely blocking transmission of nerve impulses to the

Table 8.3   Opioid use in the dog

	Trade name	Dose rate	Duration of action	Comments
Morphine		0.1–0.2mg/kg SC or IM	2–4 hours	Gold-standard analgesia; cheap
Methadone	Physeptone	0.1–0.5mg/kg IM	2–3 hours	Less vomiting and sedation than morphine
Pethidine	Pethidine	3–5mg/kg IM 5–10mg/kg SC	Up to 1.5 hours	Sedative
Papavaretum	Omnopon	0.2–3mg/kg IM or SC	4 hours	Can calm aggressive dogs
Fentanyl	Sublimaze	2–5µg/kg IV	15–20 minutes	Used as bolus during surgery
Buprenorphine	Vetergesic	0.01mg/kg IM	6–8 hours	Potent but slow-onset
Butorphanol	Torbugesic	0.2–0.8mg/kg IV or IM or SC	30–40 minutes	Poor analgesia, better sedative

Table 8.4   Opioid use in the cat

	Trade name	Dose rate	Duration of action	Comments
Morphine		0.1–0.2mg/kg SC or IM	6–8 hours	Vomiting seen
Methadone	Physeptone	0.1mg/kg IM	2–3 hours	
Pethidine	Pethidine	5–10mg/kg IM 10–15mg/kg SC	1.5–2 hours	
Buprenorphine	Vetergesic	0.01mg/kg IM or PO	6–8 hours	Excellent analgesic
Butorphanol	Torbugesic	0.05–0.6mg/kg IM or SC	3 hours	

central nervous system. A variety of regions can be desensitised:

- Entire limbs, e.g. brachial plexus block in the axilla of the forelimb.
- Specific joints, e.g. instilling local anaesthetic into the joint cavity following surgical exploration.
- Distal limbs, e.g. ring blocks around the circumference of a distal limb to facilitate minor surgery such as toe amputation, or intravenous regional analgesia (IVRA) whereby a tourniquet is applied to a distal limb, then local anaesthetic injected directly into a congested vessel distal to the tourniquet to localise the blockade. This is short-lasting, and is quickly reversed once the tourniquet is released

Commonly used local anaesthetics are lignocaine (1–2mg/kg) and bupivicaine (2–3mg/ kg). The former has a faster onset but shorter duration of action of up to a couple of hours, whereas bupivicaine will provide 4–6 hours of analgesia. Cardiac and CNS toxic side-effects of dysrhythmias and behavioural changes such as restlessness and sedation can be seen with higher doses or intravenous administration.

NSAIDs

These drugs suppress the inflammatory response and limit the amount of inflammatory mediators such as prostaglandins produced in response to injury. This will reduce not only localised pain but also the transmission of this pain through the spinal cord to the brain. These drugs can usually be combined safely with other forms of analgesia (e.g. opiates) to provide comprehensive pain relief for the patient. A single dose of a NSAID can be administered preoperatively before the onset of surgical stimulation to reduce pain for up to 24 hours (Table 8.5).

Inhibition of prostaglandins, however, occurs not just in inflammation, but also in other normal physiological processes. This accounts for some of the side-effects of NSAIDs, such as;

- reduced kidney blood flow which is often worsened by hypotension and hypovolaemia seen in general anaesthesia or shock
- reduced production of gastric mucus plus altered gastric acid production leading to stomach and intestinal ulceration, bleeding and vomiting
- liver damage – reported in Labradors following carprofen (MacPhail et al 1998)
- clotting abnormalities or anaemias.

POSTOPERATIVE CONSIDERATIONS

Drug therapy

The most frequently prescribed drugs following orthopaedic surgery are antibiotics and analgesics. Indications for antibiotic drugs have been described and are used commonly whenever implants have been used or in the case of contaminated or infected wounds or fractures. Course length depends on the sterility of the surgery, results of bacteriological testing, clinical improvement, or radiological resolution of bony changes associated with infection.

Providing analgesia in the recovery period relies on detecting behavioural signs such as vocalisation, hunched posture, inactivity, anorexia, aggression and rigidity to assess postoperative comfort. An increased respiratory or heart rate compared to preoperatively may also be seen when an animal is in pain.

- *Opioids.* Five days of postoperative opiates usually provides sufficient analgesia for most patients depending on the surgery performed. Doses of full agonist opioids can be repeated as frequently as necessary, whereas use of partial agonists in the premedication will limit which opioids can be given on recovery. Fentanyl as a continuous rate infusion (CRI) or a transdermal patches should provide continuous postoperative analgesia.
- *NSAIDs.* Several days of NSAIDs should be given following even minor surgery if there are no obvious contraindications. Where NSAIDs are used to encourage use of the affected limb or to provide analgesia during periods of physiotherapy or rehabilitation, several weeks at a time are prescribed.
- *Local anaesthetics.* These are rarely used following orthopaedic surgery although local intercostal nerve blocks for rib fractures in trauma patients can dramatically reduce the discomfort seen with breathing. These are short-acting lignocaine blockades and need repeating every 6–12 hours dorsal and ventral to the fracture just caudal to the affected rib and one rib either side.

Other drugs may be required depending on specific patient needs, e.g.

- acepromazine may be used to sedate patients following surgery to allow for a calmer hospitalisation and recovery period

Table 8.5 Preoperative data for NSAIDs		
Drug	Dog dose	Cat dose
Carprofen (Rimadyl)	4mg/kg IV or SC	4mg/kg IV or SC
Meloxicam (Metacam)	0.2mg/kg SC	0.3mg/kg SC
Ketoprofen (Ketofen)	2mg/kg IV or IM or SC	2mg/kg IV or IM or SC
Phenylbutazone	2–20mg/kg IV or IM	6–8mg/kg IV or IM

Note: Increased toxicity has been seen in animals under 6 weeks. NSAIDs should not be given to pregnant animals.

- diazepam may be used as a muscle relaxant to treat pain from back muscle spasm in patients with intervertebral disc disease
- drugs may aid the management of urinary incontinence (see below).

Support dressings

Dressings are used either to support and rigidly immobilise limbs or joints as a form of external co-aptation, or else to offer limited protection and comfort for a shorter period following internal fixation of a fracture. Dressings used to immobilise the limb (and often the patient) include Robert Jones, moldable or plastic splints, and casts.

Robert Jones dressings

Robert Jones dressings can be used effectively for distal limb injuries, plus elbow and stifle support depending on the breed and conformation of the dog. The potentially damaging nature of these dressings must be stressed and the pressures generated beneath a poorly fitting or uneven Robert Jones dressing can become incredibly high. They can cause ischaemia and death of large areas of skin in only a few hours with subsequent extensive tissue sloughing (Fig 8.13) (Anderson & White 2000). The heavy cotton-wool padding can also absorb large volumes of exudate, becoming

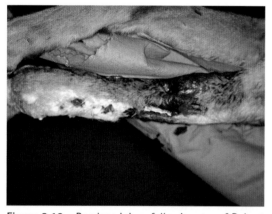

Figure 8.13   Bandage injury following use of Robert Jones dressing which was applied too tightly. Photo courtesy of Dr R A S White.

sodden and allowing wounds to become macerated or infected. Loose fitting, slipped or soiled dressings should be removed or replaced immediately, with close inspection paid to the tissues beneath.

Some debate exists over whether Robert Jones dressings should be used to support stifle surgeries postoperatively. Although a well placed dressing will provide comfort and reduce swelling, significant complications can be seen with a poorly placed or maintained dressing acting as a heavy weight on the distal limb, causing increased pain. The decision is normally down to surgeon preference but if in doubt the limb should be left undressed.

Casts

Casts are commonly used for incomplete fractures, non-displaced paediatric fractures, e.g. fracture of the tibia with ulna intact, and immobilisation of joints, e.g. to allow joint fusion following arthrodesis, or to remove tension from ligament or tendon repairs to encourage healing. The animal should ideally be hospitalised for at least the first 24 hours following cast application. The central two toenails should be left exposed to ensure there are no early signs of the cast being too tight such as toe swelling or visible discomfort (Fig 8.14). Casts are typically in place for up to 8 weeks and client education about home care is vital. The owners should be instructed to look out for cast rubbing, skin infection, unexpected lameness, inappetance, signs of fever, toe swelling or necrotic smells coming from the cast. Nibbling or pawing at the cast (Fig 8.15) is another sign of possible discomfort and is normally associated with a break in the skin. These normally arise from insufficient padding in the secondary layer allowing movement and friction, especially over pressure points (Fig 8.16). Extra padding should be placed in the depressed area either side of the pressure points or padded 'donuts' placed over pressure points to prevent rubbing of the cast on the exposed prominence (Fig 8.17).

Once the cast has been set and dried it should be cut immediately with an oscillating cast saw on opposite sides into medial and

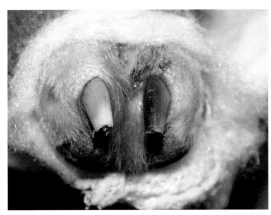

Figure 8.14 One of the earliest signs of an overly tight cast or dressing is the toes becoming swollen and beginning to 'splay'.

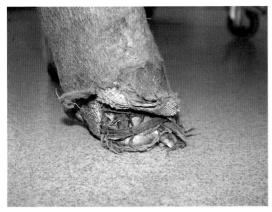

Figure 8.15 Self-trauma to the cast is an early sign of an underlying problem.

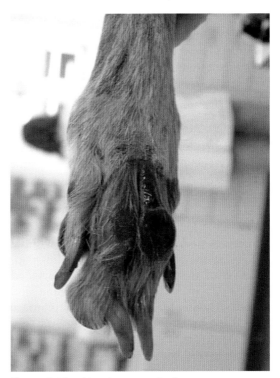

Figure 8.16 Abrasions over the bony interphalangeal joints in the foot in Figure 8.15 which was causing the irritation.

Light compressive dressings

Light compressive dressings can be applied at the end of surgery to reduce postoperative swelling when rigid support is not required. Typical examples include minor distal joint surgery or internal fracture fixation where

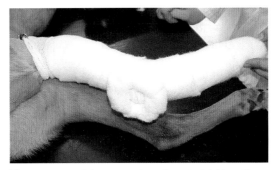

Figure 8.17 A home-made soft material 'donut' over pressure points beneath casts or dressings helps prevent sores.

lateral or dorsal and palmar/plantar halves. This 'bivalving' is 'repaired' by wrapping adhesive tape around the two halves. The technique weakens the cast slightly, but more importantly allows the primary and secondary layers of the dressing to be rapidly changed by removing the tape and opening the cast. The inner layers often become soiled or worn, especially in the first week as the surgical wound exudes and heals, and these can be replaced without requiring the cast to be completely destroyed and replaced. It is important to redress the limb with exactly the same amount of secondary padding to avoid looseness or skin ischaemia.

there has been considerable tissue manipulation. These are three-layered supportive dressings that should never be left on for more than 24 hours before replacing them to take into account postoperative swelling and wound exudate.

External fixator application

Following external fixator application, protective dressings are placed between the frame construct and skin to reduce swelling in the short term. Sponges removed from disposable scrubbing brushes and sterilised with ethylene oxide make for good versatile soft dressings that can be packed beneath the frame without damaging the skin. These are held in place by covering the frame itself in secondary and tertiary layers to help reduce swelling and absorb exudate. Once the pin–skin interface has sealed and the tissue swelling has subsided, these dressings can be removed and the clamps covered with an adhesive tertiary layer (e.g. Vetrap, 3M) to protect the patient's skin from rubbing when walking or the owner's furniture from scratches when mobile.

Management of surgical wounds

Surgical wounds and the surrounding skin should be cleaned of all blood whilst in theatre and the area dried. An adhesive protective dressing (e.g. Primapore) should be placed over the wound if applicable to provide additional protection whilst fibrin seals the wound over the next few hours. Most wounds will be sealed by 6–12 hours after surgery and the dressings may be removed at that point. Wounds should then be inspected at least twice daily in the immediate postoperative period for signs of erythema, swelling, seroma or breakdown. The sutures should be loose enough to allow for anticipated wound swelling without 'cutting in' – one of the commonest reasons for animals to start worrying their wounds. The wound should be gently handled and additional analgesia given if painful.

It is imperative that gloves are worn when handling or cleaning non-sealed or discharging wounds as nosocomial pathogens are still the most likely source of a postoperative wound infection. Multi-resistant organisms such as methicillin-resistant *Staphylococcus aureus* (MRSA) are becoming increasingly common in busy veterinary hospitals and basic hygiene procedures of washing hands before and between patients or wearing gloves should be a standard principle of care. Surgical wounds should be gently cleaned with non-spirit-based preparations such as dilute povidone solutions. Any wound which deteriorates or fails to behave as expected should be swabbed for culture and sensitivity. If a wound is very exudative then the skin ventral to the wound can be protected from maceration by applying petroleum jelly daily.

No compressive dressing should be left on a limb in the immediate postoperative period for more than 24 hours without the bandage being removed and the wound inspected. The primary dressings may need to be replaced as the skin overlying fractures can often be very bruised and exudative.

Management of surgical drains

Drains are not commonly required in orthopaedic surgery but are used whenever dead space exists, contaminated tissue is closed, or if fluid production would create serious complications e.g. septic arthritis, septic osteomyelitis, amputation. Choice of whether to use a passive or active drain is based on anticipated fluid type and volume, dead space present, location of surgical site, availability of drain types, and surgeon familiarity.

Passive drains

Passive drains (e.g. Penrose) allow fluid to exit under gravity by capillary action around the drain and so they must be placed dependently in the wound. They are typically only in place for 1–3 days but are a potentially direct path for bacteria to enter the wound. This is especially true in areas of high motion, such as the axilla, where air and bacteria are often sucked back into the wound as the patient moves. A large area of hair should be clipped around the wound, especially dependently, and the stoma (drain exit hole) and skin surrounding the drain should be cleaned regularly. The drain needs to be covered with a sterile dressing (e.g. Primapore) or light bandage if feasible or if it is likely to become contaminated when the animal is recumbent. When the drain is removed the stoma should be left open but covered with a small dressing to absorb continuing discharge.

Active drains
Active drains are a closed system and allow an accurate assessment of the volume and nature of fluid produced. The stoma tends to remain dry and the greatest consideration is keeping the vacuum primed in the collection bottle. These bottles can be bulky but can be easily held in place beneath a body stockingette. Pain and irritation caused by drains is often overlooked, which may account for premature drain removal by the patient – additional analgesia may be needed in these cases. Simply inserting a drain should not be a reason for antibiotic therapy postoperatively, but the indication for the drain itself may well be, e.g. large dead space, fluid accumulation, infected tissues.

The urinary/faecally incontinent patient
Urinary and/or faecal incontinence in orthopaedic patients is typically neurogenic. The nerve supply to the bladder, urethra, terminal colon and rectum is the pudendal nerve (voluntary), pelvic nerve (parasympathetic) and hypogastric nerve (sympathetic) – all of which arise from the three sacral nerves off the spinal cord (S1, S2 and S3). The spinal cord, however, terminates at L6 in the dog and L7 in the cat, so the sacral nerves travel inside the vertebral canal for a short distance (along with the coccygeal nerves – together forming the cauda equina) before exiting the vertebral column in the sacrum.

Damage to the individual sacral nerves after they have left the spinal cord can therefore arise following pelvic, sacral or sacrococcygeal trauma – so-called lower motor neurone

(LMN) injury – which leads to flaccid paralysis of the bladder and urethra plus lack of anal or rectal tone and little perineal sensation. The bladder and rectum fill with no attempt made by the patient at emptying, and the bladder can be expressed easily through a relaxed urethra on abdominal compression. An overflow urinary incontinence is typically seen.

Injury to the spinal cord before the sacral nerves have left (typically cranial to L6/7) will interrupt higher feedback from the brain – so-called upper motor neurone (UMN) injury. This is seen following trauma or compression of the spinal cord, for example concussion from a road traffic accident or disc prolapse, compression from a tumour, or iatrogenic following spinal surgery. UMN injury of the bladder and urethra allows bladder filling but abnormally increased urethral tone prevents emptying. Manual expression will therefore be met with significant resistance and urinary retention incontinence is typically seen.

Care of the incontinent patient
In cases of LMN or UMN injury the bladder should be periodically emptied. This will prevent the bladder becoming irreversibly flaccid from excessive stretching causing damage to the muscular network of the wall. Conversely, if the bladder is emptied too frequently it remains small and so removes the stimulus for the animal to attempt to urinate voluntarily.

LMN injury
Manual expression of a LMN bladder twice daily over a floor drain or into a kidney dish is sufficient but care must be taken to avoid urine scalding. The hair around the penis or vulva should be clipped and the area inspected regularly. Daily bathing or washing with a dilute chlorhexidine solution will prevent skin infection. Application of petroleum jelly will add further protection. Incontinence pads should be placed under the patient when recumbent to draw urine away and reduce urine–skin contact. Examination of perineal and preputial reflexes, tail tone and anal tone should be carried out daily to monitor progress

and identify signs of return of neurological function to these areas. Improvements here are likely to correspond to an improvement in bladder function. Following tail traction injuries in cats and resulting LMN urinary incontinence, the patient is unlikely to fully recover if there has been no improvement in voluntary urination after 1 month.

UMN injury

Manual expression of a UMN bladder with urinary retention can be uncomfortable for the patient as initially pressure is being applied against a closed urethral sphincter. Alternatives include intermittent catheterisation or indwelling catheterisation with a closed collection system. A closed system has several advantages:

- the bladder is normally fully emptied
- no painful expression is required
- there is less chance of urine scalding.

The major disadvantage is that there is an increased risk of a urinary tract infection because the catheter bypasses the local defences of the urethral papilla and sphincter. Infection, however, can be seen regardless of the technique used to empty the bladder and debate exists whether antibiotics should be used routinely in cases of urinary incontinence, both for LMN and UMN. Immediate use of broad-spectrum antibiotics may reduce the likelihood of infection and the pain and discomfort seen with cystitis, but may also result in the development of resistant bacterial strains. Ideally, antibiotics are not used and frequent urinalysis is performed for signs of infection such as degenerate neutrophils and intracellular and extracellular bacteria. If systemic signs arouse suspicion of an infection, urine can be cultured and antibiotic therapy given based on sensitivity.

The technique adopted to empty the bladder is normally based on the practicalities of a given clinical setting, including the availability of staff to offer high intensity nursing. Bladder palpation every 4–6 hours with at least twice daily manual expression may reduce the chance of developing an infectious cystitis

with all the associated complications, but care must to be given to ensure the bladder is emptied sufficiently each time, with intermittent catheterisation performed if necessary.

Drug therapy

Bladder emptying can be encouraged by the addition of the parasympathomimetic bethanecol (Myotonine, 1–2mg/kg BID or TID), which increases bladder wall muscle detrusor tone. Reduction in urethral spasm can be achieved with the sympatholytic phenoxybenzamine (Dibenyline, 1mg/kg TID) or diazepam (1.25–2.5mg/kg), although care should be used with the latter in cats due to liver toxicity. Both bethanecol and phenoxybenzamine take several days to reach full effect so immediate improvements should not be expected.

Faecal retention in these patients is very uncommon but can be managed with stool softeners (e.g. Isogel), laxatives (e.g. Klean prep) or enemas (e.g. Micralax or Fletchers Phosphate enema). Patients will often defecate following the use of a rectal thermometer, which appears to stimulate this action.

Decubital ulcers

Disease mechanism

Recumbent or debilitated patients are prone to developing decubital ulcers. These are pressure sores most commonly seen over bony prominences, although even large areas of skin subjected to long periods of increased pressure may eventually necrose. Pressure generated from the animal's body weight against the ground is greater over bony prominences as there is less subcutaneous tissue to absorb and re-distribute it and focal areas of tissue ischaemia develop. In normal situations, this ischaemia is temporary because as the animal moves or changes position blood flow to this vulnerable tissue is restored. However, prolonged periods of increased pressure, as seen in recumbent orthopaedic patients, may cause areas of cell death and subsequent necrosis. Large areas of necrosis coalesce to form an ulcer. Typically medium/large breed dogs are affected – especially thinner, heavier dogs, e.g. greyhounds or Irish Wolfhounds.

Management of decubital ulcers
Key points:

- comfortable environment
- regular turning
- massage
- soft bedding
- care of skin over pressure points.

Decubital ulcers can be labour-intensive, frustrating and expensive to manage, often requiring treatment long after the cause of the recumbency has been resolved. Nursing of the debilitated patient includes proactively preventing ulcer development. Patients should be placed in large kennels for easy access for examination and treatment – the larger space will also encourage them to voluntarily move when able. Air temperature should be controlled thermostatically to provide a comfortable environment. Patients unable to turn themselves should have their position changed every 2 hours from lateral recumbency, to sternal, to the opposite lateral recumbency if their injuries allow. Gentle massage and rubbing of at-risk areas following rolling will encourage return of blood to the area. Frequent turning also reduces the risk of developing hypostatic lung congestion, which predisposes to pneumonia.

Proper bedding is vital with the patient lying on thick duvets or thick fleecy acrylic mats (Vetbed). These should be changed regularly to keep them clean and dry and to avoid urine or faecal scald or skin maceration. Extra padding either side of bony prominences may be useful. Beneath the blankets should be a supportive rubber-coated foam mattress which adds more support and helps distribute the patient's weight. Pressure points should be inspected twice daily – including the point of the elbow and the lateral epicondyle of the humerus, the sternum, the greater trochanter of the proximal femur and the ischium of the pelvis. The bony points of the carpi and hocks are less commonly affected, presumably due to less pressure being exerted by the lighter

limbs. Early signs include hair loss and reddening, thinning and flaking of the skin.

Early skin changes (Fig 8.18) mean more frequent checks are needed and if concerned the affected area should be bandaged. The patient should be assessed for any predisposing cause to ulceration such as poor hydration or nutritional status, drug therapy, endocrinopathies, cardiovascular, hepatic or renal disease etc. Any break in the skin allows the skin and environmental bacteria to communicate directly with ischaemic tissue – use of topical antibacterials is indicated in addition to standard wound care such as cleaning the surrounding skin, sterile lavage and dressing the wound. Debriding dressings, such as the wet-to-dry, are often used in the early stages to remove all necrotic soft tissue. When ulcers have become established (Fig 8.19) or conservative therapy is failing, surgical debridement with wound closure or reconstruction may be required.

Fluid therapy

A properly hydrated patient will have a shorter recovery and hospitalisation time compared with a dehydrated animal. Anticipated surgical losses should be replenished by the intraoperative fluid rate of 10ml/kg/h but if blood loss during surgery is in excess of 10% of circulating volume (blood volume estimated

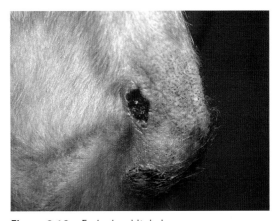

Figure 8.18   Early decubital change over a pressure point. This elbow should now be bandaged and inspected daily to prevent progression.

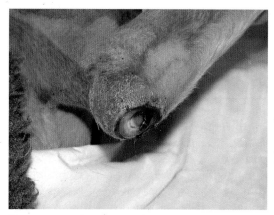

Figure 8.19   Decubital change can rapidly lead to full thickness ulceration that requires complex surgery to repair.

at 66ml/kg in the dog, 90ml/kg in the cat) then intravenous fluids should be continued after surgery until losses have been replaced. Crystalloids should be adequate (e.g. 0.9% saline or Hartmann's) if the loss is in the region of 10% and the animal is clinically bright, but greater losses may require colloids or even blood products.

Physiotherapy

Short-term problems of recumbency include urine or faeces scald, pneumonia and urinary tract infection. Chronic recumbency leads to muscle loss, joint stiffness and limb oedema – physiotherapy to encourage joint flexibility and prevent muscle atrophy should start as soon as the patient is comfortable enough to tolerate it. Different techniques include:

- *Gentle massage*: rubbing and stroking of skin and soft tissue helps warm tissues and disperse oedema and congestion. Kneading (petrissage) compresses muscle groups and encourages circulation.
- Alternate warm and cold *compresses* will promote vasodilation and vasoconstriction to help disperse swelling and oedema and ease muscle spasms. Both can be used in the early stages but cold is used more in the long-term to reduce joint pain and effusion.

- *Passive exercises*: each joint in turn, starting distally, is flexed and extended to the limit of its range of motion. This is repeated 15 times, three times daily. This is repeated on all limbs. These passive exercises can be painful and opioid analgesia or even muzzling may be required when first working on stiff joints.
- *Active exercises*: the weight of the animal is supported off the ground and gently lowered towards the floor. When the feet touch the ground they are encouraged to gently resist and push against being lowered. This is repeated 15 times, three times daily. Similar exercises can be performed with the animal in lateral recumbency by repeatedly pushing the foot and encouraging the patient to resist limb flexion.
- When more mobile, *sit to stand* exercises improve hind limb strength and co-ordination. This can progress to stair walking when confident.
- *Hydrotherapy* for dogs through swimming is an excellent way to promote joint movement and muscle use. Dogs that are non-weight-bearing lame on one limb will often use it to swim with when in the pool. Swimming can start postoperatively once the wound has sealed, but is normally delayed until any skin sutures are removed. The first sessions are normally used to acclimatise the patient to the pool and harness and are only 5–10 minutes long, but when confident 2–3 sessions a week of up to 30 minutes can be given. The pools use underwater jets to create a current for the dog to swim against.
- Devices consisting of a small battery pack and electrodes can be used daily to give muscle groups low intensity *neuromuscular stimulation* to improve the tone and development of atrophied muscles.
- Walking aids such as *slings* suspend the patient with all four toes touching the ground and encourage them to pull themselves forward with a paddling motion.
- Patients with hind limb weakness only can be walked on the lead with a *towel sling* underneath the caudal abdomen. Care

should be taken when towel-walking on hospital floors as these can be slippery when wet and inco-ordinated patients can easily loose their footing.

- Any outdoor exercise or activity should ideally be performed on clean grassy areas to encourage the patients to walk and urinate.

Special nutrition to meet increased needs

The increased calorific needs of most in-patients reflect the hypermetabolic states created through the stresses of illness, surgery and hospitalisation. Loss of body mass in hospitalised patients is caused by protein and fat breakdown to compensate for decreased calorie intake or an increased calorie requirement. If this is allowed to continue, wound breakdown, acquired infections and a more prolonged recovery are all more likely. Long-term in-patients should therefore have their weight checked and recorded daily.

Many elective orthopaedic patients, however, spend only 24–48 hours in hospital and few problems arise through lack of food intake. Any that are anorexic after surgery usually resume eating once they are back in familiar surroundings, so if they are otherwise comfortable it is worth considering discharging them back to their owners to see if their appetite improves at home. Animals which have sustained fractures often have concurrent soft tissue injuries which will either increase calorie requirements (e.g. large effusive shear injuries, bladder rupture and peritonitis), or make eating slower (e.g. altered mentation) or more painful (e.g. broken teeth, mandibular or maxillary fractures, split hard palate). Attempts should be made to prevent malnutrition by predicting the increase in requirement and feeding accordingly (hyperalimentation). Basal energy requirement (BER) is dependent on body weight:

$$30 \times \text{body weight in kg} + 70 = \text{BER (kcal/day)}$$

BER is then multiplied by an 'illness factor' – such as cage rest (1.00–1.25), postsurgical stress (1.25–1.35), or trauma (1.35–1.50) – to give the maintenance energy requirement (MER) in kcal/day which needs to be supplied. Wherever possible this should be given by mouth as this is the safest, cheapest, easiest and most physiological route. However, trauma and injury to the mouth or an inability to achieve an increased nutritional intake orally may mean tube feeding is introduced. Naso-oesophageal, oesophagostomy, pharyngostomy, gastrostomy or enterostomy tubes all provide additional enteral feeding options, but require increasing amounts of surgical intervention to place, and nursing care to maintain. Parenteral nutrition, whereby a pre-prepared solution containing energy substrates, protein and micronutrients is administered intravenously, is useful for patients anorexic for several days, malnourished or with profound ongoing protein losses. Venous access is either obtained centrally (i.e. jugular catheter) or peripherally (e.g. cephalic catheter), depending on whether the solution will provide 100% of energy requirements (central) or whether 50% in combination with oral or tube feeding (peripheral).

SURGICAL PROCEDURES AND THE ROLE OF THE ASSISTANT

Few surgeries are easier performed alone and a scrubbed assistant will reduce operating time, complications and therefore morbidity. Although the surgeon will be leading, the more preparation the assistant can do, the smoother surgery will be. This includes understanding the anatomy and aim of the surgery (Table 8.6), the surgical plan (e.g. size of implant to be used, type and configuration of external frame to be applied) plus potential intraoperative complications. It is often useful for the assistant to scrub ahead of the surgeon to familiarise themselves with the instruments and get the trolley ready prior to patient draping to minimise delays under anaesthesia. The general role of the surgical assistant is to hand instruments to the surgeon from the trolley, swab the surgical field, use suction and occasionally diathermy, retract tissues under the direction of the surgeon, and cut suture

Table 8.6   Common surgeries (excluding fractures) which require a scrubbed assistant

Surgical site	Procedure	Diagnosis/indication	Surgical aim
Carpus	Arthrodesis	Carpal hyperextension	Debride carpal cartilage and apply a bone plate to fuse the carpus
Antebrachium	Ulnar osteotomy	Poor joint conformation	Ulna is cut to improve elbow joint congruency and 'fit'
Elbow	Arthrotomy	Osteochondrosis	Remove abnormal joint cartilage
Humerus	Cancellous bone graft harvest	Non-unions or failed fracture repair	See below
Shoulder	Arthrotomy	Osteochondrosis	Remove abnormal joint cartilage
Shoulder	Bicipital tenodesis	Bicipital tenosynovitis	Inflamed biceps tendon cut and re-attached into humerus with screw to reduce rubbing over bone
Tarsus	Arthrotomy	Osteochondrosis	Remove abnormal joint cartilage
Tarsus	Calcaneo-quartal arthrodesis	Proximal intertarsal joint subluxation	Debride cartilage from tarsal bones and apply bone plate to stabilise joint
Stifle	Wedge osteoplasty Tibial tuberosity transposition	Patella luxation	Deepen the groove the patella runs in and straighten the line of pull of the quadriceps
Stifle	Arthrotomy	Osteochondrosis	Remove abnormal joint cartilage
Stifle	Lateral imbrication suture	Cruciate disease	Stabilise joint externally
Stifle	Fascia lata graft	Cruciate disease	Stabilise joint internally
Stifle	Tibial plateau levelling osteotomy (TPLO)	Cruciate disease	See below
Hip	Femoral head and neck excision	Arthritis, fracture	Femoral head and neck removed
Hip	Total hip replacement (THR)	Hip dysplasia with hip arthritis	See below
Pelvis	Triple pelvic osteotomy (TPO)	Hip dysplasia without hip arthritis in young dogs	Rotate the acetabulum over the femoral head to 'tighten' joint

material. More specific orthopaedic roles include holding joints stable, keeping fractures reduced with bone holding instruments, lavaging joints, and keeping instruments clean during surgery, e.g. removing bone debris from drills bits and bone taps.

Once the skin is breached, warm saline-soaked swabs should cover all exposed tissue not currently being dissected. Occasional wound irrigation to remove blood clots and debris can be performed with a 20-ml syringe plus suction. Commonly used suction tips for orthopaedic surgery are Frazier or Yankauer.

Hand-held retractors such as Senn, May-dering, Langenbeck and Hohmann are all frequently used in orthopaedic procedures and are placed by the assistant to provide more exposure for the surgeon. Self-retaining

Gelpi retractors are also useful but may need stabilising by hand during bone or joint manipulation.

When repairing fractures, it is normal for at least two pairs of bone holding forceps to be needed to reduce the fragments. These are often held by the assistant whilst the surgeon applies the bone plate.

Whenever surgical implants have been used, a postoperative radiograph is taken at the end of surgery to assess their position, along with fracture reduction and alignment. This will serve as a comparison when healing is assessed in the future. Whilst the animal is being radiographed, it is sensible for the surgical assistant to remain scrubbed and to cover the surgical trolley with a sterile drape in case the animal needs to return to surgery for adjustments to the implants to be made.

SPECIAL CONSIDERATIONS PERIOPERATIVELY

Clipping of the patient is normally performed when anaesthetised in the theatre prep room. Long haired dogs can be roughly clipped the day before surgery but a fine surgical clip causes an increase in the skin flora population and so should only be done when anaesthetised immediately before an antibacterial skin prep is applied. A size 40 blade is used and a generous clip should be performed for all procedures to take into account complications and a change of surgical plan.

The skin should be scrubbed in the prep room with a chlorhexidine based solution on either cotton wool or gauze swabs. If open wounds or mucosal surfaces are in the surgical field then any alcohol containing solutions should be avoided. The surgical field should either be covered by chlorhexidine soaked swabs during transfer to theatre, or the area scrubbed for a second time once positioned for surgery.

Procedures such as carpal arthrodesis or foot exploration are usually performed under tourniquet – this is placed prior to the second scrub. An Esmarch tourniquet is used whereby thick rubber tape is tightly wrapped around the limb from the foot proximally, exsanguinating the tissue as it goes. The strapping is then clamped proximally at a wider part of the limb where nerves are protected against direct compression. The distal wrapping is then unwound from the foot to the clamp, leaving an exsanguinated limb. The limb is then surgically re-prepped. The tourniquet needs releasing within 90 minutes to minimise hypoxia of muscles and nerves.

Many orthopaedic procedures benefit from having the affected limb vertically suspended for 5–10 minutes whilst being re-prepped and draped. This is achieved by attaching a rope tie around the metacarpals or metatarsals, looping it over a drip stand or theatre light and tightening until the body just begins to leave the table surface. This also helps overcome some of the muscle contracture associated with fractures, making intraoperative reduction easier.

Draping is usually achieved with a four quadrant technique. Disposable sterile drapes are recommended over reusable cloth drapes to avoid complications such as holes or strike-through. Whilst the patient drapes are being placed, the foot is held by a non-scrubbed member of the team, directed into a sterile polythene bag or towel being held by the surgeon, then secured with sterilised string or a towel clip. The foot is then covered with sterile Vetrap or other water-resistant layer. Whenever fenestrated drapes are used, the foot should be placed in a sterile wrapping before passing it through the drape hole. Some procedures (e.g. total hip replacement) also warrant an additional protective barrier to minimise local contamination and a plastic adhesive drape (e.g. Opsite) is applied to the skin and surrounding drapes. When the skin is covered with an adherent plastic dressing, it can easily overheat under the theatre lights – superficial burns and erythema will develop within 24 hours of surgery. Moist swabs should protect the periphery of the wound but the angle and direction the lights shining on the wound should be altered every 15 minutes.

Patient warming aids such as circulating warm-water beds, heat pads or warm-air devices may be used, especially in anticipation of a prolonged time under anaesthesia. All must be serviced regularly as a malfunction can cause severe patient burns (Fig 8.20). Other techniques to counter hypothermia include tying Bubble-Wrap around the remaining limbs and warming the intravenous fluid line. Attention should also be paid to the theatre air temperature – although air-conditioning will keep the theatre personnel comfortable, it can significantly lower the patient's temperature.

Once positioned in theatre, ophthalmic lubricant (e.g. Lacri-lube) should be placed in both eyes to prevent exposure keratitis caused by the corneas drying out.

ADVANCED ORTHOPAEDIC SURGICAL PROCEDURES AND TECHNIQUES

Bone grafts

Cancellous bone within the medullary cavities ('marrow') is rich in bone growth factors. When medullary bone chips are extracted and transplanted elsewhere, they release growth factors locally – which will encourage bone healing if placed near a fracture site. The graft itself also acts as a scaffold for bone healing. Uses of bone grafts include: improving the healing of fractures, both recent or poorly heal-

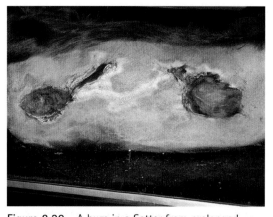

Figure 8.20 A burn in a Setter from prolonged dorsal recumbency on an incorrectly maintained heat pad.

ing chronic ones; arthrodeses; osteomyelitis; filling bone cysts.

Donor bones commonly used are the proximal humerus, iliac crest, medial tibia or greater trochanter. Ideally harvesting is delayed until the primary surgery is completed, although the donor site should be clipped in readiness. New gloves and clean surgical instruments should be used, and a small surgical approach is made over the donor bone and a hole drilled through the tougher outer cortical bone with a hand drill. A Volkmann spoon is then used to scoop out the softer 'crunchier' cancellous bone. This is wrapped in a blood-soaked swab and placed on the trolley for later use, or packed immediately around the fracture site and soft tissue closed over it. The donor hole is closed routinely.

Total hip replacement

Replacing the ball-and-socket joint of the hip with prosthetic implants (total hip replacement – THR) is considered if the hips are very arthritic and painful and the dog is still suffering despite weight loss, sensible exercise and analgesia. If both hips are affected, then the worse is operated on first. This normally gives the patient sufficient mobility that in only about 20% of cases is the second side subsequently replaced. The femoral components are made from cobalt chrome, and the acetabular cup from UHMWPE (ultra high molecular weight polyethylene) with a wire ring around the rim so it can be identified on radiographs (Fig 8.21).

Before surgery the patient should be thoroughly examined for any signs of infection, e.g. skin, ears, teeth, urine. Bacteria settling out from the blood onto any of the implants used and establishing an infection can be catastrophic – requiring the implants and bone cement used to hold them in place to be removed. All infections should therefore be treated prior to surgery. Owners of overweight animals should also be encouraged to slim their animals as much as possible. This will make surgery easier and reduce the likelihood

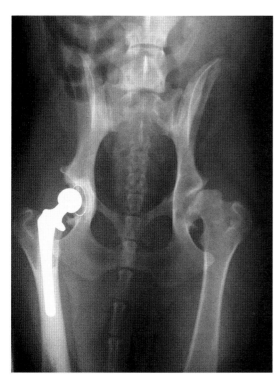

Figure 8.21   Total hip replacement: radio-opaque metallic femoral stem plus wire ring surrounding acetabular implant.

of complications postoperatively. Radiographs of the pelvis and hips are taken to allow the size of the femoral and acetabular implants to be inserted to be decided before surgery. To minimise dermatitis, it may be wise to avoid rough-clipping the patient 24 hours before surgery and perform the entire clip once anaesthetised.

Once anaesthetised a purse-string suture is placed in the anus and an epidural given. In theatre the patient is placed in lateral recumbency and carefully positioned so the pelvis is exactly perpendicular to the table top. The instrumentation for a THR set is often different between systems, but it is normal for each practice to keep to one system to avoid confusion. The large range of additional equipment means it is ideal to have the same scrubbed assistant for every THR to reduce

delays during surgery. A typical instrument list (in addition to the general kit) is outlined here:

- Gelpi retractors
- Broad and Blunt Hohmann retractors
- Maydering retractor
- Senn retractor
- Langenbeck (medium, large) retractor
- Periosteal elevator
- Suction – Frazier tip
- Lavage bowl
- Bulb syringe
- Air driver with oscillating saw attachment
- 3.5mm drill bit
- 3.5mm drill guide
- Air hose
- Hip disarticulator
- Volkmann's curette
- Rongeurs
- Cement gun
- 20g/40g polymethylmethacrylate cement
- 50ml catheter tip syringes
- Sterile bowl and spatula
- Cold saline for flush
- Plus system-specific instruments (e.g. Biomedtrix cemented hips)
- Femoral drill, tapered reamer, broach and finishing file – these hollow out the proximal femoral shaft and prepare it for the femoral implant
- Acetabular reamer and cup positioner – once the acetabular joint surface has been reamed (which removes soft tissue and bone to make it deeper) the cup can be precisely held in place in the cement relative to the landmarks of the ilium and ischium whilst the cement in the reamed acetabulum hardens.

Postoperative care revolves around a quiet recovery period with minimal activity, using acepromazine and opioid sedation if necessary. Towel walking may be enforced for several days to reduce stress on the hind limbs, and to guard against hip luxation from slipping and doing the splits on the floor. The commonest postoperative complications are loosening of the implants, dislocation of the new hip or infection around the foreign materials implanted. Signs of these are monitored for either by radiographs or clinical examination until the dog returns to normal exercise a few months postsurgery.

Tibial plateau levelling osteotomy

Tibial plateau levelling osteotomy (TPLO) addresses cruciate disease in the dog. Whereas other techniques aim to increase the stability of the joint by using loops of thick wire, nylon or even fascia to mimic the torn ligament, no attempt is made to replace the damaged ligament in a TPLO. Instead a TPLO aims to reduce instability in the joint by altering the dynamics and forces in the joint when the dog is walking. It has been noted in dogs with cruciate rupture that many have tibial plateaus that slope more caudally than unaffected dogs; this is corrected by cutting and rotating a circular section of tibial plateau, or cutting and removing a triangular wedge in the cranial tibia and repairing it with a bone plate to make the tibial joint surface in the stifle more horizontal.

Robert Jones bandaging is required after surgery to limit swelling and provide comfort. In essence a tibial fracture has been created and repaired, so postoperative exercise is restricted until sufficient radiographic evidence of bone healing is present at 6–10 weeks.

External skeletal fixators

An external skeletal fixator (ESF) consists of pins going through the skin and muscle into the bone, all connected on the outside to a bar to form a rigid frame. Their many uses include open fractures, comminuted fractures, minimally displaced fractures, angular limb deformity corrections, jaw fractures and joint immobilisation. The component parts of an ESF are described in the next section.

After surgery the limb should be bandaged for 2–3 days until postoperative swelling has subsided. After this time the frame should be left uncovered so the owners can check the pins daily. The pin–skin interface should be left alone to form a scab, which seals the entry point from contamination. Any discharge on

the skin, however, can be cleaned away with a cotton bud and warm dilute iodine solution.

Arthroscopy

Arthroscopy refers to joints being explored by fine cameras through 'keyhole' incisions. The elbow, shoulder, hip, stifle and tarsus have all undergone arthroscopy. The technique avoids large open joint surgeries (arthrotomies) and so causes less tissue damage and pain postoperatively. Camera systems are only a few millimetres thick and can allow a much more thorough examination of the joint. The camera system also magnifies the images and often small, subtle lesions can be identified which would be missed with standard arthrotomy – especially in the elbow joint when looking for early signs of cartilage fissures and softening associated with osteochondrosis.

The commonest veterinary arthroscopes are 1.9–2.7mm diameter and the end lens is angled down by 30°. The angling allows more of the joint to be examined when the scope is rotated 360°. The scopes are inserted into the joints through hollow metal tubes called cannulae, down which saline also flows in and out to inflate the joint capsule and improve the visibility. The flush also helps disperse capillary bleeding during surgery. Extra 'keyhole' sites are made into the joint to introduce instruments such as curettes, probes and motorised burrs/cutters called shavers.

The patients are anaesthetised, clipped, prepared, positioned and draped in very similar fashions to performing an open arthrotomy. Postoperatively, however, most can be discharged the day after surgery on a short course of anti-inflammatories.

SPECIALISED SURGICAL INSTRUMENTATION

General orthopaedic instruments

Jacobs chuck

This is the standard instrument for pin insertion, although it can be laborious as pins are driven in by hand. With a lot of use the teeth can become worn, making it more difficult to tighten sufficiently and allowing the pins to slip and rotate in hard bone.

Hand drill

This drill requires two hands, but may still wobble, so should not be used to drill accurate screw holes. It is very useful to drill through the bone cortex when collecting cancellous bone grafts.

Power drilling

These allow more control as only one hand is needed, allowing the other to stabilise the bone or retract soft tissue. Only a slow drill speed should be used (100–150rpm) as too high a speed will lead to thermal necrosis and bone death. When in use the drill bit should have sterile saline gently dripped onto it to keep it cool. Between each hole drilled the flutes of the bit should be cleaned of bone debris.

- *Battery drills* are heavy and cannot be sterilised, so they must be covered in a sterile fabric shroud before use. They can, however, be used at very low speeds – which is suitable for insertion of pins for external skeletal fixators. The battery should be recharged between procedures. They are also fairly cheap to buy and maintain.
- *Air drills* (Fig 8.22) are fully autoclavable, but need bottles of compressed air for operation. Their main advantages are their light weight, lack of shroud, and high speed settings. The systems tend to be more expensive.

Power saws/burrs

These can be expensive but are invaluable for cutting bone. Careful use allows the surrounding soft tissue to be undamaged. They can be classified according to the direction of blade movement relative to drive shaft.

- *Oscillating saws* (Fig 8.23) use a circular blade which moves in an arc of 5–6 degrees at right angles to the drive shaft. These are most commonly used as cast saws, although they could be used for superficial bone work if placed in a shroud.

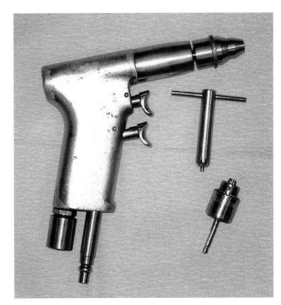

Figure 8.22   Air drill with chuck and key. Photo courtesy of Dr T R Sissener.

- *Sagittal saws* (Fig 8.24) have the blade working parallel to the drive shaft. It only moves by 5–6 degrees but can be used to cut deep bone, for example in femoral head and neck excisions.
- *Burrs* (Fig 8.25) are used in both spinal surgery and orthopaedics (e.g. to remove joint cartilage in an arthrodesis procedure). They operate at very high speeds (up to 100 000 rpm) and so irrigation to cool the burr and tissue is required. Burr guards help protect the burr from breaking.

Gigli wire

This is a braided metal wire with a handle each end which cuts through bone with a sawing motion. It is useful to cut inaccessible bone, e.g. ulna or ischium. Excessive soft tissue need not be removed from the bone, the wire can be passed around the back of the bone and then sawing can start towards the operator.

Bone cutters

These are available in a range of different sizes, for use in e.g. femoral head and neck excision, tibial crest transposition, amputations.

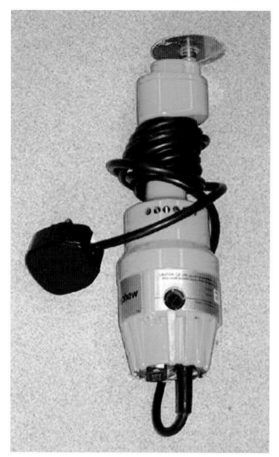

Figure 8.23   Oscillating saw most commonly used to remove casts. Photo courtesy of Dr T R Sissener.

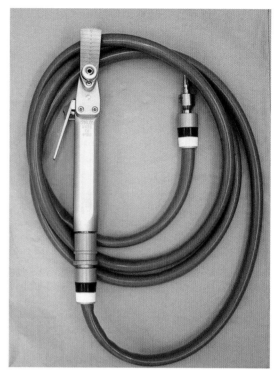

Figure 8.24   Sagittal air saw useful for most procedures. Photo courtesy of Dr T R Sissener.

Bone rongeurs

Available in single or double action, straight or angled, these are used in spinal surgery, e.g. nibbling away bone in laminectomies.

Osteotomes/chisels

An osteotome is bevelled on both sides to create a sharp cutting edge – useful in femoral head and neck excisions. A chisel has one flat edge and one bevelled edge and is usually heavier.

Periosteal elevator

These are useful for lifting periosteum or soft tissue off bone, e.g. to clear an area of bone either side of a fracture to apply a plate.

Retractors

Retractors allow maximum exposure of the wound whilst minimising soft tissue trauma. The tip of a Hohmann retractor can be inserted under a bone and the flat blade will hold back soft tissue, or can be inserted into a joint to improve visibility, e.g. when checking the meniscal shock-absorbers in the stifle. The 'cat's paw' of the Senn can be used to retract specific structures, e.g. the fat pad in the stifle (Fig 8.26).

Internal fixation

This is the use of pins, wires, screws and plates to repair fractures. The decision about which combination of implants to use will be made by the surgeon once several factors have been taken into account, such as the type of fracture, the patient, the bones involved, the forces acting on the fracture (e.g. bending or twisting), availability of advanced equipment, and surgeon experience.

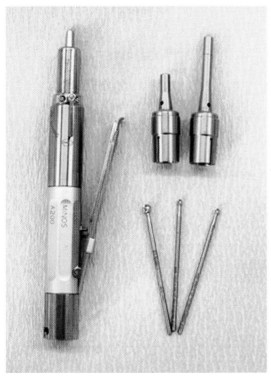

Figure 8.25   High speed air burr with guards. Photo courtesy of Dr T R Sissener.

Intramedullary pins

The pins are inserted down the middle of the bone with a Jacobs chuck and can be used alone (if very stable fractures) or with wire or

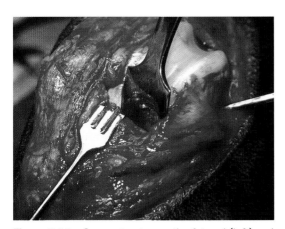

Figure 8.26   Senn retractor on the fat pad (left) and larger Hohmann retractor used to examine the stifle joint during surgery.

plates. Steinman pins come in varying sizes but all are over 2mm in diameter. They have taper point ends to help drive them into bone. Kirschner wires (K wires) are less than 2mm in diameter and are used in cats or to attach small bone fragments. The ends of small K wires are often bent over at the point they exit bone to avoid sharp points damaging soft tissue, or to help hold wire in place when used in combination (Fig 8.27).

Cerclage wire

This is a soft malleable wire which comes in varying diameters. It can be placed around the bone shaft to help stabilise fracture fragments, or used in conjunction with K wires to reattach bone fragments under tension (called Tension Band Wire). Typical sizes used are 22G (0.8mm diameter) in cats and small dogs, 20G (1.0mm diameter) in medium dogs and 18G (1.2mm diameter) in large dogs.

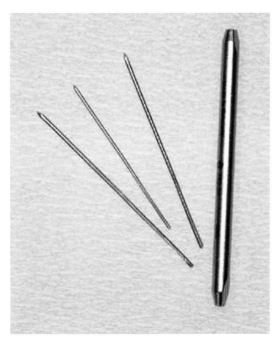

Figure 8.27   Selection of fine Kirschner wires and cylindrical pin bender. Photo courtesy of Dr T R Sissener.

Rush pins

Rush pins have a flattened end to allow for easier insertion and a curved head which fixes into the bone surface (Fig 8.28). They are used in epiphyseal fractures or those affecting the cartilaginous ends of long bones, and inserted up the bone shaft using a mallet, typically in a pair, one each side of the bone.

Bone screws

There are two main types of bone screw, those made by AO/ASIF, and Sherman screws.

AO/ASIF screws

- Designed by surgeons for human fracture repair
- Thread design makes it more difficult for screw to pull out
- Screws do not cut into bone, instead they need to be inserted into predrilled hole which has then had the treads cut in with a bone tap ('tapped'). This ensures a very close fit.
- Rounded head
- Hexagonal hole in screw head requires special screwdriver for insertion
- Either cortex screw, for use in hard cortical bone (e.g. mid-shaft fractures), or cancellous screw, for use in cancellous bone found at either end of the long bones. Cancellous screws have deeper threads to get better purchase in soft bone (Fig 8.29), and are either fully threaded or partially threaded. The sizes available are listed in Tables 8.7 and 8.8.

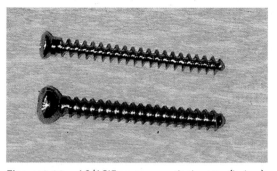

Figure 8.29   AO/ASIF screws; cortical screw (below) and cancellous screw (above) with narrower core and deeper threads for insertion into softer bone. Photo courtesy of Dr T R Sissener.

Table 8.7   Cortical screw sizes available

External diameter	Core diameter (drill bit required)
1.5 mm	1.1 mm
2.0 mm	1.5 mm
2.7 mm	2.0 mm
3.5 mm	2.5 mm
4.5 mm	3.2 mm

Table 8.8   Cancellous screw sizes available

External diameter	Core diameter (drill bit required)
4.0 mm	2.0 mm
6.5 mm	3.2 mm

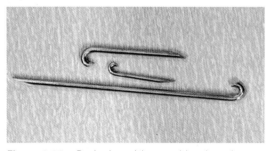

Figure 8.28   Rush pins with curved heads and flattened tips for easier insertion. Photo courtesy of Dr T R Sissener.

Sherman screw

- Sharp end with groove running down screw shaft – allows threads to cut into bone without drilling or tapping beforehand ('self-tapping' screw). Although quicker, this creates more micro-trauma around the screw, making loosening more likely.
- Flat screw head
- Slotted screw head – allows use of standard screwdriver
- Sizes (in inches) include 7/64, 9/64, 5/32.

All screws can either be used in a plate (plate screw) or alone to re-attach bone fragments with or without compression (position screw or lag screw).

Position screw These hold two pieces of fractured bone together without compression. The threads of the screw grip the near and far cortices of the bone.

Lag screw Lag screws hold two pieces of fractured bone together with compression. Threads only grip the far cortex of the bone. As the screw is tightened the threads pull the far bone fragment towards the screw head – once in contact with the near side of the bone, this generates inter-fragmentary compression. To achieve this effect, either a partially threaded screw is used with no threads near the head, or else before inserting the screw the near side fragment is 'overdrilled' with a hole equal in size to the external diameter of the screw so there is no screw–bone contact (so-called 'glide' hole). The sequence of events to insert a fully threaded lag screw is:

- glide hole (external diameter of screw) drilled through near fragment up to fracture line
- insert guide placed in glide hole and narrow pilot hole (core diameter of screw) drilled in far fragment
- countersink used to widen hole in near cortex to let screw head sit deeper into bone for increased contact
- depth of combined hole measured with depth gauge
- threads cut into far fragment with bone tap
- screw inserted – threads only engage in far fragment, screw head beds down into counter-sunk hole and compression achieved as screw tightened.

Bone plates

The types of plate available include:

Dynamic compression plate (DCP) The DCP is unique in having oval screw holes. As a screw is tightened the holes force the spherical screw head towards the centre of the plate – the bone fragment the screw is in is forced

towards the fracture site, achieving compression. The drill guide used has two ends:

- green (neutral) where the pilot hole is drilled in the centre of the plate hole and the fracture is compressed by only 0.1mm per screw
- gold (loaded) where the pilot hole is drilled eccentrically in the plate hole away from the fracture line, which allows more screw head movement on tightening – this allows fracture compression of 1mm per screw (total of four loaded screws possible per plate).

Plates sizes are 2.7mm, 3.5mm broad or narrow, and 4.5mm. Mini plates are also available which are used with 2mm cortex screws – these can be straight, angled or T-shaped for use in small bones in cats and small dogs. DCPs use AO screws.

Acetabular plate Designed for accurate repair of the acetabulum – uses AO screws.

Cuttable plates These come as long sheets and a plate of the desired length is cut according to requirements. Sizes include 1.5mm, 2.0mm and 2.7mm – uses AO screws.

Lengthening plate A sturdy plate with no holes in the central portion. This is used in unreconstructable comminuted long bone fractures to avoid the problem of having empty screw holes at the fracture site – which tends to concentrate stress and lead to plate breakage. Uses AO screws

Reconstruction plate Notching between holes in the plate allow it to be bent and twisted in three dimensions to fit uneven bone surfaces such as the pelvis, mandible or scapula. Uses AO screws.

Sherman, Lane, Venables and Burns plates These plates have been largely superseded by the AO/ASIF plates described above, although good results are still possible if the correct principles are applied. These plates use self-tapping Sherman screws.

Plate function

Regardless of plate type, its use can be described further as a compression plate, neutralisation plate or buttress plate. *Note: this refers to the function only – any plate can be used as a compression, neutralisation or buttress plate.*

Compression plate   The fracture fragments are under compression to encourage healing. This is either static compression, through the use of a DCP, or dynamic compression, when the plate is applied to the tension side of the bone so the fracture is compressed as the animal walks (e.g. lateral side of the femur). Most of the weight-bearing forces are transmitted across the fracture site.

Neutralisation plate   The plate is applied to overcome forces acting on the fracture to allow healing to progress unhindered, or to splint other compression devices such as lag screws. Lag screws can be placed through screw holes or they can be separate. Some of the weight-bearing forces are transmitted through the plate rather than the bone.

Buttress plate   The plate helps support fragments or spans an area of bone loss. All of the weight-bearing forces are transmitted through the plate and so when used, these are often larger and broader than the above two for the same sized bone.

External fixation

The components of an ESF are the pins, the connecting bar and the clamps to join the two together.

Pins

These can be smooth or threaded. The thread is either cut into the pin (Ellis, negative profile) or added onto the pin (Imex, positive profile) (Fig 8.30). Negative profile pins have the threads on the end of the pin only, whereas the more expensive positive profile pins have the thread either on the end or in the central portion of the pin. A full-pin goes through the skin, through the bone and out the skin the other side and is attached to a connecting bar on both sides. A half-pin goes into the bone on one side, crosses both bone cortices, but does not exit the skin on the far side.

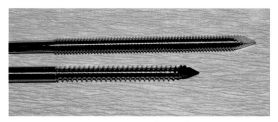

Figure 8.30   Positive profile (above) and negative profile (below) external fixator pins with trochar tips. Photo courtesy of Dr T R Sissener.

Connecting bar

These bars connect all the pins on one side together. They are typically stainless steel rods (Fig 8.31), although lightweight alternatives such as aluminium and carbon fibre are available. Polymethylmethacrylate acrylic (PMMA) can also be used as a more versatile alternative when the pins cannot easily be arranged in a straight line down the bone as it can be moulded to the correct shape before hardening.

Clamps

The Kirschner Ehmer system (KE) is the commonest veterinary system used (Fig 8.32). Clamp sizes are small (<5kg), medium (5–30kg) and large (>30kg) (Table 8.9). The clamp joins the pin from the leg to the connecting bar. Double clamps are available which connect two connecting bars to allow the frame to change direction, e.g. at joints.

Other clamp systems available include the Meynard, KE Plus, hinged clamps, Secur-U and IMEX SK. These offer a range of sizes and ease of use and versatility, e.g. to add or remove clamps without having to remove the connecting bar as with the KE system.

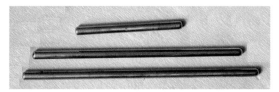

Figure 8.31   Smooth ended stainless steel connecting bars. Photo courtesy of Dr T R Sissener.

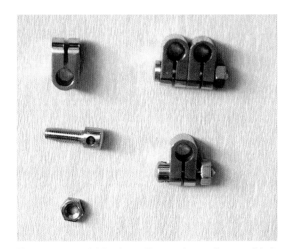

Figure 8.32 A Kirschner Ehmer clamp disassembled (left) showing the U bend, bolt and nut. Assembled double and single clamps are also shown (right). Photo courtesy of Dr T R Sissener.

Table 8.9 Implant sizes for use with KE clamps

Clamp size	Connecting bar size	Ideal pin size
Small	3.2mm	2.4mm
Medium	4.8mm	3.2mm
Large	8mm	4.0mm

The type of frame constructed will be decided on by the surgeon, depending on fracture type. One, two or even three connecting bars can be used depending on whether the frame is just on one side of the leg (unilateral), or both sides (bilateral).

Instruments required to construct an ESF include a drill (either Jacobs chuck or battery drill), a spanner to tighten the clamp bolts, and pin cutters to cut the pin ends flush with the connecting bar.

References

Anderson D M, White R A S 2000 Ischaemic bandage injuries. A case series and review of the literature. Vet Surg 29(6):488–498

Buffa E A, Lubbe A M, Verstraete F J M, Swaim S F 1997 The effects of wound lavage solutions on canine fibroblasts: an in vitro study. Vet Surg 26(6):460-466

MacPhail C M, Lappin M R, Meyer D J, Smith S G, Webster C R L, Armstrong P J 1998 Hepatocellular toxicosis associated with administration of carprofen in 21 dogs. J Am Vet Med Assoc 212(12): 1895

Chapter **9**

Pre- and postoperative nursing

Sandra Whiting, Deborah Smeeton, Lucy Goddard and Joanne Ewart

---

CHAPTER OBJECTIVES

■ Preparation of patient
    Consent forms and legal implications
    Types of surgical preparations and
       methods of aseptic preparation
    Methods of aseptic preparation
    Clippers and clipping the surgical site
    Positioning for surgery
    Preparation for surgery
    Preparation of paediatric patients
    Preparation of geriatric patients
    Preparation of exotic species
    Enemas and catheterisation of the
      bladder
    Presurgical antibiotic administration
    Analgesia
    Intravenous fluid therapy
    Blood transfusions

■ Care of the anaesthetised patient and
  postoperative recovery
    Maintenance of patient airway
    Maintenance of body temperature
    Perioperative care and postoperative
      recovery

■ Postoperative bandaging
    Wound dressings and bandage
      components
    Types of casting materials
    Complications relating to bandaging

■ Wound management
    Stages of healing
    Aseptic surgical wounds
    Surgical preparation of infected wounds
    Barrier nursing
    Protection of wound from patient
      interference
    Types of surgical drain

PREPARATION OF PATIENT

Consent forms and legal implications

Consent forms are a legal requirement for all patients who are, or may be, undergoing a local or general anaesthetic. By signing the form the owner or agent is confirming that they understand and consent to the procedures explained to them (Jones 1999). The form should include:

- details of the patient concerned (name, age, species, breed, case number etc)
- details of the owner/agent (name, address, contact details)
- an easily understandable list of procedures likely to be performed, including which limb/eye; abbreviations should not be used.
- an estimate of costs involved
- a statement that outlines the risks associated with anaesthesia and that indicates the

possibility of further procedures being necessary.

The form could also include:

- a list of medications the patient is currently taking
- a note of when the patient was last fed or offered water
- any problems, perceived by the owner, following previous anaesthesia.

The veterinary professional admitting the patient should ensure:

- the patient has, or will, undergo a full pre-anaesthetic clinical evaluation.
- the owner/agent understands the consent form and the procedures they are consenting to.

Consent forms should be kept for a minimum of 2 years.

Types of surgical preparations and methods of aseptic preparation

The type of surgical preparation selected for the patient needs to be appropriate for the area being prepared. Each preparation has certain properties that may make it more suitable in certain situations. The ideal properties of a surgical scrub solution are:

- a wide spectrum of antimicrobial activity
- rapid reduction in microbial count
- not deactivated by organic matter
- long residual effect
- safe and causes minimal irritation
- fast application time
- economical.

The most commonly used surgical preparations are chlorhexidine solutions, iodophors, chlorinated phenols (with or without detergents) and isopropyl alcohol preparations.

Chlorhexidine gluconate
- causes cell wall disruption and protein precipitation
- effective against most bacteria, *E. coli* and Pseudomonas
- viricidal, fungicidal and sporicidal activity

- residual activity is longer than iodophors and is not affected by organic material
- irritant to the cornea
- binds to keratin and has a quick onset of action
- available with or without detergent

Iodophors – povidone–iodine solutions
- cause cell wall penetration and oxidation
- broad antibacterial, viricidal, fungicidal and some sporicidal activity
- residual activity is shorter than with chlorhexidine
- efficacy impaired by organic matter
- microbial activity is achieved with 2 minutes contact time; sporicidal activity requires 15 minutes contact time
- detergent-free solution is appropriate for ocular preparation

Chlorinated phenols – Triclosan
- causes disruption of the cell wall
- broad spectrum of antibacterial activity
- onset of action is slow, and affected little by the presence of organic material
- less irritant for use with sensitive skin

Isopropyl alcohol
- effective against a wide range of Gram-negative organisms and fungal spores at 70% strength
- cannot penetrate surfaces; skin needs to be degreased prior to use
- chlorhexidine or iodine are often added to increase efficacy
- irritant to mucous membranes and open wounds, causing tissue necrosis

Methods of aseptic preparation

To ensure aseptic preparation of the patient, the following protocol has been developed.

- Ideally the patient will present in a clean and mat-free condition. Bathing of the patient has been advocated to remove dirt, loose hair and skin scurf prior to surgery. However, this is not always possible or practical, and may in fact cause a stirring up of bacteria on the skin.

- The nurse should wear either sterile or non-sterile gloves whilst performing the primary preparation of the surgical site
- Hair is clipped around the surgical site (see below for clipping protocol)
- Loose hair is vacuumed
- Empty the patient's bladder where possible
- Flush male dog's prepuce with dilute surgical preparation if within the surgical field
- Dampen hair at the peripheries of the surgical site to avoid adherence to the scrubbed area (see Chapter 10 for types of skin preparations)
- Gauze swabs are more suitable as cotton wool tags can adhere to the skin stubbles
- Avoid abrasive materials and scratching with fingernails when preparing the site
- Scrubbing should commence at the intended incision line moving in an outward direction, either in a circular motion or in straight strokes
- The first stroke is along the incision line and then strokes are continued on alternate sides until the border of the clipped area is reached
- Once the peripheral edge is reached the swab is discarded
- Avoid any pooling of fluid and run-off onto the patient – a dry sterile swab can be used to wipe away any residue
- Degreasing of the area can be performed using isopropyl alcohol – painting of solutions is more effective than spraying
- Ideally sterile forceps should be used or sterile gloves worn, especially for the final preparation

Clippers and clipping the surgical site

Clipping the surgical site is necessary for most surgical procedures. There are advantages and disadvantages for clipping before or after induction of anaesthesia:

- there is an increased risk of postoperative wound infection the longer the interval between clipping and surgery
- if the animal is in a critical condition the majority of clipping can be performed just

prior to induction of anaesthesia to reduce the anaesthetic time
- the proposed surgical site should be confirmed with the clinician prior to clipping.

The use of electric clippers is the preferred method of hair removal as the use of razor blades will cause microlacerations and irritation. A number 40 blade is the standard blade size but dense fur may require use of a courser blade first.

Rechargeable battery clippers with a narrow head are useful for intricate clipping, e.g. around the eye and paws. Blunt blades will increase the incidence of clipper rash and self-trauma postoperatively. All clippers should be regularly serviced and in good condition – after each patient ensure the blades are cleaned and sprayed with a proprietary antimicrobial and lubricating product. Blades should be sterilised appropriately after clipping a contaminated area.

Perform clipping away from the theatre area and remove loose hair and debris prior to surgical preparation. The prepared area should allow for extension of the incision if necessary and prevent hair migrating into the surgical field. Neat clipping will support owner satisfaction.

Ointment should be placed in the eyes to prevent irritation to the cornea and conjunctiva if the proposed surgical site is either the head or neck. Open wounds should be packed with saline-soaked gauze swabs or a water-based lubricating jelly to prevent further contamination of the wound with hair. For orthopaedic surgery, clip the limb circumferentially to allow manipulation during surgery and bandage the distal limb with a cohesive bandage to prevent contamination.

Positioning for surgery

Patient positioning is usually chosen by the surgeon, but it will normally fall to the assisting nurse to position the patient correctly. The patient is positioned once anaesthesia has been stabilised. Many procedures will have a standard position, with which the nurse should be familiar; when positioning a patient in a less common position certain factors should be considered:

- a patent airway must be maintained – kinking or occlusion of the endotracheal tube may occur if the neck is excessively flexed
- the need for access to the patient for monitoring purposes and intravenous access
- prevent heavy abdominal contents impeding respiratory effort and venous return by tilting the table (cranial end higher) and rotating the patient axially.

A variety of positioning aids are available – troughs, vacuum bags, sandbags, ties and foam pads will all be useful in securing the patient in the correct position.

Ensure that adequate circulation is maintained throughout the period the patient is positioned. Ties especially may need to be repositioned or loosened on peripheries. Padding should be used for areas that will be under excessive pressure to prevent myopathy and nerve damage, especially in larger patients.

Preparation for surgery

Upon admission:

- the patient should be clearly identified
- vital signs should be recorded
- accurate weight measurement should be obtained
- report abnormalities to the veterinary surgeon, should further investigations prove necessary
- food should be withheld from adult dogs and cats for 12 hours and water for up to 2 hours prior to general anaesthesia.

A premedicant is administered prior to general anaesthesia and surgery. It is often a combination from two or three different classes of drug including tranquillisers, opioids and anticholinergics. The type and combination is chosen by the veterinary surgeon and depends on procedure, personal preference, species, physical status and temperament.

Premedication might not be administered to debilitated patients as it may cause further depression of the central nervous system.

Routine premedication is administered up to 30 minutes prior to induction depending on drug and route used. Following administration, the patient should be left in a warm, quiet kennel to allow optimum drug responsiveness. The aims of premedication are (Torrance & Serginson 2004):

- to calm and control the patient, facilitating handling and reducing the levels of circulating catecholamines which may cause cardiac dysrhythmias
- to provide analgesia – an opioid administered with a tranquilliser such as acepromazine maleate will also have a synergistic effect
- to reduce the amounts of anaesthetic induction and maintenance agents and their associated side-effects
- to assist with a smooth recovery from general anaesthesia.

Preparation of paediatric patients

Paediatric patients are classified as those up to 12 weeks of age. This age group is considered to be at increased surgical risk compared with an adult patient due to the immature development of the critical organs, the reduced ability to maintain thermoregulation, and increased susceptibility to hypoglycaemia. Consideration should be given to which anaesthetic drugs are administered as these patients have a reduced ability to metabolise and excrete them (Holden 1999). With these factors in mind, consideration needs to be given to the following:

- Accurate weighing of the patient to allow precise drug dose calculations. If small volumes are required, it is recommended to dilute the drug to allow for accurate administration.
- Securing venous access for fluid and drug administration and for emergency situations. The jugular vein is probably the most accessible vein for venepuncture.
- Blood glucose analysis is advisable to establish a baseline. Fasting of patients is not recommended for longer than an hour prior

to anaesthesia – blood glucose levels can decrease dramatically due to liver immaturity and rapidly depleted glycogen stores.

- An inherently increased oxygen requirement may necessitate pre-oxygenation and supplementation during the recovery period (Holden 1999).
- Reduced renal function leads to the patient being less able to cope with large quantities of rapidly infused intravenous fluids, therefore the use of a burette or syringe driver is advisable.

Preparation of geriatric patients

A geriatric patient is one who has reached 75% of the expected life span for that species and breed. The normal physical, physiological and pharmacological changes in geriatric patients influence the care they receive and increase the risks associated with anaesthesia and surgery (Litwack 1995). Geriatric patients have reduced function in the heart and cardiovascular system, the respiratory system, the kidneys and liver and in responding to stress.

There is also an increased probability of concurrent disease being present, e.g., diabetes mellitus, mitral valve insufficiency and the resulting congestive heart failure or chronic renal disease. Obtaining a full history from the owner and performing a thorough physical examination is very important. For example, exercise intolerance could indicate heart disease and polydipsia could indicate renal failure. Further investigations may be warranted, such as haematology and biochemistry analysis, urinalysis, thoracic radiography and electrocardiography.

Specific requirements of the geriatric patient include:

- minimal period of hospitalisation to minimise stress
- maintaining the patient's normal routine as much as possible
- paying consideration to comfort and bedding, nutrition, exercise, mental stimulation and physiotherapy to help maintain joint mobility

- regular monitoring and recording of vital signs
- water should be withheld for no longer than 30 minutes prior to general anaesthesia to prevent excessive dehydration.

Preparation of exotic species

Preparing exotic species for surgical procedures is, in many ways, similar to preparing the more frequently encountered species, such as:

- routine acquisition of blood for haematology and biochemistry analysis to aid identification of systemic disease
- accurate weighing for calculation of drug doses
- provision of fluid therapy – oral, subcutaneous or, preferably, intravenous or intraosseous
- preventing hypothermia
- preoperative fasting.

Preoperative fasting can range from zero to 72 hours depending on species. Small avian patients need as little as an hour without food, whereas larger birds require up to 8–10 hours. Small mammals can warrant even less as several cannot vomit and others have high metabolic rates and are at risk of hypoglycaemia. Conversely, most reptiles need anything from 24 to 72 hours to limit enlarged intestines compromising respiration. Please consult relevant texts for information on specific species (Girling 2003).

Enemas and catheterisation of the bladder

Enemas
Enemas are performed to reduce the amount of faecal matter within the patient's colon and rectum. Preoperatively, they are performed for several reasons:

- to prepare the patient for contrast radiography as poor preparation can result in non-diagnostic radiographs
- prior to colonoscopy
- prior to gastrointestinal or anal surgery

to prevent faecal soiling of the patient during surgical procedures (although the placement of a purse string suture around the anus is more effective and less time consuming).

Warm water is commonly used to perform an enema, although there are various proprietary brands available – these include micro-enema tubes that are useful in cats. Approximately 5–10ml of warm water per kilogram body weight can be administered per rectum. This can be performed using a lubricated Higginson syringe, urinary catheter or 50ml syringe nozzle. The patient should be cleaned and dried thoroughly afterwards (Chandler 1999).

Catheterisation of the bladder

Catheterisation of the bladder is most commonly achieved via the urethra (male and female), although percutaneous catheterisation can be performed in the instance of urethral tear or obstruction. In this situation, a cystostomy tube can be left in situ for several days whilst the patient is stabilised. Preoperatively, the bladder is catheterised for several reasons:

- to empty the bladder of urine prior to contrast radiography, e.g. pneumocystogram
- to identify the urethra during surgical procedures, e.g. perineal urethrostomy
- to allow urine production to be assessed – this information can be used to evaluate kidney function and therefore, adequate blood pressure and perfusion
- to minimise risk of urine soiling during surgery
- to allow surgical access to deep abdominal structures.

Catheter placement, protocol and principles

Catheters should be inserted and maintained using a strict aseptic technique. This minimises the possible development of bacteraemia or septic complications.

Intravenous catheterisation   Common sites of placement include cephalic, lateral and medial saphenous, pinnae and jugular veins:

- an area over the vein is closely clipped, loose hair is removed
- the area is aseptically prepared
- an assistant occludes and rotates the vein (if required) to visualise the vessel
- an appropriate size intravenous catheter is advanced at an angle of approximately 25–30° through the skin and into the vein, until a flash of blood is seen in the hub of the catheter
- the catheter is advanced proximally into the vein whilst the stylet is held stationary
- the stylet is removed and occlusion of the vein is released.

Arterial catheterisation   Common sites for placement are the dorsal metatarsal, femoral and superficial palmar artery:

- the area over the artery is prepared as per intravenous catheterisation
- the artery is palpated (by locating the pulse) to confirm its location, and the area is aseptically prepared
- a transcutaneous incision is made over the artery using a scalpel blade
- occlusion of the vessel is not required
- a catheter is inserted through the incision into the artery as previously described.

Catheterisation of the jugular vein may be performed to provide venous access when access to a peripheral vein cannot be achieved. In smaller patients a standard 18 gauge intravenous catheter can be placed into the jugular vein and sutured in place. A central venous catheter is placed into a jugular vein and positioned within the anterior vena cava, so that the tip lies close to the right atrium. Central venous catheters can be used to monitor central venous pressure and provide venous access. Catheters often have multiple lumens, thus providing multiple ports for fluid administration and blood sampling.

Central venous catheter placement – Seldinger technique

- the patient is positioned in lateral recumbency
- the neck is extended slightly and elevated by placement of a support beneath the neck

- an area over the vein is aseptically prepared
- a transcutaneous incision is made over the jugular vein with a scalpel blade
- the introducer needle is inserted into the raised jugular vein
- the guide wire is fed through the introducer needle into the vein, and the needle is removed
- the vessel dilator is fed over the guide wire to enlarge the cutaneous puncture site and is then removed
- the tip of the central venous catheter is passed over the guide wire and advanced into the vein
- the guide wire is withdrawn and the catheter aspirated via each port to remove residual air, end ports are attached and each port is flushed with sterile heparinised saline
- the catheter is secured in place with sutures.

Care of catheters

All catheter placements should be performed in an aseptic manner. This may include the donning of sterile gloves and the formation of a sterile field (especially relevant in the placement of central catheters):

- catheters should be secured in place with clean adhesive tape or sutures
- a sterile dressing should be applied to prevent contamination of the insertion site and provide protection from patient interference
- patency of the catheter should be maintained by flushing all ports with sterile heparinised saline every 4–6 hours for venous catheters and every 30 minutes for arterial catheters
- if collecting blood samples via a catheter, discard the initial sample drawn to avoid contamination, obtain sample and flush catheter after collection
- ensure only compatible preparations are administered via the catheter to avoid precipitation
- do not allow air to be administered through any ports or attached lines

- store connectors in a sterile container, and ensure all open ends of catheters and connectors are treated in an aseptic manner
- venous and arterial catheters should be replaced in a different site after 72 hours
- central venous catheters may be left in situ for up to 7 days, if cared for correctly
- if a catheter-related infection is suspected (pyrexia, localised pain, swelling or irritation) remove the catheter in an aseptic manner and submit it for bacterial culture; re-address your catheter protocol
- remove catheters as soon as they are no longer required.

Presurgical antibiotic administration

Presurgical prophylactic antibiotic use is controversial and should always be the surgeon's decision. Antibiotics are generally overused and antibiotic-resistant micro-organisms are becoming a major problem. Antibiotic therapy should be:

- correctly administered
- based on the probability and degree of microbial contamination, i.e.
  - cases with a high risk of postoperative infection (anal/perianal surgery, open fractures and intestinal surgery)
  - in the presence of pre-existing infection; a bacteriology swab should be taken for culture and sensitivity to ensure appropriate antibiotic therapy.

Antibiotics should never be used as a substitute for poor aseptic technique and postoperative hygiene. There should be no need for administration if it is a clean surgical wound. A broad-spectrum antibiotic may be administered to provide cover against the most likely pathogens, e.g. *Staphylococcus intermedius*. If administered, antibiotics need to be given at the correct time to ensure plasma concentration is at its peak level at the time of the surgical incision – when bacteria are likely to enter the wound. Subcutaneous antibiotics should be given approximately 2 hours before surgery; intravenous antibiotics should be administered 30 minutes before surgery.

Analgesia

Analgesia can be achieved through a variety of different classes of drugs including opioids, non-steroidal anti-inflammatory drugs (NSAIDs) and local analgesics. Different classes of drugs used in conjunction are more effective than either drug administered alone. Pre-emptive analgesia makes the patient more comfortable during recovery and reduces the overall analgesic requirement. With severe, established pain a 'multimodal' analgesic regime provides the most effective relief (Nolan 2000).

Opioids

Opioids act centrally by binding to receptors located within the brain and spinal cord, which limits the input of nociceptive information into the CNS. The receptors are classified as mu (μ), kappa (κ) or delta (δ); μ- and κ-receptors are responsible for analgesia, sedation and respiratory depression and δ-receptors are thought to be responsible for the adverse side effects, e.g. dysphoria, excitement and restlessness. Opioids may have activity at one or more receptor. They are classified as pure agonists, pure antagonists or partial agonists. Individual opioids vary in their potency, duration of action and side effects. All opioids are metabolised by the liver and excreted by the kidneys so lower doses should be administered in patients with hepatic or renal disease. Uses of opioids:

- treatment of pre-existing pain
- assist with sedation
- pre-emptive analgesia – administered so they are active at the receptors at the time of surgical stimulation
- reduce the amount of anaesthetic maintenance agent required
- control postoperative pain.

Pure agonists   Pure agonists stimulate all receptors. They are the most potent opioids, provide excellent analgesia and have dose-dependent effects. The most commonly administered pure agonists are morphine sulphate, pethidine, methadone and fentanyl citrate. All pure agonists are classified as Schedule 2 drugs because of the potential for human abuse. Effects of pure agonists:

- analgesia
- sedation ± excitement
- reduced gut motility and sphincter spasm
- bradycardia
- respiratory depression – dose-dependent
- euphoria/dysphoria
- potential for dependency

Morphine sulphate
- very effective analgesic
- moderate to severe pain
- slow intravenous, intramuscular, subcutaneous or epidural routes
- intravenous administration can result in hypotension
- causes sedation in the painful patient but can cause excitement in the non-painful patient
- gastrointestinal stimulation can result in vomiting
- duration of action is 3–4 hours (duration is longer in cats)

Pethidine
- only pure agonist licensed for veterinary use
- intramuscular or subcutaneous
- intravenous administration results in massive histamine release
- used:
  - as part of a premedication regime
  - in animals with hepatic disease because of its short duration of action (1–1.5 hours)
  - in animals with cranial abdominal pain, as it is thought to have good visceral effects

Methadone
- synthetic drug
- similar to morphine
- intramuscular or subcutaneous route
- administration is less likely to cause excitement or vomiting
- duration of action is 3–4 hours (duration is longer in cats)

Fentanyl
- potent, fast-acting, short-lasting analgesia
- onset of action is 2–3 minutes

- duration of action is 20 minutes dose dependent
- intravenous injection (bolus or infusion), intramuscular, subcutaneous or transdermal
- very good intraoperative analgesic (intravenously)
- side effects of intravenous administration are bradycardia and respiratory depression (prepare for IPPV)

Partial agonists   Partial agonists block one receptor and stimulate another. They have a ceiling of activity – higher doses can result in reversal of effect. Partial agonists will antagonise the effects of pure agonists. They are less potent than pure agonists and have fewer side effects. The most commonly administered partial agonists are buprenorphine and butorphanol.

Buprenorphine
- mild to moderate pain
- slow onset of action (40–60 minutes)
- long duration of action (6–8 hours)
- intravenous, intramuscular or subcutaneous routes
- very effective when given sublingually in cats
- good sedation when combined with acepromazine maleate
- schedule 3 drug

Butorphanol
- quicker onset of action and a shorter duration of action than buprenorphine
- ineffective against severe pain
- produces less dysphoria, sedation and respiratory depression than other opioids
- intravenous, intramuscular or subcutaneous routes
- also available in tablet form – usually prescribed as an antitussive
- more suitable perioperative analgesics available

Pure antagonists
Naloxone
- antagonises the effects of pure and partial agonists in cases of overdose, severe respiratory depression or bradycardia
- displaces opioids from the receptors and, therefore, blocks their effects

- short duration of action (30–60 minutes)
- repeated doses necessary at frequent intervals until the opioid has been metabolised
- expensive and has a short shelf life.

Non-steroidal anti-inflammatory drugs (NSAIDs)
- analgesic, anti-inflammatory and antipyretic
- act peripherally by suppressing inflammation and swelling
- for mild to moderate pain when administered on their own
- for moderate to severe pain when combined with an opioid
- no sedative effects
- if administered preoperatively they provide good analgesia in the postoperative period
- onset of action is 30–60 minutes when administered by any route
- examples include carprofen and meloxicam.

Arachidonic acid (released from cell membranes when they are damaged) is catalysed by the enzymes lipo-oxygenase and cyclo-oxygenase (COX) and results in the formation of prostaglandins in damaged tissues, which causes pain and inflammation. NSAIDs inhibit cyclo-oxygenase, resulting in decreased prostaglandin production, therefore preventing pain and inflammation.

Two forms of COX have been identified – COX-1 and COX-2. COX-1 synthesises prostaglandins that help maintain normal physiological functions, e.g. protection of gastric mucosa, maintenance of renal blood flow and platelet aggregation – inhibition of COX-1 is thought to be the cause of NSAID side effects. COX-2 synthesises prostaglandins that cause pain and inflammation. Toxic side effects can be seen and include:

- *Gastric ulceration.* Prostaglandins present in the gastric mucosa decrease acid secretion and increase mucus production. If prostaglandin levels are reduced these effects are reversed and can result in ulceration.
- *Renal toxicity.* NSAIDs have the potential to reduce renal blood flow if prostaglandins are inhibited – this can result in acute renal

failure. Intravenous fluids should be administered and arterial blood pressure monitored in anaesthetised animals because they are predisposed to hypotension and reduced renal blood flow.

- *Impaired platelet aggregation*. There is potential for prolonged bleeding times at surgery but this has never been reported.

NSAIDs do have some advantages over opioids:

- they are not controlled
- no potential for human abuse
- oral administration is effective
- no cardiovascular or respiratory side effects
- they do not depress the central nervous system, so there is no sedative effect.

Local analgesia

Local analgesia is used as part of a balanced general anaesthesia protocol as it prevents transmission of pain impulses into the CNS. This reduces the amount of maintenance agent required and also provides good postoperative analgesia. It can also be used if the animal is debilitated and a high anaesthetic risk as procedures can often be performed on conscious animals or those under mild sedation. Local analgesic drugs temporarily block sodium channels so nerve depolarisation cannot occur, resulting in loss of nerve conduction. Motor and autonomic nerve fibres are affected as well as sensory fibres.

Different drugs vary in tissue penetration, onset of action and duration of action. Lignocaine and bupivicaine are the commonly used drugs in veterinary medicine. Lignocaine has a rapid onset but a short duration of action; bupivacaine has a slower onset of action but a longer duration. A vasoconstrictor, such as adrenaline, is often added to increase the duration of action. There are several ways to prevent and treat postoperative pain; listed below are the three methods commonly used.

Infiltration A local analgesic is infiltrated into the tissues in close proximity to the nerve that is to be affected. This is commonly used for surgery involving superficial tissues, e.g. subcutaneous mass removal, or to block intercostal nerves following thoracic surgery to provide good postoperative analgesia.

Intra-articular Injection of a local analgesic into a joint following surgery provides good postoperative pain relief for up to 8 hours. The drug used should not contain adrenaline.

Epidural A local analgesic or, more often, an opioid is injected into the epidural space. Unless motor paralysis is required for surgery, administration of an opioid is more advantageous because it provides excellent analgesia without loss of motor function to the animal's hindquarters. Preservative-free morphine sulphate should be used and acts directly at the opioid receptors within the spinal canal. This provides profound and long lasting analgesia without the systemic side effects (Waterman-Pearson 1999).

Intravenous fluid therapy

Fluid therapy is indicated for the treatment and prevention of hypotension, hypovolaemia and electrolyte, metabolic and acid–base disorders. Intravenous fluid therapy is essential for all surgery to ensure normovolaemia and normotension and minimise alterations in acid–base and electrolyte balance. Normal maintenance rates for fluid therapy are 2ml/kg/h – these are increased for surgery to compensate for fluid lost through evaporation and third spacing, which occurs during any surgical procedure. Third spacing is an abnormal accumulation of fluid in extracellular locations. It is caused by expansion of the interstitial fluid space, ascites, hydrothorax or accumulation around traumatised tissues, i.e. during surgical manipulation. The greater the tissue damage, the greater the fluid loss.

Crystalloids

Crystalloids are divided into hypotonic, isotonic and hypertonic. The main constituents of crystalloids are sodium and chloride; they may also contain other electrolytes and buffers.

Hypotonic fluids are prepared as isotonic solutions prior to the addition of glucose. A hypotonic solution is left once the glucose has been metabolised. They are generally administered as a maintenance fluid with potassium chloride supplemented.

Isotonic crystalloids maintain plasma volume, expand vascular and interstitial compartments, replace deficits in dehydrated patients and restore third space losses. They are inexpensive and readily available. The infusion must be continued to maintain volume expansion as they rapidly redistribute into extracellular space. For most routine surgical procedures a balanced isotonic crystalloid solution, such as compound sodium lactate, is suitable – administered at a surgical maintenance rate of 10ml/kg/h. This will prevent hypotension from the vasodilation and myocardial depression caused by anaesthetic agents and replace fluid lost through evaporation and third spacing. Any patient predisposed to low blood glucose levels, e.g. a paediatric patient or an animal with an insulinoma or portosystemic shunt, will benefit from a fluid containing glucose being administered concurrently.

Hypertonic crystalloids are administered as a plasma volume expander in the treatment of hypovolaemia. They must be followed with an isotonic fluid to avoid further dehydration.

Colloids

Indications for the use of colloids include hypoalbuminaemia, blood loss, hypovolaemia, hypotension and third space losses. They contain large molecules that do not readily cross the capillary walls so have a more sustained effect on the animal's plasma volume. A similar volume to what has been lost should be administered, up to a maximum volume of 20ml/kg 24 hours; the administration of excessive amounts can lead to clotting disorders. The potential for circulatory overload is another disadvantage of colloid administration because of the delay in fluid redistribution (Battaglia 2001).

Blood transfusions

Identification of blood groups in dogs and cats

Blood group determination in the dog is recommended prior to a transfusion. Typing the patient at a non-critical time can help in any future emergency situation (Fig 9.1). Generally, dogs will tolerate an initial unmatched transfusion – the antibodies formed due to an incompatible transfusion will prevent further unmatched transfusion being administered. In cats, blood group determination is more critical as an unmatched transfusion could lead to a life threatening systemic anaphylactic reaction.

Canine blood groups

Canine erythrocytes contain on their surface specific antigens, termed 'DEA' – dog erythrocyte antigen. Eight known antigens have been identified, forming the eight common blood groups: DEA 1.1, 1.2, 3, 4, 5, 6, 7 and 8. Of these, the most significant are DEA 1.1 and 1.2, with DEA 7 also important. Most reactions occur when DEA 1.1 positive blood is given to a DEA 1.1 negative recipient; less severe reactions can occur when DEA 1.2 is mismatched.

- a DEA 1.1 positive dog can receive both DEA 1.1 positive and negative blood

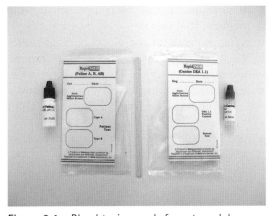

Figure 9.1   Blood typing cards for cats and dogs.

- a DEA 1.1 negative dog should not receive DEA 1.1 positive blood
- the ideal blood to be transfused would be DEA 1.1 and 1.2 negative.

Feline blood groups

The blood group system in cats consists of two antigens, Type A or Type B (there is a Type AB combination, but this is rare). Blood group incidence varies among breed and with geographic location.

- Type A cats also have a low titred naturally occurring anti-B antibody
- Type B cats also have a high titred naturally occurring anti-A antibody.

A Type B cat that is transfused with Type A blood will show an immediate anaphylactic reaction due to the high level of naturally occurring anti-A antibody. A Type A cat transfused with Type B blood will show a less severe reaction due to the lower level of anti-B antibody (Abrams-Ogg 2000).

Blood collection

Animal blood banks are not currently available. Donors may be available from staff animals, where the blood group may already be known. The ideal canine donor:

- is friendly, calm natured, no older then 8 years, and weighs over 28kg
- is of known blood type, compatible to the recipient
- is fully vaccinated, but not within the previous 10–14 days
- is free of parasites and blood-borne diseases
- is not receiving any medication at the time of donation
- has not received any transfusions themselves
- has a high packed cell volume (PCV) if transfusion is for RBC
- has a lower PCV if plasma and platelet products are being used.

The ideal feline donor:

- is as above, but weighs over 4.5kg
- preferably has a high PCV
- is negative for feline infectious diseases.

A maximum donation volume for a dog is 16–18ml/kg – a standard donation is about 450ml. Dogs can donate every 3 weeks providing their nutrition status is monitored; donations every 2–3 months require no nutritional supplementation. Ideally the donor should be starved for 12 hours prior to donation, to allow for sedation if required. In emergency donation, post-prandial lipaemia seems to have no effect on the product transfused.

Collection is normally from a jugular vein, but cephalic veins may be used in larger patients. Aseptic preparation and collection should be adhered to:

- human blood collection packs are most commonly used for canine donors
- collection bags with satellite bags are suitable for plasma and platelet collection
- feline blood donation can be collected in a 60 ml syringe into which anticoagulant/preservative solution had been measured.
- the collecting bag should be gently rocked as the blood is collected to ensure adequate mixing of anticoagulant and preservative solution.

Infusion routes and rates

Blood is an excellent medium for bacteria and needs to be handled correctly to avoid contamination. Blood transfusion giving sets include filters that prevent thrombi (microclots) or large contaminants from entering the bloodstream. Inline filters can be added to syringes for smaller donations. Infusion pumps that administer blood are designed not to damage the red blood cells.

It is generally not necessary to warm blood, even when stored in the refrigerator, as it should be at room temperature by the time it gets from the bag to the patient. The patient's thermodynamics will warm the blood when it reaches the circulation. Care should be taken if the patient is already hypothermic.

Blood that has been stored in the refrigerator can be warmed in a warm water bath to room temperature; haemolysis can occur if warmed to over 38°C. Blood should never be warmed in a microwave oven as there is a risk of overheating, leading to haemolysis and potassium release. Administration of blood is ideally through a wide bore peripheral or central intravenous catheter. If venous access can not be achieved it can be administered intraosseously, or intraperitoneally – the latter taking up to 24 hours for absorption.

Care should be taken when administering additional fluids simultaneously – solutions containing calcium will cause precipitation of the citrate in the anticoagulant while those containing dextrose will cause haemolysis.

The rate at which the blood is administered will depend on the condition of the patient, but generally initial administration should be 0.25ml/kg/h for 30 minutes. If no reaction is seen then the infusion should be increased to a rate such that the transfusion is completed within 4 hours. When the transfusion will take longer than 4 hours the risk of bacterial contamination is increased – it may be advantageous to divide the blood and keep the remainder refrigerated until it is required. The maximum rate of infusion should be no more than 22ml/kg/h, and this should only be used in emergency situations. Plasma can be administered at a faster rate, 4–6ml/kg/h.

Transfusion reactions

Transfusion reactions can occur even if the correct blood type is administered. Most reactions will occur within a short time of the transfusion commencing, although a reaction can still occur hours or days after the transfusion (Rubens 2004). Reactions can be divided into immunological and non-immunological.

- Immunological reactions (acute or delayed) can lead to an acute haemolytic crisis, caused by:
  - incompatibility reactions
  - reactions to WBC and platelets.
- Non-immunological reactions (acute or delayed) can occur from excessive volumes or rates being administered, or from changes occurring during storage:
  - anaphylactoid reactions – usually due to a fast transfusion rate

- circulatory overload – more common in small animals, or animals with concurrent cardiac or renal failure
- microbial contamination leading to transfusion associated sepsis
- poor storage or administration – hyperkalaemia due to RBC leaking potassium during storage
- pretransfusion haemolysis – contamination, poor storage, rough handling and over-heating may all damage the blood.

Clinical signs that may indicate a transfusion reaction are:

- a rise in body temperature; can be minor as little as 2°C
- heart rate and respiratory rate may increase or decrease
- tremors, agitation, urination
- vomiting and/or diarrhoea
- weakness
- collapse and seizures.

CARE OF THE ANAESTHETISED PATIENT AND POSTOPERATIVE RECOVERY

Maintenance of patient airway

Maintaining the patency of a patient's airway whilst anaesthetised is paramount. Various factors put the patient at risk of airway obstruction, such as (Johnson 2003):

- relaxed muscles within the pharynx, leading to potential airway collapse
- relaxed sphincters in the oesophagus, leading to an increased risk of gastric reflux
- loss of swallow reflex and the resultant accumulation of saliva.

Masks

Masks can be utilised to provide a source of oxygen both in the pre- and postoperative period. However, they do not protect the patient's airway and hence should only be used when the patient can maintain its own airway.

Endotracheal tubes (ETTs)

ETTs are used to maintain a patient's airway during anaesthesia and when the patient is unable to protect their own airway. They protect the airway from refluxed gastric contents, saliva, and blood or lavage fluids. ETTs provide a means to administer inhaled gaseous anaesthetic agents and intermittent positive pressure ventilation (IPPV) when necessary.

A well fitting ETT can prevent inhalational agents becoming environmental pollutants. To help the ETT fit better, some have inflatable cuffs to create a seal within the trachea. To ensure the correct level of inflation once in situ, gently squeeze the reservoir bag and inflate the cuff until escaping gas is no longer audible.

Over-inflation of the cuff can result in pressure necrosis and/or rupture of the trachea, and may even occlude the lumen if the sides of the tube are pressed together. Under-inflation of the cuff results in environmental pollution, the patient breathing 'around' the tube and poorly inflated lungs if performing IPPV. ETTs should also be of the correct length – too long and there is increased dead space and an increased risk of intubating one bronchi; too short and the tube may slip out of the trachea. There are a number of types of ETT:

- Magill
  - no 'eye' at the tip
  - cuffed and non-cuffed available
  - inflation pipe attached to the side of the tube
- Murphy
  - similar to the Magill
  - has an eye at the tip (Murphy's eye) that allows gas to flow, even if bevel end is occluded (Fig 9.2)
- Armoured
  - incorporates metal spiral within the tube to prevent kinking and occlusion when the neck is in flexion (e.g. during cisternal puncture myelography) (Fig 9.3)
- Streamlined
  - similar to the Magill
  - the inflation pipe is incorporated within the tube to make a smaller outer diameter.

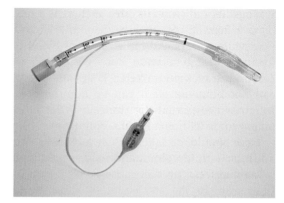

Figure 9.2 Murphy's endotracheal tube.

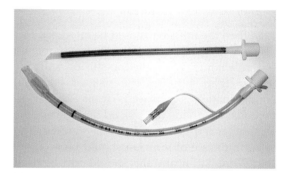

Figure 9.3 Armoured endotracheal tube.

To protect a patient's airway during oral surgery an ETT can be placed percutaneously via a pharyngotomy. This allows the surgeon excellent access to the oral cavity – useful during multiple facial fracture repair. If the airway needs to be protected postoperatively, a tracheostomy tube can be placed and maintained. This is useful in patients following complicated airway surgery, e.g. pharyngeal mass removal.

Maintenance of body temperature

Normothermia should be maintained – especially for small animals and paediatric patients due to a large surface area to bodyweight ratio. Several factors contribute to this:

- clipping and skin preparation result in heat loss – alcohol evaporation cools the skin

- anaesthetised animals are unable to generate heat through shivering or muscle activity and metabolic rate reduction results in poor heat generation
- exposure of viscera results in evaporation and cooling
- certain pre-anaesthetic drugs and maintenance agents cause vasodilation, contributing to heat loss
- inspiration of cold, un-humidified anaesthetic gases.

Hypothermia slows drug metabolism, increasing the potency and length of action, and resulting in a slower recovery from anaesthesia. Constant electronic temperature monitoring can be obtained via oesophageal or rectal measurement. Alternatively, intermittent rectal temperature readings should be obtained every 15 minutes. Prevention of hypothermia should begin immediately after induction of anaesthesia as temperature loss is greatest in the first 20 minutes. Methods to help maintain body temperature include:

- warm ambient temperature
- minimal hair removal
- avoid excessive wetting of the animal during skin preparation or lavage
- avoid the use of alcohol in small animals and paediatrics.
- avoid delays that will result in prolonged anaesthesia.
- incorporate heat:moisture exchange units or use re-breathing anaesthetic circuits to avoid heat loss through respiration (Fig 9.4)
- warm intravenous fluids and fluids for lavage
- insulate extremities and areas away from the surgical site with bubble wrap and foil
- thermostatically controlled water beds and hot air blankets are very effective at maintaining body temperature; heated pads should be avoided because of the associated risk of burns
- in the postoperative period, incubators can be used for small patients to provide both an ambient temperature and an oxygen enriched atmosphere when necessary (Fig 9.5).

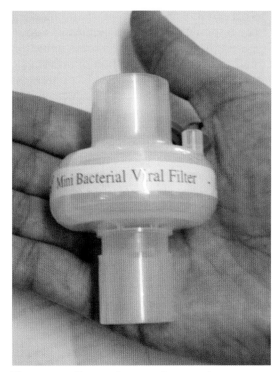

Figure 9.4   Heat:moisture exchange unit.

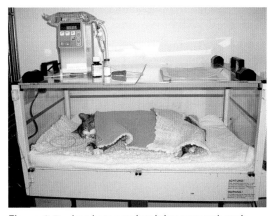

Figure 9.5   Incubator maintaining normothermia.

Perioperative care and postoperative recovery

Paediatric patients

There are certain aspects to consider when approaching paediatric surgical patients.

- Some anaesthetists prefer to induce anaesthesia by the use of inhalation gases only.

This avoids using injectable drugs, allowing the respiratory system to eliminate expired gases. The advantages are a rapid induction and recovery with reduction of anaesthetic time. However, some schools of thought advocate the prudent use of diluted injectable agents to avoid the occurrence of apnoea and release of environmental pollutants during inhalational induction.

- At induction, a laryngoscope is required to aid the visualisation of the larynx due to its reduced size.
- Monitoring and maintenance of anaesthesia requires close observation as paediatric patients are susceptible to the effects of drugs, especially in cases where cardiac output is compromised, as bradycardia and hypotension can develop.
- Hypothermia should be prevented as this can decrease metabolic rate, thus augmenting the effect of drugs.
- Paediatric patients are susceptible to hypoglycaemia and regular blood analysis is recommended. A dextrose saline solution should be available if required. Minimise the risk of hypovolaemia by obtaining the smallest volume required.

Postoperatively, paediatric patients specifically require:

- a warm environment to recover in, preferably one that is oxygen enriched; shivering can increase oxygen consumption considerably
- maintenance of normothermia or gradual return to it
- adequate analgesia to ensure a rapid return to feeding
- recognition that paediatric patients react differently to pain and therefore the nurse should not assume that it feels none
- if the patient is not weaned, removal of surgical preparations from the skin will help the mother recognise her young's smell.

Geriatric patients

Degenerative changes are a normal part of the ageing process and may potentially affect anaesthesia, surgery and recovery:

- geriatric patients have a reduced ability to distribute, metabolise and excrete drugs
- cardiovascular changes result in a reduction in hepatic and renal blood flow, so drug metabolism and excretion is reduced
- anaesthesia produces depression of the already compromised functions of the cardiovascular and respiratory systems
- close monitoring is essential to detect and prevent difficulties – this, ideally, would include measurement of:
  - blood pressure, either directly or indirectly
  - ECG
  - pulse oximetry
  - capnography to assess ventilatory function
  - temperature
- intravenous fluid therapy provision
- prevention of hypothermia, which can prolong the recovery time and increase oxygen consumption
- when positioning for surgery, use extra padding and avoid tugging on extremities to avoid placing excessive pressure on muscles, bones and joints.

When nursing geriatric patients postoperatively consider that:

- geriatric patients are likely to have a prolonged recovery because of hepatic and cardiovascular insufficiency and reduced renal blood flow resulting in prolonged drug clearance
- normothermia should be returned
- shivering, caused by hypothermia, will also increase the patient's oxygen requirement and necessitate supplementation
- intravenous fluid therapy should be continued until the patient is able to maintain its hydration status and electrolyte balance
- regular turning will avoid atelectasis and resultant pneumonia
- once the patient is fully recovered, physiotherapy will help to keep the joints mobile
- geriatric patients will have increased susceptibility to infection and an aseptic technique is vital during nursing interventions

patients should be encouraged to eat as quickly as possible to promote tissue healing and recovery.

Exotic patients

The mortality rate for exotic patients undergoing surgical procedures is considerably higher than that of dogs and cats undergoing similar surgery. Therefore, thorough planning prior to induction and during the recovery period can greatly enhance the outcome of surgery. Special attention should be taken to secure the patient's airway and monitor vital signs, and close observation is necessary during the postoperative period. Species-specific considerations may include the following.

- Reptiles
  - the use of artificial tears to lubricate the corneas of reptiles with no eyelids
  - most reptiles can survive anaerobically for long periods of time and therefore preparation for IPPV is necessary if inhalational anaesthetic agents are to be used
  - strict aseptic technique is vital with reptiles as they are prone to abscesses and septicaemia
  - postoperatively, the patient should continue to receive IPPV until good ventilatory effect has returned
  - close monitoring is necessary until the patient is able to right themselves
  - if housed in a vivarium, ensure there is adequate ventilation to avoid the accumulation of expired anaesthetic gases (Malley 1999)
- Avian
  - rapid return to feeding to prevent hypoglycaemia
  - crop feeding may be necessary once fully recovered, if not eating
  - recovery is aided if the patient is in a darkened, quiet area away from predators
  - wrapping the bird lightly in a cloth may minimise the risk of self-trauma during recovery (Forbes 1999)

- Small mammals
  - provision of fluid therapy by intravenous, subcutaneous or intraperitoneal route
  - local anaesthetic cream can be applied to pinnae prior to intravenous catheter placement
  - postoperatively, a rapid return to feeding will improve recovery times
  - care should be taken when choosing bedding material as sawdust will adhere to surgical wounds.

Spinal surgery

Patients undergoing spinal surgery have a variety of preoperative needs. For patients that have undergone myelography, these are:

- maintenance of normothermia, as the procedure can be time consuming.
- ensuring the non-ionic contrast media is prevented from flowing intracranially – this is achieved by maintaining the patient's head in a raised position whenever possible to minimise the risk of seizure postoperatively
- administration of intravenous fluid therapy to prevent dehydration, maintain blood pressure and kidney function, and replace fluid losses.

For patients undergoing cervical spinal surgery measurement of arterial blood pressure is helpful as positioning for a ventral surgical approach can result in hypotension. This is caused by the extreme extension of the patient's neck. Equipment to prevent or correct hypotension should be available. Postoperatively, spinal patients require:

- action to maintain or return the patient to normothermia
- close monitoring during recovery to observe for signs of seizure activity; anti-seizure drugs should be made available.
- maintenance of intravenous access to administer intravenous fluids and drugs
- nursing care for recumbent patients.

Orthopaedic procedures

Pre- and postoperative care for patients undergoing orthopaedic procedures includes:

- adequate pre-emptive analgesia
- temporary immobilisation of joint/bone if necessary
- provision of antibiotics to ensure sufficient level in systemic blood supply prior to surgery
- adequate postoperative analgesia
- care of dressings, including bandages and external fixators
- use of a sling or hoist to assist mobility and prevent falls/slipping
- observations of limb use/mobility/pain level.

Airway surgery

Patients undergoing airway surgery have a number of similar requirements, regardless of the procedure planned. Preoperatively, these include:

- placement of an intravenous catheter at admittance for emergency use if necessary
- careful use of premedicants to enable a calm induction
- calm, cool and quiet environment prior to induction
- pre-oxygenation to optimise haemoglobin saturation at induction
- use of a well-fitting endotracheal tube to limit the risk of aspiration and to allow effective intermittent positive pressure ventilation if required
- a range of endotracheal tube sizes available, in preparation for a narrowed airway/difficult intubation
- packing the pharynx prior to surgery.

Postoperatively, the patient's requirements include:

- removing pharyngeal packing
- delayed removal of the endotracheal tube ensuring laryngeal function has returned
- suctioning upper airway/pharynx
- monitoring haemoglobin saturation (via pulse oximetry or arterial blood gases)
- providing oxygen supplementation

- recovering the patient in sternal recumbency in a cool, calm environment
- have resuscitation equipment available, including tracheotomy tubes, to prepare for upper airway occlusion.
- use of sedatives to prevent patients barking or becoming distressed
- feed 'balls' of tinned food – a bolus is less likely to be inhaled than individual pieces.

Close observation of the patient at all times is vital before and after surgery to ensure immediate response to a patient deteriorating. There is a specific protocol for the care of patients following placement of a tracheotomy tube, including (Hamilton 2003):

- constant monitoring
- instilling 2–5ml sterile saline into the tube to dilute thick mucus secretions, followed by suctioning of the tube's lumen to remove secretions
- pre-oxygenation prior to suctioning will limit the occurrence of hypoxia
- suctioning should be performed every 20 minutes initially
- some tubes contain an inner sleeve that can be removed for cleaning, whilst maintaining the patient's airway
- regular cleaning of the skin around the insertion site
- ensure the patient does not occlude the lumen with skin folds, bedding or through body position – care should be taken to prevent the inhalation of foreign objects.

Thoracic surgery

Patients undergoing thoracic surgery have similar requirements to that of airway patients, therefore, their care is very similar. In addition, they also require:

- frequent opportunities to urinate if on diuretics
- thorough preparation of emergency equipment and procedures prior to induction
- adequate caudal thoracic skin preparation to allow aseptic placement of a thoracic drain at the close of surgery

- adequate analgesia for optimal respiration during the postoperative period
- thoracic drain management (p 118)
- use of Elizabethan collars to prevent thoracic drain interference (Fig 9.6)
- close monitoring of respiration rate, depth and quality – a change may indicate pain, an accumulation of gas or fluid within the pleural cavity or displacement of the thoracic drain; immediate action is necessary to rectify the situation.

Ophthalmic patients

All patients, not just ophthalmic patients, should be monitored for corneal drying whilst under anaesthesia or sedation. Sterile lubricant eye preparations can be applied to the cornea to prevent this. Patients with an injury to the eye that renders the eye delicate can be at risk of spontaneous rupture of the globe. In these patients it is important not to raise the intra-ocular pressure within the globe. Observe the following:

- handle patients gently, keep restraint to a minimum
- avoid occlusion of the jugular veins – obtain blood samples from peripheral veins; exchange collars and leads for a harness
- intubation and extubation should occur under deeper plane of anaesthesia, where the laryngeal reflex is not present

- prevent the patient from barking, vocalising or coughing
- avoid the use of any drug that may induce vomiting
- an aural thermometer may be less stressful to the patient than struggling to obtain a rectal temperature
- self-injury due to a 'stormy' recovery should be avoided – human contact and gentle restraint is often sufficient; sedation may need to be implemented in some cases
- postoperatively the patient should not be allowed to play with toys, as this can lead to shaking and pulling movements of the head.

Self-trauma must be prevented; the use of Elizabethan collars can be counter-productive with some patients. Shaking of the head and collision with objects may only increase the possibility of damage to the eye. Foot bandages that include the dew claw are often a preferable option. Cleaning of ocular discharge should be performed gently using gauze swabs soaked with sterile saline. Direction from the surgeon should be sought when treating patients postoperatively; a discharge could indicate complications.

If bilateral ocular surgery is being performed, care should be taken of the contralateral eye – avoid contamination from loose clipped hair and from preparation solution run-off and avoid excess pressure on the eye when positioning the patient.

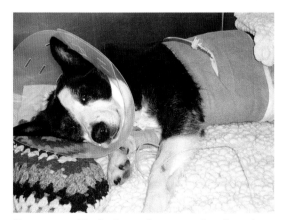

Figure 9.6 Elizabethan collar preventing thoracic drain interference.

Estimation of blood loss

Estimation of blood loss during surgery and the postoperative period is invaluable to ensure that the correct fluid type and volume is infused. During any surgical procedure carried out under a general anaesthetic, crystalloid fluid should be infused at a rate of 10ml/kg/h. Generally this fluid replacement is sufficient to cover the animal's losses during 'normal' surgical situations. The primary goal of fluid therapy is oxygen delivery. When a large amount of blood is lost at surgery the choice of fluid replacement will depend upon the estimated amount of blood lost, the speed of blood loss and the amount of haemoglobin that has been lost (Moon 1999). To calculate this certain factors can be measured:

● Swabs can be weighed to calculate the amount of blood they contain. Dry gauze swabs can be weighed; an approximate weight for a small 10-ply swab is 2g, and 10g for a large laparotomy swab. By weighing wet swabs and subtracting the dry weight, a volume of blood in millilitres can be determined:

$$1g \text{ of blood} = 1ml \text{ of blood}$$

● Suction bottle (Fig 9.7) contents can be measured. The volume of flush used is measured in millilitres (A), the volume of the suction bottle is measured in millilitres (B):

$$(B - A) = \text{volume of blood.}$$

● Other losses – onto drapes, under the patient and on the floor.

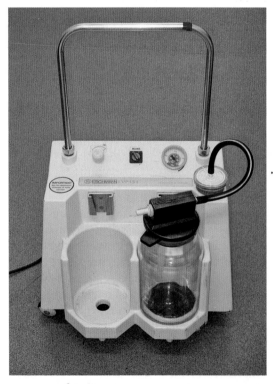

Figure 9.7 Suction bottles can be used to estimate blood loss.

All of the above calculations will provide an estimate of the total amount of blood lost in millilitres. Normal blood volume is 80–90ml/kg for dogs, 60–70ml/kg for cats – total blood loss can be determined as follows:

$$\% \text{ blood loss} = [\text{total blood loss (ml)} \div \text{normal blood volume (ml)}] \times 100$$

A guide to fluid replacement dependent on blood loss is:

● under 10% blood loss – give crystalloids
● over 10% blood loss –give colloids
● over 20% blood loss –give whole blood.

Monitoring of blood pressure and heart rate during surgery can give an indication of blood loss. A packed cell volume (PCV) reading should be performed prior to surgery. Blood typing and a donor on 'stand by' will save time if blood is required.

Dressings used postsurgically can be weighed as per above, to estimate any continued blood loss, and repeat PCV readings 12–24 hours later. Usual monitoring of pulse strength, mucous membrane colour and capillary refill time are all essential in the postoperative period. Please consult relevant texts for further information.

POSTOPERATIVE BANDAGING

Wound dressings and bandage components

The functions of a bandage and dressing are to:

● exert pressure to minimise dead space and reduce haemorrhage and seroma formation
● provide protection from environmental bacteria
● immobilise the wound and support bones
● provide comfort
● provide wound debridement
● absorb exudates
● hold drains and catheters in place.

The majority of bandages consist of three basic component layers:

● Primary (contact) layer. This is a sterile wound dressing applied directly to a broken area of skin. The type of dressing used depends on the type of wound involved.

- Secondary layer. A layer of padding providing comfort, support and protection. The padding layer is followed with a conforming bandage that compresses and holds the padding layer in place and contours well to the area being bandaged.
- Tertiary layer. The final layer provides protection and added support to the bandage. Commonly used are cohesive bandages - these have the advantage over adhesive bandages in that they do not stick to hair and skin.

Wound dressings

A correctly chosen primary layer will allow for optimal healing of the wound. Optimal healing will take place under the following conditions:

- moist but not too wet or macerated
- no infection or necrosis
- temperature 35–37°C
- undisturbed.

The primary layer must be sterile and remain in close contact with the surface of the wound at all times. It is, therefore, essential that this layer conforms to the body contours. If the wound is producing a large amount of exudate the dressing must allow this fluid to pass through to the secondary, absorbent layer of the dressing. All dressings should be frequently changed to allow assessment of the wound and the progression of healing.

Adherent dressings

- used in the early stages of wound healing to aid debridement of an open wound
- used when there is a large amount of necrotic tissue or debris present
- daily dressing changes necessary until a bed of granulation tissue has formed
- wet-to-dry dressings
  - indicated when there is a high viscosity exudate, necrotic tissue and debris
  - the contact layer (usually a gauze swab) is moistened with sterile sodium chloride to provide a moist environment
  - softens the necrotic tissue and dilutes

and thins the exudate, which makes absorption by the secondary layer easier
  - the contact layer should not be too wet as this can result in tissue maceration and bacterial strike-through
  - debris and necrotic tissue adhere to the dressing as it dries through evaporation; this is then removed when the dressing is changed.
- dry-to-dry dressings
  - indicated when there is a low viscosity exudate, necrotic tissue and debris
  - dry gauze swabs are placed directly on the wound
  - the contact layer and secondary layer absorb fluid and the dressing is removed when the contact layer has dried out
  - removal results in debridement of the wound.

Disadvantages of adherent dressings include removal of viable as well as necrotic tissue and pain for the patient on removal – therefore, sedation is often necessary.

Non-adherent dressings

- used in the repair stage of wound healing
- examples include postoperative surgical wounds or open wounds with a bed of granulation tissue
- newly formed tissue is not removed or damaged during removal because the dressing does not adhere to the wound
- mostly semi-occlusive – they absorb any exudates but retain some moisture to provide a moist environment to promote wound healing
- perforated film dressings
  - have a tendency to adhere to the wound
  - local dehydration can occur due to evaporation resulting in adherence.
  - a sheet of plastic is applied to one side of the dressing to reduce adherence
  - microscopic holes in the plastic film allow exudate to pass through into the dressing and absorbent layer
  - mainly used for clean postoperative wounds
- foam dressings
  - non-adherent

- excellent adsorptive capacity and maintain a moist, well-oxygenated environment for optimal wound healing
- more expensive than perforated film dressings.
- used mainly to dress granulating wounds because of the minimal risk of adherence
- hydrocolloids
  - used for open wounds where a large deficit is present
  - provide a moist environment, rehydrate the wound, debride through a normal autolytic process and absorb necrotic debris
  - alginates, derived from brown seaweeds, are considered as hydrocolloids because of the way they work.

Specific bandages

Bandaging techniques are well documented in veterinary nursing texts. However, points for consideration for each specific bandage will be discussed.

Bandaging of the head/neck

- commonly placed following aural surgery to prevent head shaking trauma to the pinnae
- occasionally the unaffected ear is left out to anchor the bandage
- neck bandages may be placed to secure jugular catheters or prevent caudal spread of subcutaneous emphysema after frontal sinus surgery
- staff should be able to place two fingers inside – an overly tight bandage can restrict breathing and hinder neck flexion
- care should be taken when removing bandage, to avoid damage to concealed pinnae

Bandaging of thorax/abdomen

- to cover wounds, drains and catheters; it is especially important that chest drains are not dislodged as this could potentially lead to a fatal pneumothorax
- care not to restrict breathing
- if used for applying abdominal pressure, it is recommended that it is gradually removed, starting from the caudal aspect, within 4 hours of placement

Bandaging of the extremities

- used primarily to reduce swelling and provide support
- can be incorporated to provide immobilisation using a splint or cast
- it is important to monitor the bandage for patient interference as this can indicate if the bandage is too tight or that the bandage has slipped
- frequently check that the distal end is not soiled, moist, chewed or showing strike-through (Hedlund 2002).

Types of casting materials

Casting materials are used to provide external support and prevent movement of the joints or long bones encased. Casts are used in specific situations, such as:

- immobilisation and support of distal limb fractures which are non-displaced
- secondary support of a fracture that has undergone surgical internal fixation
- to maintain a limb in extension, e.g. after an Achilles tendon repair
- secondary support of the distal limb following arthrodesis surgery.

The application of a cast immediately postoperatively is not common. A soft dressing can be applied to maintain a degree of support and provide gentle pressure around the surgical site. Once the risk of swelling has passed and the wound discharge is minimal, a cast can be applied. This is usually 24–72 hours after surgery.

There are three general categories of casting material available. Plaster of Paris has long since been superseded by its more modern counterparts because it is heavy and less comfortable for the patient. The application can be messy and time consuming due to the long drying time. More commonly used is fibreglass or polyester fabric impregnated with water-activated polyurethane resin. These types are preferred as they are light and quick drying but they are more expensive than Plaster of Paris. Both types of cast are best removed using an oscillating saw. Considerations for applying a cast correctly are as for soft bandages:

- adequate padding of bony prominences
- monitoring colour and warmth of toes
- non-adherent dressing covering surgical wound
- regular assessment of cast condition, e.g. chewed, damp, odorous.

Splints

Splints can be used to immobilise limbs but are not classed as casts. Aluminium and plastic varieties are available. They are cheap, quick and simple to apply. The support they provide may be quite weak depending on their location and size of patient. Similar care is necessary when applying splints to assess their application and efficacy.

Complications relating to bandaging

Injuries are frequently caused by improper bandage application or care. Examples of the causes are:

- being too tight or too loose
- becoming soiled/damp
- not being changed frequently enough
- inadequate selection of materials
- inappropriate application, e.g. femoral fractures when the fracture is not immobilised and the bandage provides a pendulum effect at the fracture site
- poor client compliance to return patient for re-assessment.

The resultant problems can range from minor irritation to major trauma leading to permanent disability. There are infinite problems depending on area of application, materials used and length of application, examples include:

- decubitus ulcers at bony prominences
- tissue necrosis due to pressure or tourniquet effect
- infection and skin sloughing
- lacerations caused during removal by scalpel blade, scissors or saws/embriotomy wire.

WOUND MANAGEMENT

Stages of healing

There are three stages in wound healing – lag phase, proliferative stage and remodelling stage. During the lag phase, haemostasis occurs; platelets aggregate and inflammatory cells infiltrate the area. Next, the proliferation of fibroblasts causes angiogenesis to occur. Granulation tissue forms, followed by epithelialisation and wound contraction. Finally, the bundles of collagen fibres remodel and healing is complete.

There are three ways a wound can heal – first, second and third intention:

- First intention healing occurs when the wound edges are closely apposed, for example sutured surgical incisions.
- Second intention healing occurs in open wounds where the skin edges are not apposed. The proliferative stage of wound healing is longer in second intention healing. Wound contraction can cause severe difficulties if it causes deformity or poor tissue perfusion.
- Third intention healing occurs when a wound is first treated as secondary intention until healthy granulation tissue is formed. Then the wound is surgically closed and continues healing as a first intention wound.

Obstacles can be encountered that hinder the wound healing process – namely, systemic factors, e.g. malnutrition, underlying disease or steroid use. More localised obstacles may include wound infection, poor perfusion, wound desiccation or wound trauma (Rutledge, 2004).

Aseptic surgical wounds

Aseptic surgical wounds are classified as clean with reference to the wound classification system. This indicates that the wound is non-traumatic, non-inflamed and does not involve the respiratory, alimentary or urogenital tract. As such, the risk of infection is reduced but relies on aseptic conditions being adhered to both by the surgeon and scrubbed assistant. An assumption is also made that the surgical patient has no hidden systemic disease which may delay healing. The use of pre/perioperative intravenous antibiotics is debatable but is generally recommended – in particular, if surgery involves the placement of implants or prostheses or the duration of surgery is prolonged.

Postoperatively, asepsis principles should be followed whilst cleaning the surgical wound. Sterile swabs, saline and gloves should be used and cleaning of the incision site be avoided as this not only disrupts the fragile fibrin clots but can potentially introduce bacteria. A sterile adhesive dressing is recommended, and should be kept in place for at least 48 hours allowing time for epithelialisation to take place.

Surgical preparation of infected wounds

Initial management of infected wounds will often include debridement and lavage. Before the surrounding area can be prepared the wound must be packed with either saline-soaked gauze swabs or a water-based lubricating jelly to avoid further contamination with hair and debris.

Eye ointment must be used if the wound is close to the animal's head. A large area around the wound must be clipped and the hair removed using a vacuum cleaner. Any hair at the edges of the wound can be removed using scissors. Once clipping is complete the swabs or lubricating jelly should be replaced and the area aseptically prepared in the usual way. The swabs or lubricating jelly are removed just prior to lavage and debridement:

- Lavage
  - reduces the bacteria count
  - removes debris and foreign material
  - best results achieved if performed under pressure, e.g. a 20ml syringe with 18 gauge hypodermic needle
  - excessive pressure is detrimental, causing bacteria and debris to enter further into the wound bed

- a sterile isotonic solution should be used, e.g. lactated ringer; sodium chloride has no buffers and an acidic pH so is considered cytotoxic.

- Debridement
  - debridement is performed following copious lavage to minimise infection, remove necrotic tissue, thus promoting healing
  - en-bloc debridement is performed aseptically and involves complete excision of the contaminated tissue
  - layered debridement removes devitalised tissue and debris using a scalpel blade until the deeper tissues are reached and haemorrhage is seen
  - following surgical debridement, wound dressings are applied.

Antibiotics

There are few advantages for topical preparations compared with systemic administration. High concentrations will already be present in the local tissue. Where *Pseudomonas* species are present in the wound, gentamicin can be used topically as this overcomes the renal side effects of intravenous gentamicin use. Tris-EDTA is a solution that, when applied topically, alters the construction of the bacterial cell wall and makes it more permeable to antibiotics and their use more effective. Broad-spectrum antibiotics can be administered until confirmation of culture sensitivity results is known. If there is no obvious infection, antibiotics should be discontinued to reduce the susceptibility to resistance and nosocomial infection.

Barrier nursing

Patients suffering from contagious infections, or those whose immunity is compromised, should be barrier nursed. Barrier nursing is the use of infection control to manage the spread and destruction of pathogenic organisms. The aims of barrier nursing are to protect the hospital environment from contamination with dangerous pathogens and to prevent transmission of infection between animals and people.

The most important measure in protecting any patient from hospital-acquired infections is adequate hand washing. Hands should be washed:

- between patients
- when they are visibly soiled
- before and after contact with each patient
- after contact with any source of micro-organism (blood or body fluids)
- before and after performing invasive procedures.

All patients should be isolated to prevent the spread of infection. Items that come into direct contact with the patient are considered contaminated and should be disposed of or sterilised before being returned to general use. The number of staff dealing with the patient should be limited to those necessary. Protective clothing (gloves, aprons/gowns, overshoes) should be donned before entering the contaminated area and disposed of after use. Wherever possible the patient being barrier nursed should be handled last after the other inpatients have been dealt with.

Protection of wound from patient interference

Patients may interfere with their wounds due to either boredom or irritation. This can lead to wound infection and dehiscence or self-removal of sutures/staples – it can be prevented by pre-emptive placement of an Elizabethan collar. Wounds should be covered with a dressing (if appropriate) and the use of a proprietary string matrix vest to hold indwelling catheters or drains. Feet can be bandaged to prevent scratching. Where there is persistent irritation, investigation is necessary to find the cause – it is common to find that sutures/staples are too tight or adhesive dressings are causing discomfort. Analgesia can aid in relieving discomfort if there is no obvious reason.

Types of surgical drain

Surgical drains are placed for three reasons: to remove dead space produced during surgery, to remove fluid/gas accumulations from body cavities and to drain infectious material from infected tissues.

Active and passive

There are two main types of drain that can be placed to allow drainage from a surgical site – active or passive. Active drains use gentle suction to remove fluid and/or gas accumulations from the wound or body cavity. Passive drainage is achieved through gravity and usually involves placing a drain distal to the wound to allow fluids to drain out – mainly used for subcutaneous wounds.

Closed wound drainage

A further way of categorising surgical drains is by describing them as closed drainage systems or open drainage systems. Closed wound drainage can be either active or passive. A passive, closed drain still uses gravity to remove fluid but keeps it enclosed by draining the fluid into a bag. An example is a Jackson cat catheter draining urine into an empty giving set and drip bag. An active, closed drainage system uses gentle suction provided either by a pump or by low pressure exerted by a vacuum. Examples would be concertina drain (Fig 9.8) or a vacutainer connected with a butterfly needle.

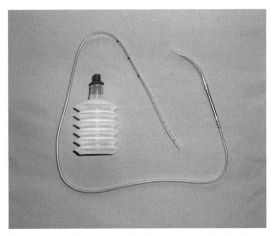

Figure 9.8 Concertina drain – an example of closed wound drainage.

Open wound drainage

Open wound drainage is always passive. It results in fluid (blood, pus or serum) draining out of a wound via gravity. The patient's skin and fur should be protected from the exudate to prevent sores and infection. A barrier cream or gel can be applied to the skin, and the end of the drain can be covered with a suitable absorbent dressing. An example of this type of drain is the Penrose.

Thoracic drainage

Thoracic drainage can be achieved either intermittently or continuously. The procedure can be as basic as an aseptically placed intravenous catheter temporarily positioned into the pleural cavity to remove gas/fluid. Alternatively, an indwelling thoracic drain can be aseptically placed. Continuous drainage of gas can be performed through the use of a Heimlich one-way valve. These are useful for a large or rapidly filling pneumothorax, but do not allow accurate measurement of product removed. Water seal drains also provide continuous drainage of gas. The intrathoracic pressure forces gas out of the pleural cavity and the water prevents air returning to the chest. These have the disadvantage of being cumbersome and need to be positioned below the patient but work well in large breed recumbent patients.

Intermittent drainage of the pleural cavity can be achieved using a syringe and three-way tap. Care must be taken to prevent the tap being opened incorrectly and allowing air into the pleural cavity. The benefit of this method is the accurate measurement of product and the removal of both gas and fluid. The disadvantage is the repeated handling of the drain, increasing the risk of sepsis. When the drain is not being suctioned, the distal end should be securely closed using a gate clamp and spigot and bandaged to the patient's body. Any uncertainty with regard to the positioning of the drain within the thoracic cavity requires a radiograph, which will confirm placement position.

Management of drains

- Dressings. All drains need to be secured safely to the patient's body to prevent them becoming entangled on cage bars and being dislodged. Aseptic technique will prevent the introduction of infection. An Elizabethan collar is vital to prevent patient interference.
- Recording of information. A record of types and amounts of fluid and/or gas removed should be made to allow comparison of daily production rates.
- Prevention of reflux. Reflux of fluid or gas travelling retrograde into the wound needs to be prevented. Introduction of infection can result in wound breakdown. This would include activating a concertina drain before the wound is sealed and thereby sucking air through the suture line, into the wound.
- Subcutaneous emphysema. Gas can collect subcutaneously around drains causing emphysema. This is identified by swelling and crepitus when palpated and is more commonly seen around thoracic drains and after surgery to the frontal sinus. Adequate bandaging can prevent or minimise the accumulation. For example, a thoracic bandage for chest drains or a neck bandage for frontal sinus drains to prevent spread along the body.
- Seroma formation. If the drain does not adequately remove fluid, an accumulation can create a seroma. Repositioning of the drain or additional drain placement may the resolve the problem.

References

Abrams-Ogg A 2000 Practical blood transfusion. In: BSAVA manual of canine and feline haematology and transfusion medicine. British Small Animal Veterinary Association, Cheltenham

Battaglia A M 2001 Fluid therapy. In: Battaglia A M (ed) Small animal emergency & critical care, 1st edn. W B Saunders, Pennsylvania

Chandler S 1999 General nursing. In: Cooper B, Lane D R (eds) Veterinary nursing, 2nd edn. Butterworth-Heinemann, Oxford

Forbes N 1999 Birds. In: Seymour C, Gleed R (eds) Manual of small animal anaesthesia and analgesia, 1st edn. British Small Animal Veterinary Association, Cheltenham

Girling S 2003 Veterinary nursing of exotic pets. Blackwell Publishing, Oxford

Hamilton J 2003 Nursing the patient in recovery. In: Welsh E (ed) Anaesthesia for veterinary nurses. Blackwell Publishing, Oxford

Hedlund, C 2002 Surgery of the integumentary system. In: Fossum T W (ed) Small animal surgery, 2nd edn. Mosby, St Louis

Holden D 1999 Paediatric patients. In: Seymour C, Gleed R (eds) Manual of small animal anaesthesia and analgesia, 1st edn. British Small Animal Veterinary Association, Cheltenham

Johnson C 2003 Breathing circuits and airway management. In: Welsh E (ed) Anaesthesia for veterinary nurses. Blackwell Publishing, Oxford

Jones R 1999 The practice of veterinary anaesthesia and analgesia. In: Seymour C, Gleed R (eds) Manual of small animal anaesthesia and analgesia, 1st edn. British Small Animal Veterinary Association, Cheltenham

Litwack K 1995 The elderly patient. In: Litwack K (ed) Post anaesthesia care nursing, 2nd edn. Mosby, St Louis

Malley D 1999 Reptiles. In: Seymour C, Gleed R (eds) Manual of small animal anaesthesia and analgesia, 1st edn. British Small Animal Veterinary Association, Cheltenham

McKelvey D, Hollingshead K W 2000 The pre-anaesthetic period. In: McKelvey D, Hollingshead K W (eds) Small animal anaesthesia & analgesia, 2nd edn. Mosby, St Louis

McKelvey D, Hollingshead K W 2000 Analgesia. In: McKelvey D, Hollingshead K W (eds) Small animal anaesthesia & analgesia, 2nd edn. Mosby, St Louis

Moon P F 1999 Fluid therapy and blood transfusion. In: Seymour C, Gleed R (eds) Manual of small animal anaesthesia and analgesia, 1st edn. British Small Animal Veterinary Association, Cheltenham

Nolan A M 2000 Pharmacology of analgesic drugs. In: Fleckwell P, Waterman-Pearson A. Pain management in animals, 1st edn. W B Saunders, London

Ruben D 2004 Transfusion medicine, administration and complications. Vet Tech 25:8

Rutledge B 2004 Obstacles to wound healing. Cosmetic Surgery Times Nov-Dec

Torrance C, Serginson E 2004 Preoperative care. In: Torrance C, Serginson E (eds) Surgical nursing, 12th edn. Elsevier, London

Waterman-Pearson A E 1999 Analgesia. In: Seymour C, Gleed R (eds) Manual of small animal anaesthesia and analgesia, 1st edn. British Small Animal Veterinary Association, Cheltenham

Williams J M 1999 Open wound management. In: Fowler D, Williams J M (eds) BSAVA manual of canine and feline wound management and reconstruction, 1st edn. British Small Animal Veterinary Association, Cheltenham

Chapter **10**

Theatre practice

Carole Martin and Jo Masters

CHAPTER OBJECTIVES

- Organising a surgical list

- Preparation of personnel
  General conduct
  General clothing
  Preparation of sterile personnel

- Surgical practice in the operating theatre
  General cleaning and hygiene
  Theatre cleaning protocol
  Equipment use, care and maintenance
  Care of specialised equipment
  Disposal of materials

- Surgical assistance
  Common surgical procedures
  Conduct as a surgical assistant
  Draping
  Tourniquets

- Patient positioning
  Patient safety

- Theatre construction
  Theatre equipment
  Management of the theatre
  Safety in the theatre

ORGANISING A SURGICAL LIST

In order to ensure surgical asepsis is maintained within the operating suite it is essential to classify each surgical procedure in relation to any degree of infection present. This can be assessed by identifying the structures involved in the surgical technique and can be simplified as shown in Table 10.1. These classifications need to be taken into account when organising the surgical list, commencing with the clean procedures first and finishing with any dirty procedures. While there is always a risk of a break in asepsis during any surgical procedure organising your surgical list correctly can effectively minimise that risk.

PREPARATION OF PERSONNEL

General conduct

All persons entering the surgical suite should follow guidelines set by the place of work as to the appropriate personal conduct. Areas that can be included in such a protocol can be as follows:

- pay attention to personal hygiene measures such as daily showering and hair washing
- keep nails short and no nail polish
- remove all jewellery
- wash hands on entry to suite
- change into appropriate scrub suit and footwear

Table 10.1   Classification of surgical procedures

Classification	Explanation	Examples of procedures
Clean	No break in asepsis present and no break in aseptic technique during surgery. The gastrointestinal, respiratory and urinary tracts are not entered	Simple tumour removal; orthopaedic procedure with no connecting traumatic wounds
Clean-contaminated	A contaminated area such as the gastrointestinal, urinary or respiratory tract is entered with no spread of contamination from its contents	Ovariohysterectomy Orchidectomy
Contaminated	No infection present but spillage of contents from viscera, thereby potential risk of spread of contamination	Cystotomy Enterotomy Urethrostomy Fresh wound caused by trauma (less than 48 hours old)
Dirty	Major break in asepsis. Area involved in surgical technique is infected, with pus present	Traumatic wound of more than 48 hours duration. Perforated viscera with pus; abscess

- anticipate and prepare for the surgeon's and patient's needs at all times
- help to organise work list to maximise efficiency and maintain aseptic approach (clean, clean-contaminated etc)
- keep theatre suite tidy
- dispose of all waste efficiently and appropriately.

General clothing

Scrub suits

When working within the theatre suite personnel should change into clothing specific to that area. Cotton mix scrub suits are ideal for this purpose. Being of natural fibre and lightweight they are comfortable to wear, easy to clean and help to reduce static electricity. These need not be sterile but clean scrubs should be worn daily and changed throughout the day if they become contaminated at all.

Footwear

This should be specifically used in the theatre suite and usually takes the form of antistatic clogs with rubber soles or similar. It is essential that the footwear is breathable and comfort-

able as personnel will be spending a considerable amount of time on their feet! Shoe covers are available but should only be used as a temporary measure as they wear through very quickly.

Headgear

Disposable masks and caps are preferable to reusable versions not only from a maintenance angle but also from an effective aseptic technique angle. Most disposable items do not allow or significantly reduce any wicking of moisture and thereby potential risk of contamination compared to that of cloth varieties. For theatre procedures longer than 30 minutes it is advisable to renew masks as their effectiveness reduces over time. While caps are available in a number of designs it is essential that whichever is chosen they effectively cover all hair present. Surgical bonnets may be worn by those personnel who have beards or sideburns.

Surgical gowns

These are available in fabric or synthetic disposable varieties. The choice may depend on many factors such as cost, effectiveness, maintenance, comfort and personal preference.

The disposable varieties tend to be less conforming and breathable due to the materials used. While these materials are naturally desirable to prevent wicking of fluids they may become unpleasant for the personnel to wear, particularly in lengthy procedures. The disposable varieties come pre-packed and pre-sterilised and should obviously be discarded after use. Fabric gowns tend to conform well but have the disadvantage of wicking fluids; the better quality fabric is preferable as it is thicker and helps to reduce risk of wicking. Fabric gowns must be laundered after each use, folded (Fig 10.1) and re-sterilised.

Gloves

There is a wide range of pre-sterilised disposable surgical gloves available, including those with and without powder. The choice with regard to powdering can be down to personal preference, allergies and the procedure to be performed. It is essential to ensure there is a good range of sizes available to meet the needs of the whole surgical team.

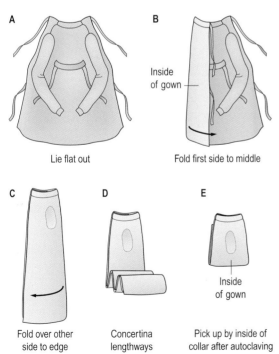

A — Lie flat out
B — Inside of gown — Fold first side to middle
C — Fold over other side to edge
D — Concertina lengthways
E — Inside of gown — Pick up by inside of collar after autoclaving

Figure 10.1   Folding a surgical gown.

Preparation of sterile personnel

The following order of preparation should be followed to meet aseptic technique:

- change into scrub suit and appropriate footwear
- don headgear – cap first followed by mask (care should be exercised to avoid touching outside of mask; it may be placed by an assistant if necessary)
- perform surgical scrub
- don a sterile gown
- don sterile gloves.

The surgical scrub

The purpose of the surgical scrub (Fig 10.2) is to ensure a high level of cleanliness of the hands and forearms. The arms and hands are in close contact with the surgical site at all times. These areas harbour both considerable resident and transient bacteria – it is therefore essential that any scrub routine is performed thoroughly and methodically. While gloves are worn it is not acceptable practice to rely on these alone. It is often possible after surgical procedures to locate small holes in used surgical gloves.

The first scrub of the day should be the longest and is usually in the region of 5–10 minutes, thereafter the timing can be reduced to 3 minutes or as appropriate for the surgical caseload. Having a clock above the scrub sink together with the method of scrubbing should help to ensure all personnel follow the same protocol. Three skin scrub solutions are currently used in veterinary theatres – chlorhexidine, povidone-iodine or triclosan. Chlorhexidine continues to be the most popular choice, having a longer residual activity than povidone-iodine, a broad spectrum of activity against viruses, bacteria, fungi and spores and providing an effective level of activity in the presence of organic matter. First scrub of the day (5–10 minutes):

- turn on water supply and adjust temperature and flow
- wet the hands and arms
- dispense some of the scrub solution into the

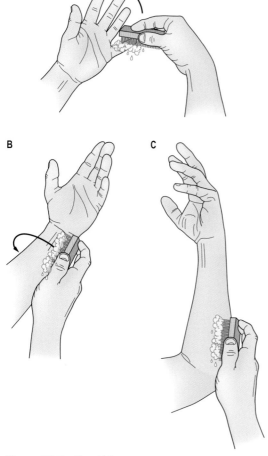

Figure 10.2 Scrubbing up.

palms of the hands and commence washing, working up a lather; check nails are clean – if necessary use a nail file
- continue to wash the arms up to and including the elbow
- rinse the hands and arms; keep the hands above the elbows to allow water to drain from the elbows
- obtain a sterile scrub brush and wet it
- dispense some surgical scrub onto brush and begin to scrub the surfaces of one hand. Scrub the palm and four surfaces of each finger; do not scrub the back of the hand excessively as this can lead to excoriation and inflammation; continue to scrub the wrist and work up the arm and include the elbow

- repeat for second arm; a new brush can be used or rinse the first brush and dispense more surgical scrub solution
- discard brush in sink
- rinse the hands and arms
- dispense surgical scrub solution into palms and wash hands and arms again – this time work to the elbow but do not include it, thereby avoiding any risk of contamination from any unscrubbed areas
- rinse the hands and arms as before
- turn off water supply or instruct an assistant to do so
- take a sterile hand towel and hold it at arms length to unfold; dry hands and arms by using a different quarter for each and discard
- keep forearms and hands raised above waist level with palms towards the chest or clasped together.

Gowning

Gowning (Fig 10.3) should be done as soon as the hands have been dried.

- The sterile gown is carefully taken out of its sterile pack. The gown is held by the neck at shoulder height and allowed to fall open. Great care must be taken not to break asepsis by touching any non-sterile surfaces.
- Once unfolded one hand is slipped into each sleeve and advanced.
- An assistant then pulls the back of the gown to fit it correctly and fasten the back ties. It is essential that the sterile person does not touch the outside of the gown in an attempt to adjust it in any way. The assistant must take great care not to contaminate the front of the gown.
- The hands should remain within the sleeves and the front ties should be grasped and pulled out to the side where an assistant can grasp the ends
- The assistant will then secure the ties at the back.

Gloving

There are three techniques for gloving – open, closed and plunge. Any of these methods is

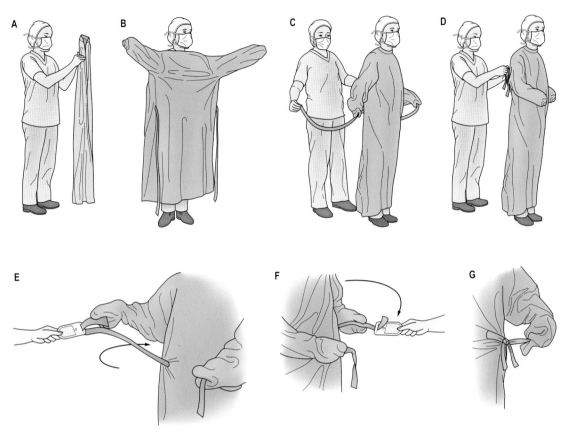

Figure 10.3   Gowning.

acceptable provided asepsis is maintained throughout. The closed method is one of the more popular as there is less risk of any contamination of, or from the hands as they are covered by the gown until gloves are donned. Plunge methods involve a scrubbed assistant holding the gloves open. This is sometimes employed if gloves require replacing during surgical procedures but is not a common method due to the greater risk of contamination from two personnel being involved.

Open gloving (Fig 10.4):

- the hands are extended out of the sleeves of the gown
- an assistant opens the glove pack
- the right hand glove is picked up at the turned-down cuff with the thumb and forefinger of the left hand

- the glove is pulled onto the right hand; the cuff is not unfolded
- the gloved fingers of the left hand now slide between the palm and folded-down cuff of the left glove and pick up the glove.
- the glove is pulled onto the left hand
- the cuff of the left glove is then pulled over the cuff of the gown, ensuring the whole circumference is included
- the gloved fingers of the left hand then slide between the palm and cuff of the right hand and pull the glove cuff over the gown cuff to include whole circumference
- the fingers are adjusted accordingly and hands remain raised above waist level.

Closed gloving (Fig 10.5):

- the cuffs of the gown should cover the hands

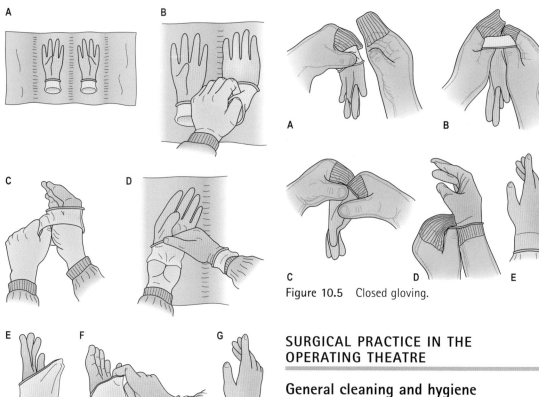

Figure 10.5   Closed gloving.

Figure 10.4   Open gloving.

- the glove pack should be opened by an assistant and turned around so that the fingers are towards the body.
- the right hand picks up the right glove by the rim of the folded cuff (the right glove will be on the left as it has been turned around)
- the glove is held at the folded part with the fingers facing towards the elbow
- the left hand then grasps the rim of the right glove and pulls it over the circumference of the right hand and cuff of the gown
- the left hand then pulls the glove on and the fingers into place by pulling down carefully on the cuff of the glove and sleeve of the gown
- this principle is then repeated for the left glove.

SURGICAL PRACTICE IN THE OPERATING THEATRE

General cleaning and hygiene

Theatre discipline

Anticipating and preparing for any surgical procedure is essential in maintaining high standards of asepsis. The four main areas involved are the patient, the personnel, the surgical area and the instruments. While all of these areas may have set protocols to follow it is still essential to have rules of conduct in the theatre to reduce the risk of contamination from ancillary equipment and general thoroughfare.

Rules of the theatre

- Only personnel involved with the surgical procedure should be present in theatre.
- All personnel must recognise their position as either sterile or non-sterile. There must be no cross contamination of non-sterile personnel touching sterile items.
- Sterile and non-sterile items should be identified and grouped separately. They should be placed with a reasonable distance between them to avoid risk of contamination.

- Personnel should concentrate on the surgical procedure and assistance and not talk excessively.
- Body movements should be restricted to avoid excessive air currents and possible contamination.
- Only the necessary equipment for the surgical procedure should be in theatre and should be removed after completion.
- All waste must be disposed of correctly and efficiently.

Theatre cleaning protocol

Before surgical procedures

At the beginning of each day and within one hour of the first surgical procedure damp dust all work surfaces using a new or sterile cloth with dilute chlorhexidine solution.

Between surgical procedures

- Remove all used surgical equipment from theatre and organise appropriately in the preparation room. Blood-stained instruments should be soaked in cold water before placing in a detergent solution. Sharps, swabs and other items to be disposed of appropriately. Soiled linen to be placed in bags ready for washing.
- Check all work surfaces for any blood or body fluids and spot clean with a disinfectant (disinfectant should be broad spectrum and be active against bacteria, spores, viruses and fungi).
- Check the floor is dry and spot clean with disinfectant.

After surgical procedures

- Remove all equipment from theatre and organise or dispose of appropriately in the preparation room.
- Wipe down all work surfaces with a detergent. Pay particular attention to joints of Mayo trolleys and operating table.
- Check all underside surfaces of trolleys and table and clean as above.
- Rinse and dry work surfaces.
- Check all other surfaces for any blood stains

or body fluids and clean with detergent, rinse and dry.
- Wipe all surfaces previously cleaned with disinfectant.
- Brush or wet-vacuum floor.
- Scrub theatre floor manually or with powered equipment with hot water and detergent.
- Use a mop specifically designated to the theatre to disinfect the floor.
- Switch off lights and clean door handles with disinfectant and close doors to avoid thoroughfare when not in use. Warning signs may also be placed on doors to avoid unauthorised entry.
- Empty mop bucket; clean and dry mop head.

Weekly and monthly cleaning of theatre

- All equipment in the theatre must be maintained as per the manufacturer's instructions.
- Operating table must be cleaned and disinfected once weekly. All joints and wheels cleaned, disinfected and lubricated.
- Mayo trolley must be cleaned and disinfected weekly. Check wheels and height adjustment parts are lubricated, freely movable and disinfected.
- Using a new or sterile cloth or sponge and disinfectant wipe down walls, ceilings, doors and door handles.
- Check all supplies that enter the theatre are in good repair, clean and disinfected as appropriate.

Equipment use, care and maintenance

General equipment maintenance and electrical safety

All electrical equipment used in the surgical suite must be maintained correctly to ensure safety of personnel and patients and to meet Health and Safety requirements. The following protocol should be adopted for all equipment used in the surgical suite:

- all equipment should be recorded in a maintenance manual stating its name, make, serial number, manufacturer details, warranty and maintenance details

- clean and maintain as per manufacturer's instructions.
- store correctly when not in use as per manufacturer's instructions
- portable appliance test (PAT) performed annually by an approved electrician
- annual service organised with supplier as appropriate to individual item
- any fault identified is reported immediately to a supervisor for actioning and the item marked 'out of use'.

Surgical instruments

Surgical instruments are precision instruments that require careful and methodical maintenance to ensure they remain in good repair and are capable of doing the job they are designed for. Following surgical procedures all blood-stained instruments should be placed in cold water to help prevent or reduce coagulation of the blood present. They should then be rinsed and placed in a suitable instrument detergent at the correct dilution and temperature. Following the allocated time they should then be thoroughly rinsed and dried. All instruments should be checked for any damage or signs of wear and dealt with appropriately. Joints should be lubricated with an instrument spray. Once thoroughly clean and dry they must then be sterilised appropriately in readiness for future needs (see Chapter 11 – instrumentation and sterilisation).

Ultrasonic cleaners This is an alternative method to manual cleaning of instruments that is often thought to be a very effective method of sanitising instruments prior to sterilisation. It should not, however, replace manual cleaning completely. An ultrasonic cleaner (Fig 10.6) consists of a metal bath with an electrical current. The bath is filled with water and the recommended detergent and the electrical current produces mechanical vibrations through water. The effect is the production of minute bubbles that rapidly form and collapse on the instrument surface, producing a cleaning and mild abrasive action. The ultrasonic cleaning process is particularly effective on joints and hinges. It also produces less wear on the instruments than scrubbing

manually. The unit should be cleaned and serviced regularly as per the manufacturer's instructions. Particular attention to detail should be taken when using this unit in relation to the electrical safety. During use:

- do not touch any of the electrical components with wet or damp hands
- wear gloves and prepare the manufacturer's recommended detergent at the correct dilution rate
- open all instrument joints before placing in basket
- do not mix different metal types
- rinse thoroughly when removed from basket.

Drying cabinet

While there may be some establishments that still use drying cabinets this is no longer common. The principle reasons for their decline in use are due to questions relating to their efficacy. Primarily, if instruments that have not been cleaned thoroughly are placed in a cabinet for drying the debris will be effectively baked onto the instruments leading to corrosion. Secondly, the cabinets are not designed with an interlocking door and therefore the drying cycle could easily be interrupted resulting in a risk of moisture remaining on the instruments and causing deterioration in quality.

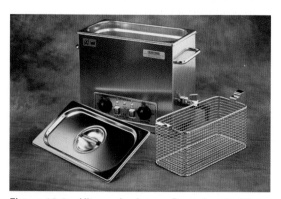

Figure 10.6 Ultrasonic cleaner. Reproduced with permission from Burtons Medical Equipment.

Care of specialised equipment

Rigid and flexible endoscopes and arthroscopes

These (Figs 10.7, 10.8) are used for a variety of techniques that require visualisation of body structures, organs, and joints. They may also be used to obtain biopsy tissue samples, perform fluid flushing and sample collection, and fragment and foreign body retrieval. The image is produced from a bundle of fibre optic cables and a light source. They are expensive, delicate precision instruments requiring careful handling and maintenance.

Handling Always handle carefully with gloved hands. Do not allow the instrument to hit any surface or be dropped and do not try to bend or twist the insertion tube.

Cleaning, maintenance and sterilisation This will vary in relation to type and make of instrument and the manufacturer's instructions should always be followed. General rules for flexible and rigid scopes are as follows.

Non-immersible flexible endoscopes

- After use withdraw from patient and ensure good flow of water from water channel.
- Clean outside of insertion tube with damp cloth.
- Examine insertion tube for any signs of damage.
- Prepare some lukewarm water and a few squirts of washing up liquid or similar and wash outside of insertion tube.
- Remove and wash biopsy cap.
- Keeping insertion tube straight, insert cleaning brush and advance beyond tip of endoscope. Gently pull brush out from tip of scope.
- Repeat until brush clean.
- Reconnect biopsy cap.

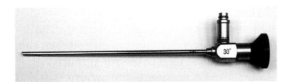

Figure 10.7   Rigid endoscope. Reproduce with permission from VES Endoscopy Services.

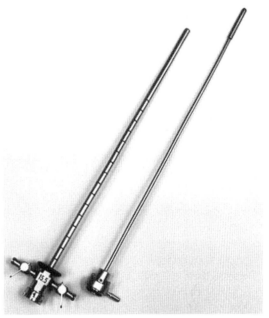

Figure 10.8   Rigid endoscope. Reproduced with permission from VES Endoscopy Services.

- Connect suction unit and aspirate the soapy water through biopsy channel until it runs clear.
- Aspirate lukewarm water with no soap until it runs clear with no soap bubbles.
- Fill bowl with recommended disinfectant at correct dilution rate.
- Place insertion tube within and aspirate the solution through the biopsy channel, making sure air does not enter the tip.
- Leave insertion tube in the disinfectant for recommended time (usually a maximum of 20 minutes).
- Rinse endoscope in clean water and aspirate clean water through biopsy channel.
- Dry insertion tube and aspirate air through biopsy channel until dry.
- Connect light source and ensure good flow of water from water channel.
- Disconnect water bottle and occlude water port with finger.
- Press water button until water from nozzle stops – pump intermittently to remove any water droplets.
- Dry insertion tube and check image is still sharp from the endoscope.

- Store in a dust-free protected case or cabinet where insertion tube hangs vertically.

Ethylene oxide or glutaraldehyde are used for sterilisation for this type of endoscope. Due to the nature of these sterilisation methods not all workplaces meet the necessary Control of Substances Hazardous to Health (COSHH) regulations, therefore the unit may need to be sent away for sterilisation. The frequency of sterilisation will depend on the manufacturer's recommendation and individual usage.

Rigid scopes

- Disconnect the light source and remove all adapters.
- Using a neutral pH enzymatic solution, immediately soak the scope (maximum 20 minutes).
- Clean outside of scope with damp cloth within the enzymatic solution to remove any contamination.
- Rinse in distilled water and dry.
- Clean optical elements with alcohol wipes to remove any residue.
- Inspect scope for any sign of damage and check it is clean and dry.
- Disinfection and sterilisation is performed with 2.5% glutaraldehyde. The scope may be soaked for a maximum of 20 minutes. It must then be rinsed thoroughly and dried (see above re COSHH regulations).
- Sterilisation by autoclaving can be performed on scopes that have 'autoclave' engraved on them
- When autoclaving a scope ensure it is clean and dry, place in sterilisation tray and autoclave for 3 minutes at 134°C. After sterilisation allow the scope to dry for one hour before removal from unit.
- Store in dust-free protected case as per the manufacturer's instructions.

NB Never immerse an endoscope in liquid unless specifically stated within the manufacturer's instructions.

When sending any endoscope away for servicing or sterilisation it is now a Health and Safety requirement to return them with a completed decontamination certificate. The

---

DECONTAMINATION CERTIFICATE

Date

Practice Name & Address:

Telephone Number:

Fax Number:

Contact:

Make & Model of Equipment:

Serial Number:

Reason for return:

Method of disinfection used:

Disinfectant product:

Any comments:

Figure 10.9   Example of decontamination certificate.

certificate should provide details as outlined in Figure 10.9.

Dental machines

A variety of dental units are available to the veterinary industry from standard ultrasonic descalers and polishers to air-driven complete units providing scaling, drilling, polishing and suction (Fig 10.10). While it is not possible to sterilise the bulk of the units, the handpieces and attachments must be cleaned and disinfected methodically after each use and, where applicable, sterilised. The manufacturer's recommendations should be followed for specific maintenance requirements and types of chemicals to use.

General care of the air-driven dental unit:

- wipe over whole of unit with clean damp cloth
- if suction has been used, prepare disinfectant at correct dilution and aspirate through suction tube into bottle for approximately 10 seconds; remove bottle, empty, dry and reconnect; autoclave suction tips as per manufacturer's instructions

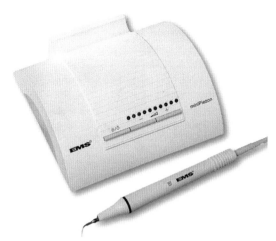

Figure 10.10 Piezon scaler and Vetair dental unit. Reproduced with permission from Burtons Medical Equipment.

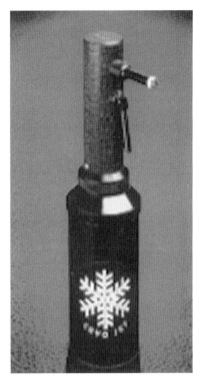

Figure 10.11 Cryojet. Reproduced with permission from Burtons Medical Equipment.

- check water container and refill with distilled water
- using dilute disinfectant wipe over scaler, polisher and drill hand pieces and leads
- remove burr from drill hand piece if used and insert greaser into hole; turn 180 degrees and remove then replace dummy burr
- remove polisher hand piece from lead; using a spray cleaner insert tube attachment into hand piece and spray; repeat with lubrication spray and reconnect hand piece; wipe with tissue
- switch off unit, remove compression hose and release pressure
- check gauges read zero and reconnect hose
- sterilisation by autoclaving can be performed for the drill and polisher hand pieces and all dental burrs
- the unit should be covered when not in use.

Cryosurgical units

Cryosurgery is performed to kill living tissue by freezing. The freezing effect is produced with the use of liquid nitrogen delivered to the tissue by means of a specially designed unit and spray or probe attachments (Fig 10.11). A combination of a succession of quick freezes and thaws produces the optimal effects and results in cellular death.

Liquid nitrogen is readily available, inexpensive and non-explosive when stored correctly. While larger veterinary establishments will have their own storage facilities, smaller premises may prefer to obtain liquid nitrogen from a local hospital or larger establishment. Handheld cryosurgery units may be used to collect the liquid nitrogen or a thermos flask can be used. If storing the liquid nitrogen within the veterinary establishment it is essential that COSHH regulations are met and a standard operating procedure (SOP) is adopted for its safe storage and use. The following guidelines can be followed for the safe use and maintenance of cryosurgical equipment:

- label all storage containers clearly with appropriate warnings
- store in a well ventilated area
- wear personal protective clothing (PPE) when handling equipment (thick or heavy duty gloves, apron, goggles)

- avoid splashing the liquid nitrogen
- avoid touching any metal areas that have been cooled with liquid nitrogen as severe burns can occur
- once procedure completed, remove probes and wash in lukewarm dilute disinfectant (e.g. chlorhexidine); gently remove any body fluid and debris from the probes
- rinse the probes, dry and sterilise as per manufacturer's instructions
- empty any unused liquid nitrogen back into storage container, ensure area is well ventilated and PPE is worn
- clean outside of cryosurgical unit with lukewarm water and clean cloth, dry and store appropriately.

Power tools – air and battery drills, mechanical burrs and saws

As with all surgical equipment, power tools are precision instruments that require correct care and handling. It is essential to always follow the manufacturer's care instructions. As a general guide:

- ensure all equipment is checked regularly for signs of damage, wear and tear
- arrange servicing or replacement as appropriate
- clean as per manufacturer's instructions
- store in dry dust-free environment
- sterilise as per manufacturer's instructions – most air drills, saws and burrs can be autoclaved; battery drills need to be sterilised using ethylene oxide
- ensure batteries for battery drills are fully charged before use and sterile sleeves are available to place over them during use.

Disposal of materials

Several regulations apply to the correct method of disposal of waste from veterinary establishments: Controlled waste regulations (1992), Environmental Protection Act (1990) and Control of Pollution Act (1974). The type of waste for disposal from theatres falls into the categories of clinical, sharps or special waste.

Clinical waste from theatre

This includes waste contaminated with body fluids during a surgical procedure and any form of animal tissue, e.g. blood-stained swabs, soiled drape material, disposable gowns and gloves, used syringes, body organs, tumours, body tissues. On leaving the theatre it should be placed within a yellow bag marked 'for incineration only'. The bag should then be sent for incineration. If it is not to be incinerated immediately it must be placed in a secure sealed container ready for collection.

Sharps

This includes hypodermic and suture needles, scalpel blades and sharp instruments for disposal. They should be discarded immediately after use into a designated sharps container. Once full, the sharps container must be closed and sent for incineration.

Special waste

This includes pharmaceutical bottles and vials and part-filled syringes that have not actually been administered and thereby are not contaminated with body fluid or tissue. These need to be stored in designated pharmaceutical bins and sent for incineration.

SURGICAL ASSISTANCE

An efficient surgical assistant must have a good understanding of surgical procedures and techniques in order to anticipate and prepare for the needs of the surgeon. Common surgical techniques can be recognised by the use of some general prefixes and suffixes (Box 10.1). Surgical procedures can be classed as either elective, i.e. involving choice (such as neutering), or non-elective, i.e. must be carried out in order for the animal to survive or regain a good quality of life (such as orthopaedic surgery).

Common surgical procedures

Examples of common surgical procedures include the following.

> **Box 10.1   Common prefixes and suffixes in surgical terms**
>
> ■ otomy – describes a temporary opening or dividing of tissue during surgery, e.g. laparotomy, cystotomy
> ■ ectomy – describes the surgical removal of all of a or part of a structure, e.g. enterectomy, ovariohysterectomy.
> ■ ostomy – the surgical creation of a stoma or opening, e.g. urethrostomy, gastrostomy.
> ■ scopy – describes examinations by various devices, e.g. endoscopy, gastroscopy

Surgery to the cutaneous system

- Suturing wounds – repairing tissue to enable it to heal quickly and return to its original function.
- Draining an abscess – removal of the pus from an abscessed area to enable healing to take place. Also referred to as lancing.

- Removal of tumours – this will include the removal of all skin tumours and tumours of the adipose tissue (lipoma). This may be as a curative measure or as palliative care.

Aural surgery

- Lateral wall resection – removal or restructuring of the lateral cartilaginous wall of the vertical ear canal to provide drainage for the ear by exposing the horizontal canal to the environment. An aural ablation (Fig 10.12) may be chosen if it is felt that the medial wall of the vertical canal could still be a source of inflammation.
- Drainage of aural haematomas – the collection of blood found in the ear pinna can be treated in a variety of ways; drainage may occur in a non-surgical fashion. Surgery will include the basic points of removing clots and preventing re-filling of the area using a device to encourage the ear to heal flat.
- Bulla osteotomy – this procedure involves gaining access to the tympanic bulla and is

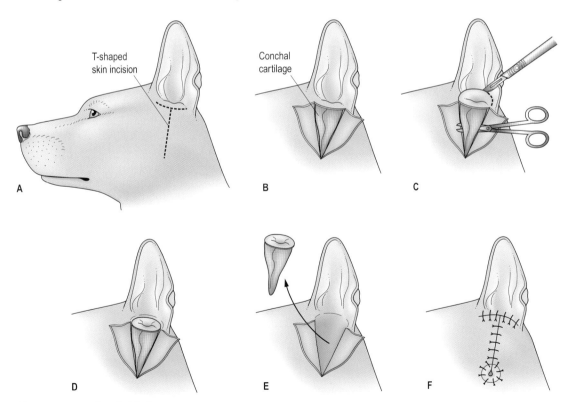

Figure 10.12   Aural ablation.

used to treat chronic cases of otitis media where all other treatments have failed. Diseased bone is removed wherever possible and the remaining structures are curetted and lavaged.

Ophthalmic surgery

- Enucleation – removal of the eye as a result of damage or disease.
- Third eyelid flap – the nictitating membrane is sutured across the cornea to allow healing to take place underneath; this procedure is known as a temporary tarsorrhapy.
- Keratectomy – the removal of some or all anterior corneal opacitation to improve vision.
- Entropion surgery – used to correct an anatomical deformity of the eyelids where the lid rolls inwards.
- Ectropion surgery – used to correct an anatomical deformity of the eyelids where the lid rolls outwards.
- Distichiasis surgery – removes the unwanted cilia from the eyelids.

Surgery to the gastrointestinal tract

- Gastrotomy – temporary opening into the stomach.
- Duodenotomy – temporary opening into the duodenum.
- Jejunotomy – temporary opening into the jejunum.

These three procedures are often carried out in an exploratory manner, possibly to locate a foreign body or diseased area, and may be termed exploratory laparotomy (opening into the abdominal cavity, until the exact anatomical area is located).

- Pharyngostomy tube placement (Fig 10.13) – placing a pharyngostomy tube through an incision (stoma) of the pharynx and into the oesophagus, terminating in the stomach.
- Gastrostomy tube placement – placing a gastrostomy tube into the stomach via a stoma in the abdominal wall.

Tubes such as these may be placed in patients who are unable or unwilling to eat in

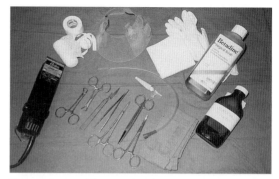

Figure 10.13 Pharyngostomy tube placement kit.

the normal way. This may be due to oral or oesophageal surgery or disease. Once the patient is able to eat properly again the tubes are removed, leaving the stomata to heal by secondary intention.

- Resection of the intestine – removal of part of the intestine; carried out when part of the intestine is unable to function.
- Anastomosis – when intestinal lumen has been removed due to resection; the two remaining ends are joined together (anastomosed) in order that the intestinal tract stays patent.

Other surgical terms used in relation to the gastrointestinal system include:

- Cleft palate repair – repairing the hard palate, enabling the patient to suckle/eat normally.
- Oesophagotomy – opening into the oesophagus.
- Oesophagectomy – removal of part of the oesophagus.
- Pyloromyotomy – relieves constriction of the pyloric sphincter.
- Surgery for gastric torsion – laparotomy to relocate the stomach; may include a gastropexy – suturing of the stomach to the abdominal wall to prevent further episodes of torsion.
- Repair of rectal prolapse – relocation of the prolapse; may include preventative measures such as purse string sutures.

Orthopaedic surgery

- External fixation – most external fixation in general practice will make use of casting materials to stabilise a fracture site so that healing can take place; however, external fixators (using pins as a scaffold around a fracture site) can be used.
- Internal fixation includes the use of implants such as pins, plates, screws and wires to align and stabilise a fracture and promote repair – this may be further enhanced with external support in the initial stages of healing.
- Reductions of dislocations/luxations – usually affecting the hip joint, dislocations are often reduced without surgery; in some cases the joint may need to be visualised in order for reduction to take place.
- Excision arthroplasty (Fig 10.14) – removal of a fractured femoral head.
- Hip toggle procedure – attachment of the femoral head to the acetabulum after recurring or long-standing hip dislocations.
- Anterior cruciate ligament repair – a common procedure is the 'over the top' method which involves the use of a graft to replace the ruptured ligament.

Surgery to the reproductive tract

- Ovariohysterectomy – removal of the ovaries and uterus; common terms include spaying, neutering, OH.
- Caesarean section – removal of the foetus or foetuses via an incision into the uterus (hysterotomy) via the abdomen (laparotomy); also referred to as a C section.
- Castration – removal of the testicles; the correct terminology for this procedure is orchidectomy but it is commonly referred to as neutering.

Conduct as a surgical assistant

A surgical assistant who is 'scrubbed in' may be responsible for:

- preparing the instrument trolley
- arranging the instruments in logical order (Fig 10.15)
- keeping a check on instrumentation throughout the procedure

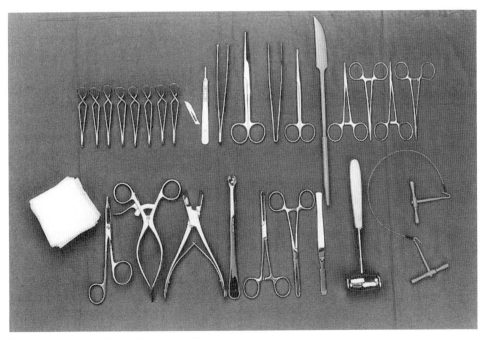

Figure 10.14 Excision arthroplasty kit.

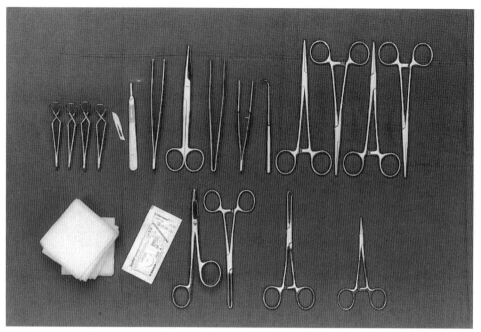

Figure 10.15 Instruments should be placed in a logical order.

- passing instrumentation and sterile items to the surgeon
- holding and utilising instruments as directed by the surgeon
- cutting sutures
- swabbing of the surgical site
- counting instrumentation and swabs at the end of a procedure.

Preparation of personnel

The surgical assistant should have donned a mask and cap, scrubbed up, and gowned and gloved in a sterile manner.

The instrument trolley

An unscrubbed assistant should be responsible for passing the packaged sterile supplies to the scrubbed surgical assistant. The surgical assistant should be handed a trolley drape which is sterile and large enough to cover the whole trolley surface. The drapes and instrumentation required for the procedure are then handed to the sterile assistant using a sterile transfer method. It will depend on how the practice packs its equipment as to which form this will take; ideally drapes should be passed

first to enable the surgeon to place them whilst the remainder of the instruments are sorted and arranged by the surgical assistant. Towel clips to secure the drapes should be handed to the surgeon individually.

The instrumentation being used should be checked and counted. Any faulty or unnecessary equipment should be either removed or removed and replaced at this stage. Do not overcrowd the trolley as equipment is more likely to be knocked from the trolley if this is the case. Any extra instrumentation can be kept in its packs and offered to the sterile assistant when required. If there is any doubt as to the cleanliness or sterility of the equipment it should be rejected and another pack sought.

Instruments will be arranged on the trolley in a manner that suits the surgeon, assistant and procedure. Usually instruments are placed in the order in which they are likely to be used, with similar instruments being grouped together. It is most important that the surgical assistant is aware of where each instrument is in relation to the trolley. This allows for quick retrieval when required and it becomes obvious when an instrument is missing. It is vital that instruments are put back in place each time they have been used.

The surgical assistant will place the scalpel blade on the blade handle using a pair of artery forceps (haemostats) and will pass this to the surgeon for the first incision to be made. An experienced surgical assistant will then follow this with the next instrument the surgeon is likely to require and so on. If the assistant is unsure then a good knowledge of instrument names should allow the correct choice when requested by the surgeon.

After each use, surgical instruments should be wiped clean with a sterile swab prior to being returned to the trolley.

Swabbing

The surgical assistant should watch and prepare for any accumulations of blood that may appear on or around the surgical site. Swabs should be counted as packets are opened and a tally kept, ensuring all are accounted for at the end of the procedure. Blood should be swabbed by blotting rather than wiping to discourage further damage to blood vessels and promote clotting.

Handling instruments

These general rules apply when handling instruments:

- the instrument handle should always be offered to the surgeon rather than the point
- the instrument should be firmly placed into the surgeon's hand to prevent it from being dropped and to prevent the surgeon from having to look up each time
- curved instruments should be passed with the concave side up.

Using instruments

- Instruments with finger rings should be held with the thumb and ring finger through the rings and the index finger along the shank (Fig 10.16). Tissue should be grasped by the tip of the jaws and locked in place by the ratchet.

- Curved instruments are applied with the concave side facing upwards.
- Rat-tooth, dressing or spay forceps (or other thumb forceps) should be held in a pencil grip.
- Retractors that are self-retaining (e.g. Gelpi) should be placed inside the incision and spread according to the surgeon's wishes. The retainer can then be locked in place. Retractors that have to be held (e.g. Lagenbeck) will require constant attention by the assistant until they are no longer required.
- Suture materials should be cut by the appropriate scissor. This should be brought to the surgical area with blades closed, then opened slightly ensuring that only the tips are used to severe the suture.

Draping

Drapes should be placed around the surgical site to ensure a sterile field. This may be achieved by using either reusable or disposable drapes – this will be down to practice policy or surgeon's preference. Drapes may be either fenestrated with appropriate sized gaps or plain four-cornered drapes. Draping may be either the responsibility of the surgical assistant or the surgeon involved.

Plain drapes

These are placed around the surgical site and held in place with towel clips. The advantage

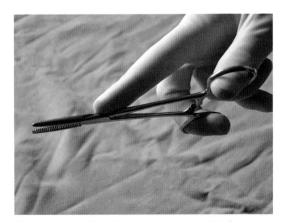

Figure 10.16   Holding an instrument with finger rings.

is that the fenestration size can be adjusted to suit the specific surgical procedure. They can be laid out using one of three methods (Box 10.2). Drapes should be large enough to drape the patient and hang over the table, ensuring a sterile field (Fig 10.17).

Fenestrated drapes

These have prepared fenestrations and a range of different sizes need to be on hand. The drape is placed over the patient with the fenestration appearing over the surgical area. The drape is then secured with towel clips. Again the drape should be large enough to cover the surgical area and its immediate environment.

Draping limbs

The method used for limb draping (Fig 10.18) will depend on both the surgeon's preference and the surgery to be performed:

- lift the foot up by attaching to a drip stand or holding via tape, ensure the limb is clear of the table and place a sterile drape underneath
- a sterile drape is attached to the limb and the limb is then allowed to drop onto the drape below it
- the limb is then draped in a normal fashion using four plain drapes.

An alternative method could be:

- take a large fenestrated drape and pull the limb through it so that the drape covers the patients body with the limb free
- apply sterile bandaging to the foot and cover with a drape or sterile boot as required
- lower the limb onto the sterile drape and continue draping accordingly.

When draping a patient for orthopaedic surgery sterile bandaging can be beneficial as it works well with the contours of the limb.

Additional draping

Additional drapes may be used for procedures which may contaminate the surgical area – such as abdominal surgery. This may involve 'double draping' to try and prevent strike through and therefore a break in sterility.

Tourniquets

Tourniquets may used in surgery to the distal limb to limit the blood loss – time of application should be noted and the tourniquet should not be left in place for more than 20 minutes.

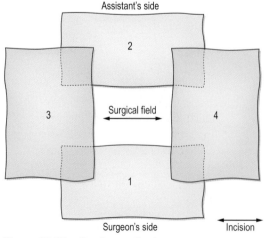

Figure 10.17   Draping methods.

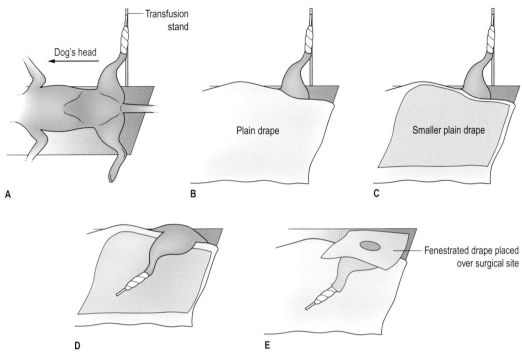

Figure 10.18   Draping a limb.

PATIENT POSITIONING

The patient needs to be positioned in such a way that facilitates access to the surgical area without compromising the safety of the patient (Box 10.3).

Patient safety

Patient safety (Box 10.4) must always come first – remember that there is no point operating on a dead patient!

Box 10.3   Factors in patient positioning

The following points will need to be taken into consideration:

- the surgical procedure and its approach
- the size of the patient
- the patient's condition – i.e. elective vs non-elective surgery

---

Box 10.4   Patient safety

Remember the following:

- The airway must be kept patent throughout the procedure.
- There must be no constrictions around the thorax – check positioning aids are not interfering.
- Maintain circulation and temperature. Ensure that ties are not constricting limbs, that pressure points are padded and that equipment to maintain temperature is considered, i.e. heat pads.
- Ensure that the anaesthetist is able to monitor the anaesthetic effectively – ensure that drapes do not restrict access for the anaesthetist. The anaesthetist and theatre staff will require access to any monitoring equipment being used.
- The position needs to afford the surgeon maximum visibility to enable the procedure to be carried out quickly and effectively.

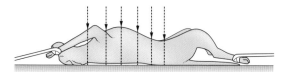

Figure 10.19   Patient positioning.

Positions (Fig 10.19)

Dorsally   This describes the patient laying in dorsal recumbency (Box 10.5) and is the commonly used position for entering the abdomen. The patient is placed on its back with the limbs secured both anteriorly and posteriorly, dependent on the surgeon's preference. It is important that the patient is correctly aligned on the table – positioning equipment such as troughs, sandbags and blocks can be used for this purpose. When correctly positioned the surgeon should have direct access to the linea alba.

Laterally   The patient is positioned in lateral recumbency for procedures such as flank spays, surgery to limb extremities, some orthopaedic procedures and some thoracic procedures. The exact positioning of the limbs will be dependent on the type of surgery; they can be extended cranially and caudally for

---

Box 10.5   Modifications in patient position
■ Modifications of the dorsal position may be used for some procedures. These can involve the patient being tilted with its head slightly down (modified dorsal position), so abdominal viscera fall into the anterior abdomen leaving the posterior abdomen clear for surgery, or the opposite (modified reverse dorsal position), to encourage the abdominal viscera to fall posteriorly. ■ Care must be taken to avoid the patient slipping in both cases; when using the modified dorsal position the surgical team must ensure that the viscera are not causing a respiratory problem by pressing on the diaphragm.

---

maximum exposure to the main body, or can be positioned in various ways to allow access to specific areas.

Sternally   The sternal position involves the patient lying on its sternum with the hind legs extended (abducted) at the hips and secured. Care must be taken to ensure that there is no obstruction to the neck – this may involve the use of a sandbag to prop the head up. This position is used for some spinal surgery and for surgery to the head and oral cavity.

THEATRE CONSTRUCTION

To maintain aseptic standards the operating theatre should be separate from all other clinical rooms and only used for surgical procedures. All patient and personnel preparation should be carried out in the designated preparation area to ensure patient safety during surgery. When taking into consideration the construction of a theatre ideally:

- the theatre should have a minimum of two doors – double doors that swing both ways are ideal as they allow the passage of sterile staff without the use of hands and arms, and give enough space to easily manoeuvre larger patients into theatre
- all surfaces in the theatre should be constructed of a non-porous material that can withstand harsh cleaning chemicals – this includes floors and walls; edges of floors should be curved to allow easy cleaning and to prevent debris from becoming lodged in corners
- ease of accessibility for cleaning should be taken into consideration when deciding on permanent fixtures such as lights
- the heating/air-conditioning of the theatre should be appropriate; bacterial filters can be a useful addition to any fans or ventilation in the room.

Theatre equipment

Permanent theatre equipment should be kept to an absolute minimum to ensure maintenance of asepsis. Basic theatre equipment (Fig 10.20) will include:

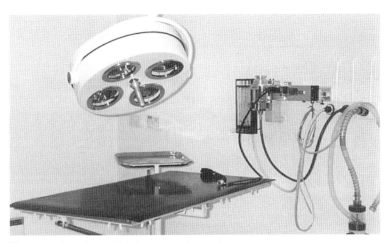

Figure 10.20   Essential theatre equipment.

- operating lights – can be free-standing or permanent and should provide good light intensity without giving out too much heat; lights that can be placed at close proximity to the patient can cause thermal burns if not monitored; lights need to be of the right size to suit the theatre dimensions and use
- operating table – again either free-standing or permanently fixed; surgical tables will usually have a hydraulic base that can be operated with the foot to allow movements up and down and tilting of the table top – the table should be constructed of a product that is easy to clean and durable
- anaesthetic trolley/machine (either wall mounted or free-standing) – the equipment kept with them should be minimal to prevent dust trapping; this includes any monitoring equipment
- instrument stand – stainless steel and of correct size and height
- kick bowl – stainless steel for theatre waste
- light box – to enable the viewing of radiographs perioperatively
- other equipment, such as suction and electro surgery units, is often brought in to theatre for specific surgeries but stored elsewhere.

Management of the theatre

Each theatre should have its own set of rules which may include the following:

- no admission to non-surgical staff
- surgical attire only to be worn in theatre – i.e. scrub suits/gowns (Fig 10.21)
- doors are opened as infrequently as possible
- all cleaning equipment used in the theatre should be specified for this use only – i.e. the theatre should have its own mops, buckets and cleaning cloths
- a maintenance/cleaning protocol should be devised that takes into account how the theatre should be cleaned, when and with which products – this protocol should take into consideration cleaning protocols for all static equipment found in the theatre.

Safety in the theatre

When using anaesthetic gases in the presence of oxygen all staff should be mindful of the dangers of fires and explosions (Box 10.6). These can be ignited by electrical sparks or static electricity and therefore the possibility of these being produced needs to be minimised in the theatre.

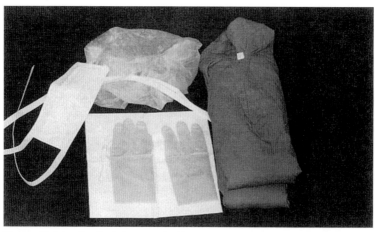

Figure 10.21   Surgical theatre clothing.

Box 10.6   Theatre safety

Methods of minimising risk include:

- Ensure that surgical attire only is worn in theatre. This should be made of an antistatic material such as cotton; synthetic fibres can give rise to static electricity.
- Theatre personnel should have their hair covered at all times and should ensure all animal hair is draped – this will also prevent static build up.
- Where electrical equipment is used it should be regularly checked for electrical safety and positioned as far away from the anaesthetic gases as possible when being used in theatre. Electrical equipment should always be used in a safe manner.

- General equipment used in the theatre, such as anaesthetic trolleys and instrument trolleys, should be on castors made of a conductive material that can disperse any static build up.
- Fire extinguishers should be maintained, appropriate and readily available.
- Smoking should be forbidden.
- Cleaning products used in the theatre should be checked to ensure they are not conducive to fire or explosion.

Further reading

Aspinall V 2003 Clinical procedures in veterinary nursing. Elsevier, Oxford

Bowden C, Masters J 2001 Veterinary surgical kits. Butterworth-Heinemann, Oxford

Lane D R, Cooper B C 2003 Veterinary nursing, 3rd edn. British Small Animal Veterinary Association, Cheltenham

Tracy D L 2000 Small animal surgical nursing, 3rd edn. Mosby, St Louis

Chapter 11

Instrumentation and sterilisation

Anne Ward

ASEPSIS AND INSTRUMENTATION

Asepsis

The mid-1800s saw a boom within the medical world with the discovery and introduction of ether anaesthesia. It was soon realised that without good hygienic practice wounds were becoming infected at the point of incision – frequently leading to patient death. Robert Koch discovered steam sterilisation for surgical instruments and dressings in 1878, which revolutionised surgical practice. Barrier techniques were introduced in 1913 by William Halstead with the use of sterile gloves. Further advances developed through Alexander Fleming's pioneering work in 1928 with the discovery of the first internal antiseptic – penicillin.

Definitions
- *Asepsis*: absence of disease-producing micro-organisms (pathogens)
- *Sepsis*: presence of bacteria (bacteraemia) or other infectious organisms or their toxins in the blood (septicaemia) or in other tissue of the body
- *Antisepsis*: prevention of infection by inhibiting or arresting the growth and multiplication of micro-organisms – antisepsis implies scrupulously clean and free of all living microbes
- *Sterilisation*: process capable of destroying all pathogenic and non-pathogenic micro-organisms – including spores

● *Nosocomial infections*: an infection acquired in a hospital that was not present or incubating prior to the patient being admitted to the hospital, but occurred within 72 hours after admittance to the hospital.

Nosocomial infections

This type of infection may or may not be a complication of the operation site alone, though it will present as a complication to the patient in general. They can be linked to a number of potential intrinsic and extrinsic risk factors:

From the patient

● overuse of antibiotics
● concurrent diseases, e.g. malnutrition
● immunisation and vaccination status
● patients currently on immunosuppressive drugs
● prolonged hospitalisation
● inherited conditions
● breed predisposition
● stress
● age
● hypothermia.

From personnel

● poor hygiene methods
● poor patient preparation
● poor nursing technique
● poor surgical technique
● excessive fluid loss, e.g. haemorrhage
● prolonged time in surgery
● misuse of prophylactic antibiotics – resulting in de-emphases of surgical asepsis, development of antibiotic-resistant bacteria, antibiotics becoming ineffective, incorrect choice/dosage of drug.

Prophylactic antibiotic therapy

Antibiotics are overused and old habits are hard to break for some. They should be used when there is a likelihood of infection, when infection would be detrimental to recovery (e.g. hip replacements), to target expected bacterial flora (e.g. *Staphylococcus* spp from the skin), to treat infections found prior to surgery or when an appropriate course of treatment is initiated prior to surgery. Whether prophylac-

tic or therapeutic, bacterial numbers should be reduced to a level that will allow the hosts defences to be effective.

Techniques of disinfection and sterilisation

Disinfection

Disinfection is a cleaning process which destroys most micro-organisms – but not the highly resistant forms such as bacterial or mycotic spores. It is also effective against some viruses, depending on the solution being used. There are a number of disinfectants available and all have different uses (Table 11.1). The general points that should be observed when using disinfectants are:

● observe current COSHH (Control of Substances Hazardous to Heath) regulations for each product
● remove gross debris prior to disinfecting
● use correct solution for the target pathogen
● wear personal protective equipment as required
● use correct dilution
● use hot water when diluting a concentrated solution
● use fresh solutions (e.g. hypochlorites deactivate in light after a while)
● do not mix two or more solutions
● rinse thoroughly
● ensure the area dries thoroughly as micro-organisms may thrive in damp areas
● phenolic disinfectants are *toxic* to cats.

Sterilisation

Sterilisation is the complete destruction or elimination of *all* living micro-organisms. It is accomplished by physical methods (dry or moist heat), chemical agents (gas plasma, ethylene oxide, formaldehyde and alcohol), radiation or mechanical methods such as filtration. Gas plasma sterilisation is a relatively new technology where hydrogen peroxide vapours are converted into gas plasma using a radio frequency – a technique currently becoming popular in human medicine. There are a number of sterilisation methods available (Table 11.2), however *autoclaving* is by far the

Table 11.1 The range of disinfectant groups and their uses

Disinfectant group	Use	Area of activity	Method of action	Examples of product	Comments
Alcohols	Skin disinfection commonly used for swabbing injection sites	Bacteria. TB. Not viruses	Coagulates bacterial protein	Ethyl alcohol Isopropyl alcohol Methylated spirit Surgical spirit	Organic compound. Evaporates quickly. Contaminated once open to the air
Aldehydes					
– Formaldehydes	Environment. Sterilant for vaccines and pathological specimens	Sporicidal. Highly irritant to skin	Fixes bacterial cell proteins making them useless	Parvocide Formula H	Specimens are stored in 10% solution. Evaporates easily
– Glutaraldehydes	Cold sterilisation	Bacteria, viruses and spores – if left in contact long enough	Protein inactivation	Cidex	Less irritant to tissue than formaldehydes
Diguanides	Skin disinfection. Surgical scrub	Gram +ve bacteria, fungi	Unknown	Hibiscrub Hibitane	Easily inactivated by organic matter. Make sure area is really clean and rinsed before use
Halogens					
– Iodines	Skin disinfection. Surgical scrub	Bacteria, fungi, protozoa, some viruses	Oxidises the cell of the micro-organism, causing inactivation	Aqueous iodine solution	Used as a 2% tincture. Can be irritant if left too long – stains brown
– Iodophors	Skin disinfection Surgical scrub Environmental if preparation includes a detergent	Bacteria, fungi, protozoa, some viruses	Oxidation	Pevidine Wescodyne	Iodine molecule is bound to organic molecules which act as carriers making them ↓ toxic but ↑ inactivation by organic matter
– Hypochlorite (bleach)	Environment	All pathogens including bacterial spores	Oxidation	Domestos Milton Chloros Bleach	Tissue irritant. Corrosive to metal. Inactivated by sunlight and organic matter

table continues

Table 11.1 continued

Disinfectant group	Use	Area of activity	Method of action	Examples of product	Comments
Peroxide	Environment Skin application	Bacteria, esp. anaerobes	Oxidation	Virkon (environment only) Hydrogen peroxide	Use as a flush for abscesses or as a control of haemostasis
Phenols					
– Black/white/clear	Environment	Bacteria, TB, viruses, fungi	Denatures protein	Jeyes fluid Izal	Strong smell, absorbed by rubber. Toxic to cats
– Chlorinated	Environment Skin disinfection	Gram +ve bacteria	Denatures protein	Dettol Ibcol	↑ irritant. Inactivated by hard water and organic matter. Toxic to cats
– Hexachlorophene	Skin disinfection	Gram +ve bacteria	Denatures protein	Phisohex	Used in soaps and detergents
Quaternary ammonium compounds (QACs)	Environment Skin disinfection	Gram +ve/–ve bacteria. Some viruses, fungi and bacterial spores	Dissolve lipids in the pathogens cell wall	Trigene Vetaclean Savlon Zephiran	Non-toxic, cheap, colourless, odourless. Inactivated by hard water, organic matter and soap

Table 11.2 The range of sterilisation methods and their uses

	Example	Advantage	Disadvantage
Dry heat	Hot air oven 150–170°C 60–180min	Kills micro-organisms incl. spores by oxidation. Does not blunt sharp instruments, i.e. drill bits, scissors, finer detail instruments (ophthalmic)	Dry heat requires ↑ sterility time to achieve oxidation, 4–5h. Needs time to heat and to cool. Not recommended. Not suitable for plastic/rubber material. Does not remove prions.
Moist heat	Boiling water	Kills micro-organisms if boiled for minimum of 30mins. Does not destroy virus/spores/prions.	Not recommended. Sterility difficult to achieve and cannot be guaranteed. ↑ potential for rust.
Moist heat under pressure	Autoclave 121–134°C 3–30min	Preferred method. Steam drives air out when introduced under pressure then kills micro-organisms. Use for instruments, cloths, swabs, drapes and some rubber articles.	Requires correct packaging or pockets of inadequate sterility may occur. Can blunt instruments due to being packaged next to each other. Tight packing will not allow steam to penetrate the articles sufficiently, failing complete sterility. Does not remove prion proteins, which raises the question as to whether autoclaving is still to be considered a safe method of sterilisation.
Chemical	Isopropyl alcohol; Ethyl alcohol; Glutaraldehyde	Does not blunt instruments. Used for scopes; suture material in cassettes or pre-package material. Emergency use.	Not reliable. Some solutions require 24h of contact for sterility usually takes 6–12h. Not all chemicals are effective against spores/prions. Toxic/carcinogenic chemical and irritant.
Radiation	Ethylene oxide – EO (Anprolene)	Useful for anything that may melt, e.g. plastic, rubber. Does not blunt instruments. Used for pre-prepared materials i.e. syringes, needles. Effective against prion proteins.	Toxic, irritant and flammable gas. Sterilisation takes 12h; 2h before removal from the cabinet and a further 24h required for airing; gas then needs to be converted to a safe gas as hazardous to the environment. COSHH regulated. Hazardous to personnel; needs to be monitored. Wet instruments produce ethylene glycol – toxic to patients.

table continues

Table 11.2   continued

	Example	Advantage	Disadvantage
Gas	Gas plasma	Safe – does not compromise the health and safety of personnel or patient. No monitoring required. Sterilisation time of 55min (quicker than EO; ↓ need for extra inventory of instruments). Can be used with heat- and moisture-sensitive instruments as uses low temperatures. By-products are safe to the environment. Available as a mobile sterilising unit. Effective against prion proteins.	Expense with regards to the equipment and replacement of working current systems in practice. Not suitable for cellulose material or fine bore instruments of more than 30cm.
Mechanical	Filtration	Liquid is passed through a filter by gravity, pressure or vacuum. Used in combination with some autoclaves.	Specialist equipment required when used alone, not commonly used in practice. Questionable efficacy in removing prion proteins.

most common method due to its size and convenience – though care must be taken to ensure that it is being used correctly to ensure 100% sterility of all articles.

Sterilisation indicators

A variety of indicators are available.

Bowie Dick tape (BDT; autoclave tape) Stripes on the tape turn brown when subjected to steam. This method does not indicate effective sterility as it changes colour when a temperature of 210°C is reached – it does not record how long that temperature is maintained.

Brownes tubes These are small glass tubes which change colour (from red to green) at a certain temperature (Fig 11.1); red indicates pre-exposure and green indicates post-exposure. Because of their reaction to heat it is important to store them in a cool, dry place. Different types work at different temperatures and are identified by a spot – black for steam (autoclaves), green for hot air ovens (Fig 11.2).

Autoclave bags The indicator spots on these bags turn from red to brown when autoclaved. Some will change from blue to yellow (Fig 11.2) when used with ethylene oxide (Anprolene).

Time, steam, temperature (TST) indication strips Strips used at specific temperatures and/or pressures produce a mark on a colour

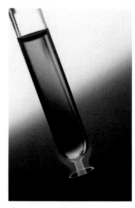

Figure 11.1   Brownes tubes.

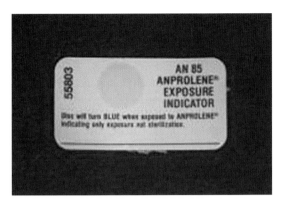

Figure 11.2   An exposed indicator spot to ethylene oxide.

bar (Fig 11.3) during exposure. Only when has it been exposed at the correct temperature and pressure will the bar read 'safe'.

Culture method   Bacteria samples are put through the sterilising process and then cultured to see if any growth occurs. This is a reliable method but can be time consuming. *Bacillus stearothermophilis* is used to test steam under pressure; *B. subtilis* is used to test dry heat, gas plasma and ethylene oxide.

Mechanical methods   Mechanical methods such as gauges, thermometers, timers and recorders are sometimes in-built with the steriliser and may have an alarm to alert to any failure with the sterilisation cycle. However, these tend to be quite large and costly, and are therefore only found in the larger hospitals.

Preparation of articles for sterilisation

Use the following guidelines when preparing/using sterile articles:

● articles should be clean, dry and free of any dirt

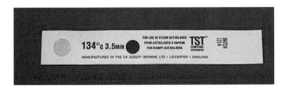

Figure 11.3   TST indication strip.

● instruments should be placed so that they are removed handles first when opened
● do not drop instruments onto the trolley as this may damage them – always open and pass gently
● cover sharp-tipped ends with a protective cover to protect packaging
● place needles in a swab or within a syringe case for security
● label with the expiry date, the name of the piece of equipment and the initials of the person who packed it
● operate a rotation system, with the earliest sterilised items at the front so that they are used first.

Wrapping material

Ideal wrapping material must be permeable to steam (or gas) but not to microbes. It should be flexible and resistant to damage when handled, e.g. muslin/cotton, paper (crepe) or nylon film.

Autoclave film bags (nylon or nylon and paper)   Double-fold the end and seal with a heat-sealer, masking tape, or autoclave tape. Some materials can be reused but beware that they can become brittle and cracks may appear; small holes may also occur.

Peelable pouches (peel and seal)   Pouches of nylon with a self-seal end make a convenient, quick and easy-to-use method of packaging. One side remains transparent; the other has a sterilisation indicator and areas to allow easy labelling. They are more expensive than other methods and can remain unsterile if sealed incorrectly

Corrugated plastic boxes   These can be used to contain sterile equipment such as gowns and hand towels to make access to larger articles easier. The boxes are sturdy and not easily damaged – they can be re-sterilised and re-used.

Autoclave drums or boxes   Both can be used as a container for kits, gowns and swabs and are particularly useful for fine instruments.

Disposable drapes or crepe paper   These provide a water-resistant material which can be cut to size.

Storage of sterile items

Once sterile, items can be stored in closed cabinets or within a designated area – ideally one that is not a thoroughfare for traffic, and is dust-free and away from contaminated articles. Correctly prepared sterile materials/instruments are considered sterile for up to 6 weeks. However, sterility may be affected if handled excessively or kept in conditions of extreme heat or humidity. Dust-bags or dust-sheets can be used to lengthen sterility expiry dates.

SURGICAL AND ANCILLARY INSTRUMENTS

Within the theatre the assistant's role is critical in ensuring the correct care, preparation and sterilisation of all equipment – failure to do so could result not only in wound breakdown but potentially place the patient at a grave risk. Instruments are usually stainless steel with qualities relating to strength, durability and resistance to corrosion. There are two types: martensitic and austenitic.

- Martensitic:
  - a solid mixture of iron and up to 1% carbon; the chief constituent of hardened carbon tool steels referred to as hardenable stainless steel
  - very strong
  - magnetic, though more susceptible to corrosion than austenitic instruments (plating reduces this)
  - used for haemostats, needle holders, forceps, cutting edge instruments, retractors, curettes and osteotomes (Fig 11.4).

- Austenitic:
  - a non-magnetic solid mix of ferric carbide or carbon in iron
  - corrosion-resistant steel due to passivation (a thin layer of chromium oxide is used in the final stages of the manufacturing process)
  - used for pans, trays, bowls, drivers, handles and surgical implants.

Tungsten carbide (TC) provides additional durability and improves function, e.g. better gripping ability in a needle holder. It is generally darker than stainless steel and is very expensive – only the area of direct workload is made of TC to keep overall costs down. A gold handle (Fig 11.5) on the instrument indicates it has a TC insert.

Titanium instruments provide a strong, low-density, highly corrosion-resistant, lightweight instrument useful for ophthalmological surgery – they allow the surgeon greater instrument control when dealing with delicate tissues. Titanium is known for its ability to withstand high temperatures and its durability – keeping instruments sharp and functional for longer. Such instruments are supplied in a distinct pale blue colour.

Care of instruments

As a general guideline:

- use the appropriate tool for the job
- Debakey tissue forceps should not be used to grasp needles

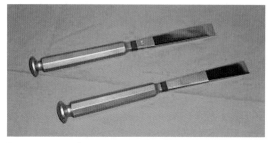

Figure 11.4   Osteotomes.

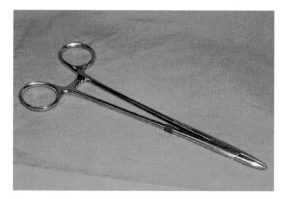

Figure 11.5   Gold-handled Mayo Needle Holders.

- needle holders are designed to hold needles and suture material only
- tungsten carbide inserts provide excellent grip and durability
- Mayo scissors are used for fascia and connective tissue only
- Metzenbaum – used for soft tissues, never for skin or suture material
- do not use scissors to cut wire
- curved scissors allow for better visibility
- ensure a good routine of maintenance for all instruments/equipment
- only traumatise the tissues being removed, if you have to!
- bandage scissors are to be used for bandages, nothing else
- *employ instruments for their intended use only!*

See Table 11.3 for examples of instruments required in specific surgical kits.

Duties of the scrubbed surgical assistant

Instruments should always be handled in an aseptic manner. Pass instruments handles first, pressing them firmly into the palm of the hand. Learn the methods of holding various instruments and employ the correct method for how the instrument is to be used. Find what is comfortable for you.

- prepare and deal with each surgeon's idiosyncrasies
- swab count – before the start and at the end of surgery
- instrument count – before the start and at the end of surgery
- sharps: correct method of attachment; removal and disposal
- place instruments out to allow easy retrieval, e.g. all forceps together (Fig 11.6)
- be aware of what the surgical procedure involves and stay one step ahead – having instruments at the ready when needed, e.g. drill, measure, tap, screw
- immediately place instruments into soak (see instrument care)
- prepare samples for biopsy/histology.

Samples for biopsy/histology

Samples are correctly prepared using the following principles.

- Obtain junctional samples from lesions/tumours, i.e. those that include the junction between normal and abnormal tissue.
- Carefully handle your sample to avoid crush artefacts; lymphoid tissue is particularly vulnerable to this type of iatrogenic damage.
- Do not remove crusts and scales from skin lesions or clean the samples as this will remove important information for the pathologist.
- Ensure you state on your laboratory submission form whether or not all of the lesion/tumour has been removed.
- Include as much description of the lesion as possible, e.g. size, shape, consistency, ulceration, discharge, appearance of the cut surface, colour. Bear in mind much of this information can be lost or distorted once the sample has been preserved.
- Use diagrams to illustrate the size, appearance and site of the tissue removed (especially when submitting more than one) to assist the laboratory pathologists further in their interpretations.
- Ensure the correct labelling and full history details are included for each sample submitted, e.g. multiple lump removals from one animal could include a sebaceous adenoma, a follicular cyst and a mast cell tumour – it is therefore important to know exactly which of these was the malignant one, especially where surgical margins need to be reviewed.
- Help your pathologist orientate the samples you send, e.g. securing skin samples onto card (it will stick to the card naturally after a few minutes) and writing the direction of hair growth on the card. If needed, you could indicate which end of a lesion is which (e.g. proximal, distal) by carefully securing a loop of suture material to the tissue and attaching a label written in pencil.
- Use an appropriate sized pot with 10% neutral buffered formalin. As a minimum

Table 11.3 Examples of instruments to be found in surgical kits

Small animal kit	Spinal kit	Ophthalmic kit	Caesarean section kit for sheep
6 × Backhaus towel clips	1 × Periosteal elevator	1 × Intraocular foreign body forceps	8 × Backhaus towel clips
2 × Needle holders	1 × Freer elevator	1 × Titanium fine St Martins forceps	2 × Needle holders – Mayo–Hegar and Thomson Walker
2 × Allis tissue forceps	1 × Daniels rongeurs	1 × Castroviejo needle holder (no catch)	4 × Allis tissue forceps
6 × Halstead-mosquito artery forceps – straight	1 × Lempert rongeurs	1 × Large St Martins forceps	8 × Halstead-mosquito artery forceps – straight
6 × Halstead-mosquito artery forceps – curved	1 × Double-action rongeurs	1 × Intraocular scissors	8 × Halstead-mosquito artery forceps – curved
1 × Straight Mayo scissors	1 × House Stapes curette	1 × Bangerter eyelid speculum	1 × straight Mayo scissors
1 × Curved Mayo scissors	2 × Dental scalers	1 × Landolt Vectis	1 × curved Mayo scissors
1 × Metzenbaum scissors	Frazier suction tip	1 × Straight scissors	1 × Metzenbaum scissors
1 × Dressing forceps		1 × McPherson–Westcott sharp scissors	1 × dressing forceps
1 × Rat tooth forceps		2 × Small curved artery forceps	1 × rat tooth forceps
1 × Jeanes rat tooth forceps		1 × Pair of Jaffe eyelid retractors	1 × Jeanes rat tooth forceps
1 × Scalpel handle No.3		1 × Gutter eye drape (Alcon)	1 × scalpel handle no.3
1 × Scalpel handle No.5		1 × Set of sterile phaco tubing	1 × scalpel handle no.5
1 × Gelpi retractors		1 × 27G Rycroft cannula (John Weiss)	2 × Gelpi retractors
2 × Gallipots		*Additional equipment:*	2 × Gallipots
1 × Mayo bowl		2 × Microscope (rubber) sleeves	1 × Mayo bowl
10 × 10 × 10cm gauze swabs		10 × Cellulose spears	1 × Scalpel blade no.23
5 × Plain surgical material drapes		15ml Balanced salt solution	8 × Spencer Wells – box joint
		2 × Operating arm-chair covers	1 × large retractor – Balfour or Gosset
		1 × Plastic drape with pouch	
		1 × medium sized fenestrated drape	
		Other i.e. Phacoemulsification probe	

These essential points will help pathologists enormously as there are many grey areas of interpretation that can be overcome by the provision of full and detailed information – an aspect commonly neglected.

Instrument care following surgery

At the end of the surgery use the following protocol (depending on the equipment used):

- place dirty instruments into a bowl of cool water as soon as possible, allowing them to soak for at least 5 minutes
- empty the cold water and refill the bowl with a proprietary instrument cleaner
- scrub the instruments with a soft bristled brush which is *only* used for cleaning instruments
- pay special attention to grooves and joints
- place the clean instruments into the ultrasonic cleaner
- clean ophthalmology instruments for 8 minutes; all other equipment for 10 minutes
- do not overload the ultrasonic cleaner
- place sharp instruments at the top of the cleaner, not under much heavier instruments
- remove basket from the solution and with the instruments still in the basket place under clean running water
- shake off any excess water and place instruments into instrument lube (*do not put hands into the lube – always wear gloves*)
- immerse instruments in solution for 1–2 minutes
- remove and shake off any excess solution
- do not wipe or rinse instruments, lube is steam permeable
- rinse basket thoroughly before placing back into ultrasonic cleaner.
- *Remember*:
  - do not leave instruments wet or dirty for longer than necessary, without proper cleaning, as this will cause rusting and damage
  - looking after instruments with care prolongs their life and better maintains good quality
  - ensure that any instruments that have been

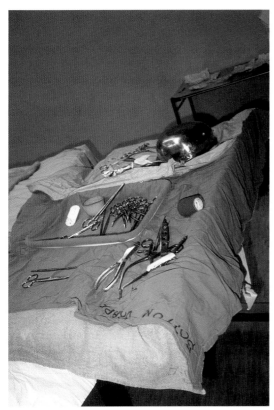

Figure 11.6   Place instruments out to allow easy retrieval, e.g. all forceps together.

use a 10:1 fixative to tissue ratio (25:1 would be ideal) and state exactly what preservative has been used on your submission form. If inadequate amounts of fixative are used, the tissue will autolyse and become uninterpretable by the time the pathologist receives it.

- A 0.5–1cm thickness allows the preservative to penetrate the sample adequately in 24 hours or so. Sections can be removed from larger samples or alternatively incompletely incised at intervals to allow penetration of fixative without losing the architecture of the tissue you submit.
- If in any doubt, check with your own laboratory for their individual requirements with regards to sample preparation, preservation and transportation as this may differ from one laboratory to another and depend on the type of laboratory testing required.

in contact with saline are always cleaned as saline will corrode the instruments

- blood will corrode the instruments, soak as soon as possible
- do not use abrasive cleaning agents on the instruments
- above all use instruments only for their intended use.

Operating instruments and other surgical equipment

Would you be prepared to start a procedure with a piece of equipment you knew nothing about? I hope your answer is no – especially if you have to deal with old equipment. Good nursing involves having knowledge of all the equipment being used – if this is not the case then your patient or other personnel could be at risk (see Table 11.4).

INTERNAL FIXATION

Indications for internal fixation include: unstable fracture, when accurate reduction is essential (joint fracture), avulsion type fracture (distracted), surgical reduction of a dislocation (i.e. open reduction) – indicated if reduction is impossible and when the joint remains unstable and dislocates recurrently. Examples of techniques include cruciate ligament repair, tibial crest transplantation, hip toggle and total hip replacement

The advantages compared with external fixation include reduced animal interference, well tolerated, no damage from external pressure, a greater range of sites, an earlier return to normal for the patient and efficient immobilisation of fragments.

The disadvantages compared with external fixation include higher risk of infection, requires experienced technical skill for the correct usage of the implant, requires specific equipment and/or materials, more expensive method (due to the materials), time and skill involved.

Complications of internal fixation include infection (strict asepsis required during surgery, bone infection is hard to get rid of), soft tissue damage (during surgery can delay healing), mal-union (wrong position of implant, mobility of fragments), weak implant (breaks or bends), reaction between implant metals (occurring when two different types of metal are used between the implants and screws), and movement of pins/screws.

Definitions

- *Union*: the successful result of healing of a fracture, in which the bone ends have become firmly united by newly-formed bone.
- *Malunion*: deformity of a bone resulting from union of a fractured end in which the bone ends are poorly aligned.

Table 11.4   Operating instruments and other surgical equipment

Do:	Do not:
Know how to prepare your equipment	Learn how to use a piece of equipment during the procedure
Know how to operate the equipment	
Know how to care and maintain for each piece of equipment	Use equipment that you are not yet comfortable with
Know how to spot a fault	Pretend to know how something works when really you don't
Have a back up for any faulty equipment	
	Use faulty or poor equipment, e.g. blunt scissors
	Knowingly use materials/equipment if its sterility is in question

- *Delayed union*: slow repair of the fractured parts.
- *Non-union*: when the fractured parts of bone will not heal, e.g. due to infection, mobility.
- *Osteomyelitis*: inflammation of the bone marrow due to infection, e.g. may follow a compound fracture.

Orthopaedic implants

Intramedullary pins

Steinman pins   A suitable sized Steinman pin (Fig 11.7) is inserted into the intramedullary cavity using a Jacob's chuck. The length of pin required is measured against an x-ray of the normal bone. Pins only are removed if they subsequently ride up and cause damage. They are suitable only for use in long bones and are available with trocar, beveled and screw tips. The advantages of these pins are the easy technique, minimal equipment required and that they are cheap. The disadvantages are rotational instability and pin movement.

Rush pins   These are small, springy intramedullary pins (Figs 11.8, 11.9) used to repair condylar fractures of the femur and/or humerus. Pins are inserted so that the 'sledge-

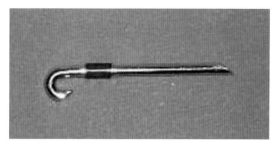

Figure 11.9   Rush pin.

runner' tip contacts the bone of the apposing cortex. Another rush pin is inserted into the other condyle in the same way. The spring action brings the bone closer together.

Kirschner wires   Kirschner wires (K-wires; see also under external fixators) are small, sharp, pointed intramedullary pins used for repairing growth plate fractures and small fragment fractures. They are inserted using a Jacob's chuck and can be used in very small animals as an intramedullary pin (Figs 11.10, 11.11).

Orthopaedic wire   This is mainly used as cerclage wire to supplement other fixation techniques, e.g. intramedullary pins (Fig 11.12).

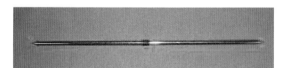

Figure 11.7   Steinman pin.

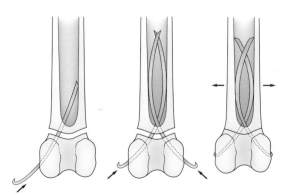

Figure 11.8   Rush pinning.

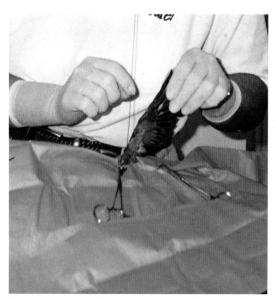

Figure 11.10   A fig parrot having an intramedullary pin placed in a humeral fracture using a K-wire.

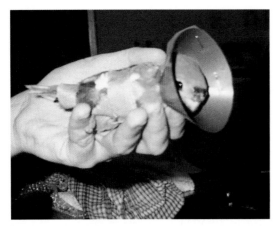

Figure 11.11   The patient made a successful recovery and was later released following appropriate rehabilitation.

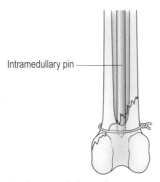

Intramedullary pin

Figure 11.12   Intramedullary pin.

The correct size of wire should be used and the wire should be twisted evenly.

Plates

Plates and screws should produce optimal stability and allow the patient to use the limb early in the recovery process. They come in a wide variety of sizes and must be of sufficient strength to support weight bearing. The screws must be of the same metal as the plate to avoid electrolyte reactions. Types include Sherman, Venables, ASIF dynamic compression plate and Lanes (similar to Venables).

● Sherman plate. This is a weak plate (Fig 11.13) and should be used for small, light animals.

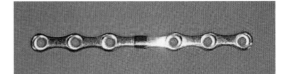

Figure 11.13   Sherman plate.

● Venables plate. A strong plate for general use, available in narrow and broad widths (Fig 11.14).
● Dynamic compression plate (DCP; Association for the Study of Internal Fixation – ASIF). These come in a wide range of sizes (Fig 11.15) to repair fractures in animals of any size. Compression of the fracture results in faster fracture repair. ASIF DC plates must be used with ASIF screws and equipment – the ASIF system is expensive.

Screws

Sherman   The Sherman is self-tapping (cutting its own channel) – a smaller hole is drilled so that the screw has a tight grip once fitted. Self-tapping screws can sometimes work loose, causing microfractures.

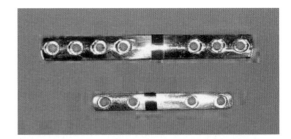

Figure 11.14   Venables plate.

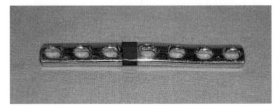

Figure 11.15   An example of a dynamic compression plate.

Partially threaded screw These are ideal for use as a lag screw – only the end of the screw (Fig 11.16) grips the bone and the fragment is squeezed back into position when the screw is tightened. When used with ASIF equipment lag screws are double drilled – first a large drill through the cortex, then the smaller drill to thread, which then compresses the fracture together.

ASIF cortical (fine thread) and cancellous (wider thread) screws Cortical screws are fully threaded and intended for use in the hard cortical bone of the diaphysis. They are not self-tapping – providing a sturdier hold. Debris must be removed from the site with a tap before the screw is placed (Fig 11.17). *Cancellous* screws are either fully or partially threaded and are intended for use in the softer cancellous bone located within the metaphysis of the bone. Cancellous screws require use of a washer in conjunction.

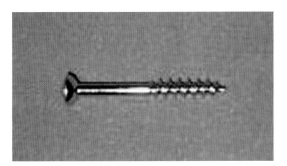

Figure 11.16 Partially threaded screw.

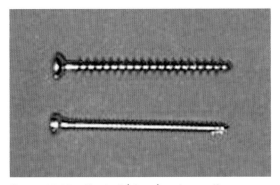

Figure 11.17 Cortical (above) and cancellous (below) screws.

Care and storage of orthopaedic implants

After use, soak instruments in cold water to remove blood and debris. Scrub instruments under running water, paying particular attention to joints, serrations and ratchets – clean with detergent solution. Ultrasonic cleaners will remove debris from inaccessible areas. Remember to lubricate movable parts. Handle equipment gently, protecting sharp points. Sort into sets ready for use and keep different instruments in divided compartments; separate and store pins, plates, screws etc into their different sizes/types. Packages should be clearly labelled for ease of recognition and with details relating to the sterility dates.

ASIF/AO

The ASIF or AO (Association for the Study of Internal Fixation or Arbeitsgemeinschaft für Osteosynthesefragen) system provides compression at a fracture site.

- *Drill bits* (Fig 11.18) must be sharp – dispose of if useless. Air drills need specific lubricating oils for general maintenance. The drill is powered by N_2O, because it is cleaner than compressed air, which also can be used. The size will be found on the end of the drill bit that connects into the drill.
- The *depth gauge* must be used before tapping – if done after tapping it could disturb the ready made thread. They cannot be re-sharpened and therefore are disposed of. Two clockwise followed by one anti-clockwise is the correct tapping technique.
- *Taps* (Fig 11.18) cut a thread into the bone to assist in securing a cortical bone screw that is not self-tapping.
- *C-guide* – used to guide the route of the drill.
- *Neutral and load drill guide* – load (yellow)

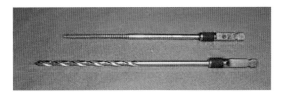

Figure 11.18 Tap (above) and drill bit (below).

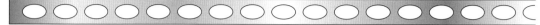

Figure 11.19   Cutable plate.

is off centre; the hole is designed for the dynamic compression plate and the green (neutral) is for straight screwing (oil regularly with ASIF oil).

ASIF equipment can include a cutable plate (Fig 11.19), a DCP Plate (Fig 11.20), an acetabular plate (Fig 11.21), a reconstruction plate (Fig 11.22; – this plate can be bent and cut to requirement), T-plates for small animals (Fig 11.23) and broad plates (Fig 11.24).

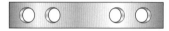

Figure 11.20   DCP plate.

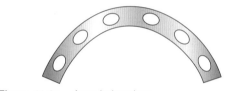

Figure 11.21   Acetabular plate.

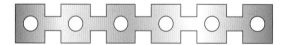

Figure 11.22   Reconstruction plate.

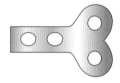

Figure 11.23   T-plates for small animals.

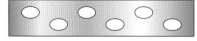

Figure 11.24   Broad plate.

Other important points to consider include:

- never mix instruments of other companies with these when sterilising, as this will cause electrolytic reactions
- when cleaning equipment always remember to dismantle all parts to clean and use specific ASIF oil
- never immerse the mini-compressed drill or the oscillating saw in water
- plate screws hold a plate in place and do not go through a fracture line, whereas a lag screw can go through the fracture line
- lubricate with proprietary instrument milk such as Downes or a spray after every wash/use and autoclave at 134°C.

For good images and implant techniques visit the various AO/ASIF websites using AO and ASIF as your key search words.

EXTERNAL FIXATION

An external fixator is applied as a first aid measure or following the reduction of the fracture, either by manual reduction or internal reduction performed under general anaesthesia. The technique is used for a fracture within a limb and occasionally for neck/tail fractures.

The advantages are that it is a less skilled technique using less sophisticated apparatus. It is also cheaper and carries less risk of infection. There are some disadvantages – they are cumbersome (can restrict limb movement) and liable to physical damage and possible interference from the animal (use an Elizabethan collar if interest is shown in either the fixator or stitches). Also, the efficacy is reduced if it gets wet, there is a risk of pressure sores and restriction of the blood supply, it may slip or fall off, it is difficult to examine wounds, and owner compliance is essential. See Figure 11.25 for the result of a cast getting wet, allowing infection to take hold for nearly 3 weeks before

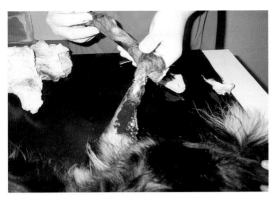

Figure 11.25   Infection as a result of a wet cast.

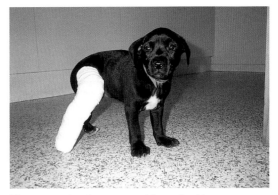

Figure 11.26   A cast on a 12-week-old Staffordshire Bull Terrier puppy.

the animal was returned to the surgery. It is essential that follow-up checks are always tracked with any non-attendance chased up. The dog pictured here made a full recovery following amputation of the limb.

Types of external fixators

A number of types exist: bandages (e.g. Robert-Jones), casts (Plaster of Paris, e.g. Gypsona, Plastrona), thermoplastic materials (e.g. Hexalite, Vetlite), resin-impregnated (DeltaCast), fibreglass tape (with resin – Scotchcast, Scotchflex), splints (Zimmer, Gutter, Thomas, inflatable), and stainless steel apparatus (Kirschner splints).

Casts
Casts are more suitable for the smaller breed of dog (Fig 11.26) or cat. There are a number of advantages and disadvantages of Plaster of Paris compared with other cast materials:

- generally heavier than other cast materials
- generally more uncomfortable
- does not dry if it becomes wet – unlike synthetic casting materials (SCMs)
- cheap
- does not require additional equipment or specialist skill, easy to apply
- has become superseded by more user-friendly SCM such as fibreglass or polyester fabric impregnated with water-activated polyurethane resin.

A cast is applied as follows:

- place adhesive stirrups on the limb
- cover with a stockinette then apply cast padding over the stockinette using an overlapping pattern
- place 4–6 layers of casting material on the limb, overlapping each layer by 50% (producing four layers on cross-section) quickly – sets within 4–6 minutes
- roll edges of the cast outward by pulling the proximal aspect of the stockinette over the end of the cast
- apply elastic adhesive or Vetwrap around the cast then stick the stirrups to this layer
- fashion a walking bar of aluminium rod into a 'U' shape and tape it to the bottom of the cast so that the animal does not weight-bear directly onto the cast.

Splints
Zimmer (finger splint)   The Zimmer:

- is a temporary measure when unable to provide long-term rigid support
- is malleable to the patient with the length being cut to requirement
- is bandaged into place with padding underneath the splint
- can have the proximal and distal ends bent over to protect the skin
- is cheap/reusable
- is available in different widths.

Gutter splint   The Gutter:

- is cylinder shaped and can be cut as required
- is made of plastic, metal or cast
- covers three sides of the limb, increasing support and strength of the splint
- can be applied to the palmar or plantar aspect of the limb
- is bandaged into place with padding underneath the splint
- is reusable for the same patient
- can be removed to allow examination of the limb
- is available in different sizes.

Thomas extension splint   The Thomas:

- is used on the hind limb involving a fracture within the lower extremity (Figs 11.27, 11.28)

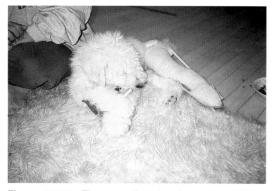

Figure 11.27   Thomas splint placed on a 6-month-old Komondor puppy.

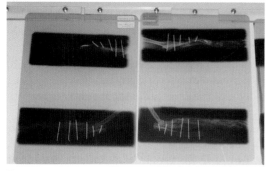

Figure 11.28   Postoperative radiographs of the patient in Fig 11.27.

- is a metal loop which is fitted around the proximal aspect and extremity of the limb
- is attached to a 'U' loop extending distally
- can be home-made with a coat-hanger covered with Elastoplast or bought as a complete kit.

Kirschner external fixator splint   The advantages of this technique are: the immobilisation of bones and joints, it is useful for open-contaminated fractures, it is well tolerated (especially by cats), it maintains stability of the fragments, it allows the patient to use the joint, it allows access for wound examination and cleaning, the surgery is quicker compared with that of internal fixation – which would be beneficial for an ill or elderly animal.

Security between the pins can be achieved using specialised stainless steel bolts (Fig 11.29). Alternatively, plastic tubing is injected with surgical cement, which will then harden and hold together – as demonstrated in a patient with an external fixator in place which was bandaged (Figs 11.30, 11.31) to protect the implants from damage and injury to others.

The disadvantages are: the pins can move or work their way out (destabilising the fracture), the pin holes may discharge, it is easier for pins to break, the splint is liable to physical damage or possible interference from the animal, and is not very aesthetic looking for squeamish owners. The differences in nursing a patient following internal or external fixation are detailed in Table 11.5.

SUTURES AND SUTURE MATERIALS

The ideal suture material would be of use in any operation, easy to handle, form knots that hold securely (without slipping, cutting or fraying), have a high tensile strength sustained in vivo, have no memory, have little elasticity, cause no tissue reaction and would not shrink in vivo. Further, it would be non-electrolytic, non-toxic, non-allergenic, non-capillary, non-carcinogenic, non-corrosive, non-pyogenic and non-thrombogenic. It would have predictable or controllable absorbability when no longer

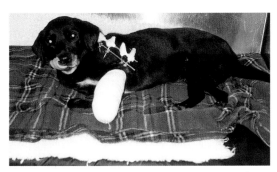

Figure 11.29   An elderly patient with a humeral fracture.

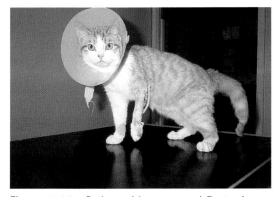

Figure 11.30   Patient with an external fixator in place.

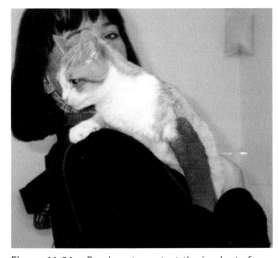

Figure 11.31   Bandage to protect the implants from damage and injury to others.

needed, good visibility in use but be inconspicuous within tissues postoperatively, have a long shelf life and be economical and easy to sterilise.

The use of sutures began some 4000 years ago in ancient India and Egypt between 1600 and 1000BC when linen or flax and hemp were described as the material of choice. Since then a variety of materials have been tried – unfortunately none of them have all of the qualities listed above. Modern synthetic materials have now replaced most of the older suture materials, but a few remain such as silk. Today's sutures are classed as: natural *or* synthetic, absorbable *or* non-absorbable, monofilament *or* braided. Refer to Tables 11.6 and 11.7 relating to the various absorbable suture materials and Tables 11.8 and 11.9 for information regarding non-absorbable suture materials.

Properties of suture materials

Generally, synthetic suture materials cause less tissue reaction (Table 11.10). Monofilament materials are less reactive and are much less likely to harbour bacteria – and thus are less likely to be associated with local suture line infections. Braided materials generally have more strength but have more tissue drag (Fig 11.32) and cause more tissue tension. Bacteria can be harboured in the spaces between the filaments. Most braided materials are now coated to reduce tissue drag – but this has the disadvantage of reducing knot security. Monofilaments do not tend to have these problems, though they do have significant memory and can be difficult to handle.

Suture material can be obtained as a cassette reel, though sterility cannot be guaranteed. Usually chromic catgut absorbable sutures or nylon non-absorbable materials are used for skin sutures. Supramid and Vetafil are used widely in veterinary practice. They are braided nylon materials coated with nylon to create a strong pseudo-monofilament suture and should only be used for skin closure, not buried in tissues. The strength of the material should be as strong as the tissue it is being placed into:

Table 11.5   Differences in nursing a patient following internal or external fixation procedure

	Internal fixator patient	External fixator patient
Bedding	Padded bedding should be available	No loose bedding material as fixator may become tangled. Lots of padded bedding should be available such as waterproof foam beds
Wound care	Incision wound to be monitored and cleaned as necessary	Pin wounds must be kept clean and bathed twice daily
Bandaging		Bandage should be applied over the pin edges to protect the patient and others
Postoperative radiography	Immediate postoperative image obtained	Immediate postoperative image is obtained and later x-rays are taken to assess healing and to see that the fracture has united before removing the pins
Physiotherapy	Leash walking is encouraged	Physical therapy to maintain joint motion and enhance use of limb as patient sometimes becomes weighed down and tends to be lazy, resulting in increased muscle atrophy and limb weakness

Strongest ⟶ *Weakest*
(skin, fascia)   (stomach, bladder, small intestine)

Choice of material by the veterinary surgeon or nurse involves: personal experience, nature and condition of the tissue being repaired, physical properties of the suture material, biological characteristics of the material, predisposition of the wound to infection and presence of tissue trauma. There are also important patient factors such as shock, stress, malnutrition, the effects of drugs and irradiation. The suture size depends on durability, handling qualities and knot security. Fascia has a minimal tensile strength of about 3kg and is the strongest soft tissue in the body; this is equivalent strength to size 0 catgut or silk and 2/0 and 3/0 in the synthetic materials (Table 11.11).

There is a tendency to use materials that are too large and will bury foreign materials. This creates a more inflammatory response, retarding wound healing – which might then result in the enhancement of infection. Correct technique in placement (not too tight), tissue handling and reduction of local swelling by gentle care, use of small, sharp swaged-on needles and use of smaller materials all help facilitate uncomplicated wound healing.

Selection of suture size

Suture materials are available in metric (Imperial) or USP (US Pharmacopeia). Metric = diameter in $\frac{1}{10}$ mm, e.g. if the actual size is 0.4mm, then metric size is 4 (multiplying the size by 10).

Needles

A wide range of stainless steel needles is available in a variety of designs (Fig 11.33). Suture material can be swaged onto the needle directly or have an eye for the suture material to pass through. Ideally, needles should be able to pass through tissues causing minimal damage or trauma – the selection of the most suitable suture material and needle is crucial. Some needles are coated with silicone to facilitate passage through the tissues. For the advantages of the different point types available see Figure 11.34 and Table 11.12.

Table 11.6   Absorbable suture materials

Suture	Surgical gut	Surgical gut 2	Polyglactin 910 (Vicryl)	Polydioxanone (PDS)
Types	Plain	Chromic	Braided	Monofilament
Colour of material	Yellowish–tan	Brown	Violet	Violet
Raw material	Collagen derived from healthy mammals	Collagen derived from healthy mammals. Treated to resist digestion by body tissues	Copolymer of lactide and glycolide coated with polyglactin 370 and calcium stearate	Polyester polymer
Tensile strength retention	Lost within 7–10 days	Lost within 21–28 days	Approximately 60% remains at 2 weeks, 30% at 3 weeks	Approximately 70% remains at 2 weeks, 50% at 4 weeks and 25% at 6 weeks
Absorption rate	Digested by body enzymes within 70 days	Digested by body enzymes within 90 days	Minimal until about 40th day. Essentially complete between 60–90 days, absorbed by slow hydrolysis	Minimal until about 90th day essentially complete within 210 days. Absorbed by slow hydrolysis
Tissue reaction	Fairly high	Moderate	Low	Slight
Contraindications	Should not be used in tissues that heal slowly and require support	Being absorbable, should not be used where prolonged approximation of tissues under stress is required	As Surgical gut 2	As Surgical gut 2
Warnings	Absorbs relatively quickly	Protein-based absorbable sutures have a tendency to fray when tied	Safety and effectiveness in neural and cardiovascular tissue has not been established	As Vicryl
Frequent uses	Ligate superficial vessels, suture sub-cut. And other tissues that heal rapidly. Ophth. sx	Used as an absorbable suture in tissues that heals fairly slow and as a ligature. Ophth. sx	Ligate or suture tissues where an absorbable suture is desirable. Ophth. sx	Intended for use where an absorbable suture or ligature is indicated such as orthopaedic and plastic sx etc
Colour code	Yellow	Beige	Violet	Silver

Table 11.7 Absorbable suture materials

Suture	Polyglactin 910 (Vicryl rapide)	Poliglecaprone 25 (Monocryl)	Polyglactin 910 (Coated Vicryl)	Polydioxanone (PDS II)
Type	Braided	Monofilament	Braided	Monofilament
Colour of material	Undyed/violet	Undyed/violet	Undyed/violet	Undyed/violet
Wound support requirement	Short	Medium	Medium	Long
Tensile strength retention	10 days	20 days	30 days	60 days
Areas of frequent use	Closure of the skin and mucosa	Closure of SC skin and soft tissue closure requiring medium–term support where a monofilament is preferred	Closure of the soft tissues requiring medium–term support where a braided suture is required	For slow healing tissues and for patients where healing may be delayed
Comments (benefit if avoiding suture removal)	e.g. minor or paediatric surgery, perineal repair, oral mucosa, scalp wounds or wounds under plaster	e.g. biliary or GI tract, urology (bladder reconstruction), peritoneum, plastic surgery or caesarean (uterus)	e.g. general surgery (ligation), gynaecology or muscle	e.g. fascia, tendon, meniscus, oesophagus, rectum or colon
Main benefit	For effective short-term wound support and no stitch removal	For unprecedented monofilament pliability and smoothness	For excellent handling and knotting performance	For extended wound support in slow healing tissue

Table 11.8   Non-absorbable suture materials

Suture	Polyester (Mersilene)	Polyester (Ethibond)	Polypropylene (Prolene)
Types	Braided monofilament	Braided	Monofilament
Colour of material	Green, white	Green, white	Blue, clear
Raw material	Polyester Polyethylene Terephthalate	Polyester Polyethylene Terephthalate coated with polybutylate	Polymer of propylene
Tensile strength retention	Indefinite	Indefinite	Indefinite
Absorption rate	Non-absorbable, remains encapsulated in the bodies tissues	Non-absorbable, remains encapsulated in the bodies tissues	Non-absorbable, remains encapsulated in the bodies tissues
Tissue reaction	Low	Low	Low
Contraindications	None	None	None
Warnings	None	None	None
Frequent uses	General, cardiovascular, plastic and ophthalmic surgery	General, cardiovascular and ophthalmic surgery	Cardiovascular, plastic and ophthalmic surgery
Colour code	Turquoise	Orange	Deep blue

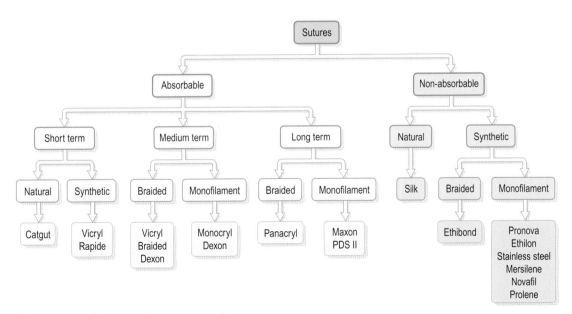

Figure 11.32   Summary of suture properties.

Table 11.9 Non-absorbable suture materials

Suture	Mersilk	Surgical linen	Surgical steel	Ethilon
Types	Braided	Twisted	Monofilament and multifilament available	Monofilament
Colour of material	Black or white	White	Metallic silver	Black
Raw material	Natural protein Fibre of raw silk spun by silkworms	Natural long staple flax fibres	An alloy of iron-nickel-chromium	Polyamide polymer
Tensile strength retention	Loses most or all in about one year	Loses 50% in 6 months, has 30–40% at end of 2 years	Indefinite	Loses 15–20% per year
Absorption rate	Usually cannot be found after 2 years	Non-absorbable, remains encapsulated in the bodies tissues	Non-absorbable, remains encapsulated in the bodies tissues	Degrades at a rate of about 15–20% per year
Tissue reaction	Moderate	Moderate	Minimal	Low
Contraindications	Should not be used for placement of vascular prostheses and heart valves	None	Should not be used when a prosthesis of another alloy is implanted	None
Warnings	Slowly absorbs	None	May corrode and break at points of twisting, bending or knotting	None
Frequent uses	For ligation and suturing where long-term support of tissue is not required	For ligation and suturing in GI surgery	Sternum closure, tendon sutures	Closure of skin, retention plastic surgery, ophthalmic, microsurgery and general surgery
Colour code	Light blue	Pink	Yellow ochre	Mint green

Table 11.10	Uses of different suture material
Location	Recommended material
Skin	Monofilament nylon or propylene
Sub-cutis	Fine; synthetic; absorbable
Fascia	Synthetic; non-absorbable PDS and Vicryl
Muscle	Synthetic; absorbable or non-absorbable. Nylon or Prolene for cardiac muscle
Hollow viscus	Synthetic absorbable or Prolene
Tendon	Stainless steel; Prolene and nylon
Blood vessels	Prolene and Silk
Nerves	Nylon and Prolene

Table 11.11	Uses of different sizes of suture
Size	Uses
7/0 and smaller	Ophthalmology and microsurgery
6/0	Face, blood vessels
5/0	Face, neck and blood vessels
4/0	Mucosa, neck, limbs, tendons and blood vessels
3/0	Limbs, trunk, gut and blood vessels
2/0	Trunk, fascia, viscera, blood vessels
0 and larger	Abdominal wall closure, fascia, drain sites, arterial lines, orthopaedic surgery

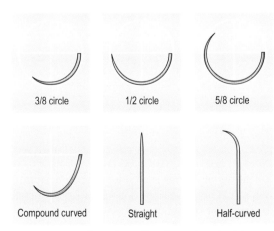

3/8 circle   1/2 circle   5/8 circle

Compound curved   Straight   Half-curved

Figure 11.33 Curved needles. Reproduced with permission from SURU International Pvt Ltd.

Suture patterns

Good wound healing relies on good suture technique – here are some of the common suture patterns used in practice.

Simple interrupted (Fig 11.35) Provides a secure anatomical closure through the complete layer of the skin; easily applied; excessive tension may cause wound inversion. Used with skin, sub-cutis, fascia, blood vessels, nerves and GI tract.

Simple continuous (Fig 11.36) Saves time and material. Allows good apposition with a good seal. Useful for layers under minimal tension as it provides less strength than the simple interrupted pattern. Puckering and strangulation of tissues will result with excessive tension. Used with intradermal skin closure.

Ford interlocking (Fig 11.37) Similar to the simple continuous pattern, though this provides greater security if broken. Used with skin, diaphragm.

Cushing (Fig 11.38) This style is a continuous inverting suture that penetrates the submucosa but not the lumen (the inner channel through which the stomach contents flow) of the bowel. Provides less inversion than the Lembert pattern. Used with closure of hollow viscera in abdominal surgery.

Interrupted vertical mattress (Fig 11.39) Appositional to everting pattern; single sutures used with tissues under tension providing greater strength than the interrupted horizontal mattress; helps to eliminate dead space. Used with skin, sub-cutis and fascia.

Interrupted horizontal mattress (Fig 11.40) Appositional to everting suture depending on the tension of the tissues; can be used for full or partial thickness; the potential for tissue strangulation can be reduced with the use of stents.

Continuous horizontal mattress (Fig 11.41) Appositional to everting suture, depending on suture tension facilitating rapid closure. Used with skin, sub-cutis and fascia.

Interrupted cruciate or cross mattress (Fig 11.42) Provides a stronger closure compared to the simple interrupted pattern; resists

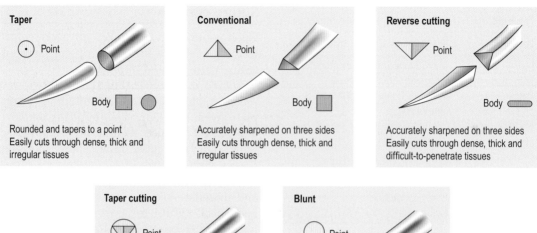

Taper

● Point

Body ▪ ●

Rounded and tapers to a point
Easily cuts through dense, thick and
irregular tissues

Conventional

△ Point

Body ▪

Accurately sharpened on three sides
Easily cuts through dense, thick and
irregular tissues

Reverse cutting

▽ Point

Body ▭

Accurately sharpened on three sides
Easily cuts through dense, thick and
difficult-to-penetrate tissues

Taper cutting

▽ Point

Body ▭

Designed to easily cut through dense
and tough tissues without damaging the
surrounding tissue

Blunt

○ Point

Body ▭

Blunt-nosed for dissection of
friable tissues

Figure 11.34   Point types and their advantages. Reproduced with permission from SURU International Pvt Ltd.

Table 11.12   Advantages and disadvantages of swaged and eyed needles

Eyed	Swaged
Re-usable	Suture material attached directly
Can be used with any type of size suture material	Reduced chance of unthreading
	Less traumatic to tissues
Cheaper	Expensive
Repeated sterilisation dulls cutting edges	Sharp, sterile, single use needles are
More bulk to go through tissues	available in each pack
	Minimum handling and preparation leading to maintenance or integrity of the suture
	Easy to locate, if accidentally dropped into tissue

tension and helps reduce eversion; easy to apply. Used with skin, amputation stumps of tail/digits.

Lembert (Fig 11.43)   An inverting suture that can be either continuous or interrupted; used to join two segments of an intestine without entering the lumen. Used with fascial imbrication (regular overlapping edges) or plication (folding) and closure of a hollow viscera. The knot (Fig 11.44) should be just to the right of the wound when tied.

Tension suture   The tension suture is used to help control low-pressure haemorrhage from small vessels and also as a secure way of

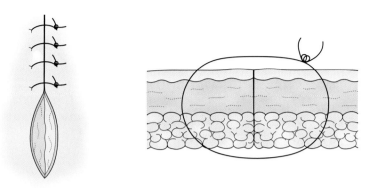

Figure 11.35   Simple interrupted suture.

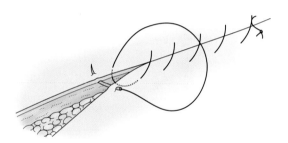

Figure 11.36   Simple continuous suture.

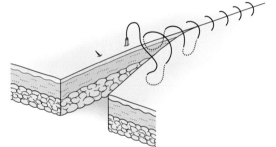

Figure 11.37   Cushing suture.

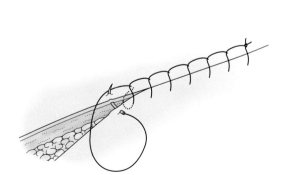

Figure 11.38   Ford interlocking suture.

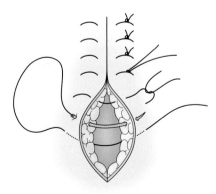

Figure 11.39   Interrupted vertical mattress.

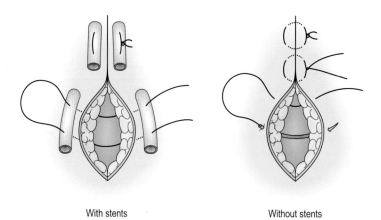

With stents   Without stents

Figure 11.40   Interrupted horizontal mattress.

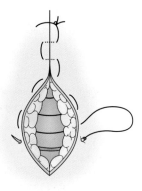

Figure 11.41   Continuous horizontal mattress.

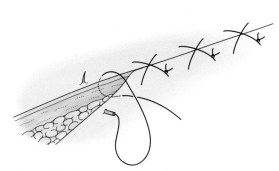

Figure 11.42   Interrupted cruciate or cross mattress.

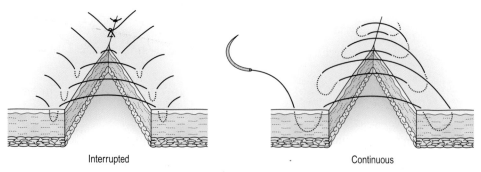

Interrupted   Continuous

Figure 11.43   Lembert suture.

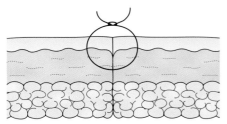

Figure 11.44   The knot should be to the right of the wound.

closing a wound, which will then be subjected to additional strain or pressure due to the location/position of the wound. The arrow in Figure 11.45 indicates a piece of gauze, swab or roll of cotton wool that can be used directly against the wound.

Pseudo–sutures

Alternatives to suture needles and materials that can be used include the following.

Tissue glue
Made from cyanoacrylate, with a similar composition to superglue, this can be used in place of interrupted or subcuticular stitches that require no other sutures. It should not be used on raw tissue as the edges should be straight and lie naturally together. Apply tiny dots of glue sparingly at intervals where the wound edges meet or with a bridge of tiny droplets over the edges; thick applications do not enhance bonding and tend to crack and loosen prematurely. Products dyed blue are much easier to see.

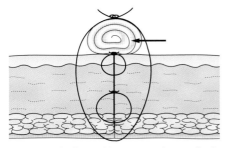

Figure 11.45   A piece of gauze, swab or roll of cotton wool can be used directly against the wound.

Use a hair dryer or fan the area for 30 seconds until the adhesive stiffens. Bathing is not contraindicated but soaking should be avoided. The adhesive should flake off in 3–7 days. Allergic reactions are rare though reports have been made of inflammation and swelling. The result is an improved cosmetic appearance due to the absence of suture marks.

Adhesive tapes
These are not used widely within the veterinary field due to their poor adhesion to animal skin.

Ligating clips
Clips that are either 'V' or 'C' shaped are designed into a similar applicator and used in the control of haemostasis of small vessels causing little tissue reaction. Again, speed is the key advantage here; allowing good security of the clip.

Staples
Disposable skin staplers are quick and easy to use, allowing precise application. Staples are tolerated well by animals and are relatively pain-free when removed. The disadvantages are that they are expensive, may cause tension and require a special staple remover. However, the advantages of speed and ability to reach difficult areas over-ride these, allowing rapid anastomosis of sections of GI tract or bowel and closure of bronchi.

Stapling devices are designed to deliver multiple staples at one time, producing a linear staple line (Fig 11.46) or producing two linear staple lines where the tissue is cut between the two. Figure 11.47 demonstrates a stapler that can produce a circular staple line – useful for anastomosing the GI track or bowel.

Diathermy and suction equipment

Diathermy
Diathermy (also called electrodiathermy, electrocautery, electrocoagulation, vascular coagulation or cauterisation) involves heating body tissues by taking advantage of their resistance

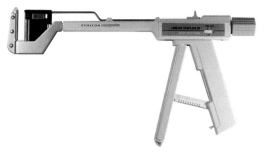

Figure 11.46 Linear stapling device. Reproduced with permission from Ethicon Endo-Surgery.

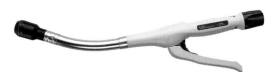

Figure 11.47 Circular stapler device. Reproduced with permission from Ethicon Endo-Surgery.

to the passage of high frequency electromagnetic radiation, electric currents or ultrasonic waves. The tissue forms part of the electrical circuit and is thus heated. Diathermy is used to either cut or destroy tissue or to produce coagulation in vessels less than 1.5–2mm in diameter (if larger, these should be ligated). In medical diathermy (thermopenetration) the tissues are warmed but not damaged; in surgical diathermy (electrocoagulation) tissue is destroyed. Good haemostasis allows appropriate tissue visualisation during the procedure and prevents life-threatening haemorrhage such as shock. Animals suffering from a condition or disease which prevents clotting must be stabilised prior to surgery.

Monopolar diathermy The electrical plate is placed on the patient (Fig 11.48) and acts as indifferent electrode. Current passes between the instrument and the indifferent electrode – localised heating is then produced at the tip of the instrument. The autoclavable electrode tips join together where the heat is being produced, with minimal heating effect produced at the indifferent electrode.

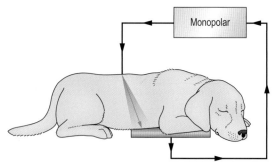

Figure 11.48 Monopolar diathermy.

Bipolar diathermy Two electrodes are combined (Fig 11.49) in the instrument (e.g. diathermy forceps) and the current passes between tips and not through the patient. A range of forceps-like autoclavable tip shapes are available for different situations. Bipolar diathermy is used for precision haemostasis or as a form of incision/dissection tool to speed up surgery time. The tips are separated to allow the passage of the current from one electrode to another.

Effects of diathermy

- depends on the current of the intensity and wave form used
- coagulation is produced by interrupted pulses of current (50–100 per second) or by desiccation and sealing of the blood vessels
- cutting action is produced by continuous current
- blend action is a combination of cutting and coagulation waveforms to increase the degree of haemostasis during cutting

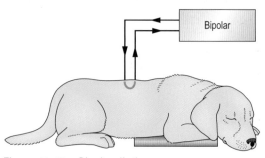

Figure 11.49 Bipolar diathermy.

- can be controlled by a handpiece or foot pedal by the surgeon/nurse

Risks and complications
- contraindicated in patients with arrhythmias
- may affect the function of a pacemaker
- full thickness burns if a spirit-based skin preparation is used
- poor positioning of the indifferent electrode may result in diathermy burns
- channelling effects possible if used on appendages
- concern over arcing with metal instruments and implants (though rare)
- can delay wound healing

Safety and user guidelines
Responsibility for safety lies ultimately with the veterinary surgeon. Alarms should be available to sound if the plate is not connected to the machine; remember – always connect patient to plate, then plate to machine. If the equipment used is not sterile then a sterile sleeve must be provided.

Patient plate Ensure the plate is not kinked or bent. Site the plate close to the operation site and ensure the current is moving away from the ECG electrodes. The skin area under plate should have a good blood supply; avoid bony prominences and scars and for good conduction shave long fur. Do not let skin fluids seep under the plate (especially if spirit-based).

Surgical points Only the surgeon wielding the active electrode should activate the machine. Secure the line of the diathermy onto the surgical drape to avoid it falling onto a non-sterile area and to ensure easy access for the surgeon. Sterilise a plastic container of a 60ml syringe and use this as a temporary holder during surgery; secure it on to the drape with tie (Fig 11.50). Always replace the electrode in an insulated quiver.

Diathermy in use
In patients with pacemakers

- use bipolar diathermy wherever possible

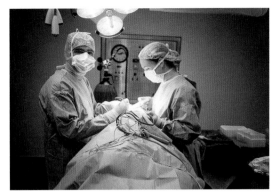

Figure 11.50   Diathermy in use.

- ensure the current flows away from the pacemaker system
- use short bursts only
- observe for arrhythmias and stop immediately if any occur.

Haemostasis, other than electrocoagulation, can also be controlled using one of the following methods:

- application of a ligature around the bleeding vessel
- direct pressure: digital pressure or pressure bandage, pressure with a sponge or gauze swab, artery forceps
- haemostatic agents: Bonewax (beeswax and a softening agent – isopropyl palmitate), Surgicel (oxidised regenerated cellulose), Gelfoam (absorbable gelatin sponge), lignocaine (causes vasoconstriction), cold saline (causes vasoconstriction)
- chemical: silver nitrate, sedative ($\downarrow$ blood pressure), platelets/clotting factors
- physical: limb elevation, tourniquet (less frequently used), pressure points
- CO_2 surgical laser
- suction.

Suction equipment

Suction allows the removal of fluids or debris using an active process by raising atmospheric pressure and can be used as a form of haemostasis. Comprising a suction chamber, suction pipeline and a reusable or disposable tip, such equipment is an invaluable tool to the surgeon in helping to maintain a clear field of visibility. Fluids can be removed in a safe and controlled manner to prevent the animal's condition being compromised. Most endo-scopes have suction abilities that can also be used to collect fluids suitable for diagnostic testing.

Suction and diathermy in use

Suction equipment can also be placed in a temporary syringe tube or a similar piece of equipment (as used for diathermy equipment) for security and safety during the operation (Fig 11.51). A range of tips is available to allow different levels of suction control. Tips can be either disposable or non-disposable. Some examples of non-disposable tips include (dis-posable versions are made of clear plastic):

Frazier suction tip For fine, delicate suc-tioning; increased suction can be controlled by the surgeon/nurse by covering the hole at the base of the tip.

Yankauer The bulb/tapered tips reduce tissue trauma and allow maximum visibility. The open tip allows access into tight spaces and permits rapid aspiration

Poole The Poole is specially designed to evacuate pooled blood, fluid or debris – the sump action allows pinpoint suctioning. This tip is useful for deep abdominal surgeries

Care and maintenance of suction tips/tubing

Equipment cleaning is integral and could act as a major source for cross-contamination:

- ensure all blood/debris is removed as soon as possible by placing tubing and tip immediately into cold water
- allow to soak for a minimum of 10 minutes

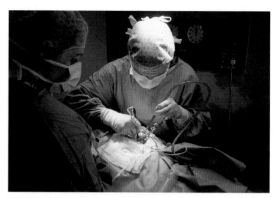

Figure 11.51 Suction and diathermy in use.

- use a stylet on the tip to ensure all debris is removed from the inside
- use a 60ml catheter-tipped syringe to force water through the tubing
- repeat process using a warm disinfection solution
- handle tubing to allow drainage of all fluids
- position tips so that fluid can drain away
- leave to dry
- re-sterilise prior to use
- use sterile equipment for every patient.

Acknowledgements

With thanks to: College of Animal Welfare, Edinburgh, Scotland; Dr Rory Brotheridge, Edinburgh, Scotland; Jo-Ann Tilley Dip AVN (Surgical) VN; Katie Dargan (Head Nurse), Veterinary Specialist Services, Brisbane, Australia; Nicola Forrest BSc, Dip AVN (Sur-gical) VN, Edinburgh, Scotland; staff at the Queen Mother Hospital for small animals, London; Southside Veterinary Surgery, Cairns, Australia

Further reading

Bowden C, Masters J 2003 Textbook of veterinary medical nursing. Butterworth-Heinemann, Oxford, 42–43
COSHH Regulations 2002 Available from: www.hse.gov.uk (accessed 28 June 2004)

Diathermy. Available from: http://www.surgical-tutor.org.uk/default-home.htm?core/preop1/diathermy.htm~right (accessed 19 July 2004)
Fossum T W et al 2002 Small animal surgery, 2nd edn. St Louis, Mosby

Manley Ventilator. Available from: www.rvc.ac.uk/
Services/Museums/Tour.cfm (accessed 27 May
2004)

MedTerms Dictionary A-Z list. http://www.
medterms.com/script/main/art.asp?ArticleKey
=5449 (accessed 12 January 2004)

On-line Medical Dictionary. Available from:
http://cancerweb.ncl.ac.uk (accessed 19 July
2004)

Orpet H, Welsh P 2002 Handbook of veterinary
nursing, Blackwell Science, Oxford

The history of penicillin. Available from:
www.hhtp://oh.essortment.com/historyofpen_
pnd.htm (accessed 12 January 2004)

Multiple choice questions

SURGICAL CONDITIONS AND INTRAOPERATIVE MANAGEMENT

1. A skin wound will heal by adnexal re-epithelialisation if damage has occurred to:
   a. dermis
   b. epidermis
   c. dermis and epidermis
   d. dermis and adipose tissue

2. In order to access the thoracic section of the oesophagus it is necessary to perform the following approach:
   a. median sternotomy
   b. ventral midline
   c. left sided thoracotomy
   d. right sided thoracotomy

3. The nuchal ligament must be spared in surgery as it plays an important role in supporting the:
   a. stifle
   b. head
   c. bladder
   d. pelvis

4. The following anaesthetic agent will greatly aid fracture repair:
   a. barbiturate anaesthetic
   b. opioid analgesic
   c. benzodiazepine sedative
   d. neuromuscular blocking drug

5. Lactate is produced in muscles when there is:
   a. aerobic hydrolysis
   b. anaerobic hydrolysis
   c. aerobic glycolysis
   d. anaerobic glycolysis

6. During wound healing new capillary growth is known as:
   a. proliferation
   b. angiogenesis
   c. migration
   d. chemotaxis

7. The process by which platelets attract inflammatory cells to the site of injury is known as:
   a. proliferation
   b. angiogenesis
   c. migration
   d. chemotaxis

8. Following two weeks of healing a wound only has which percentage of its final strength:
   a. 3%
   b. 10%
   c. 15%
   d. 20%

9. The most effective method of obtaining accurate culture from an infected pocket is:
   a. Fine needle aspirate
   b. Impression smear
   c. Biopsy of wall
   d. Exudate collection

10. The bacterium species *Clostridium* is often associated with infected wounds involving the:
    a. gastrointestinal tract
    b. urinary tract
    c. reproductive tract
    d. respiratory tract

OPHTHALMOLOGICAL SURGERY

11. Tonometry measures:
    a. tear production
    b. retinal function
    c. retinal detachments
    d. intraocular pressure

12. The type of local anaesthesia required for corneal surgery is:
    a. regional
    b. topical
    c. infiltration
    d. retrobullar

13. Normal intraocular pressure in the dog is:
    a. 0–9mmHg
    b. 10–25mmHg
    c. 26–30mmHg
    d. 31–50mmHg

14. The monitoring equipment used to determine degree of paralysis following administration of a neuromuscular blocking agent is:
    a. oximetry
    b. electrocardiogram
    c. Doppler flow
    d. train of 4 muscle stimulator

15. In cataract extraction the instrument used to incise the cornea and anterior capsule is:
    a. keratome
    b. beaver blade
    c. paragon handle
    d. diamond knife

16. The preferred suture material for conjunctival sutures is:
    a. Polydioxanone
    b. Polyglactin
    c. Polyester
    d. Polycaprone

17. The preferred type of needle for corneal suturing is:
    a. reverse cutting
    b. tapercut
    c. round bodied
    d. spatula tipped

18. A congenital absence of eyelids or lens is known as:
    a. ankyloblepharon
    b. lagophthalmos
    c. polymyositis
    d. coloboma

19. Abnormal swelling of the optic disc is known as:
    a. optic neuritis
    b. papilloedema
    c. symblepharon
    d. descemetocoele

20. Direct pressure on the globe or manipulation of the eyelids may initiate the:
    a. oculocardio reflex
    b. palpebral reflex
    c. corneal reflex
    d. pedal reflex

SURGERY OF THE ABDOMINAL CAVITY

21. The most superficial muscle of the abdominal wall is the:
    a. transverse
    b. internal abdominal oblique
    c. rectus abdominus muscles
    d. external abdominal oblique

22. The most suitable suction tip for abdominal surgery is the:
    a. Poole
    b. Gosset
    c. Balfour
    d. Kelly

23. Abdominal lavage should be carried out with:
    a. warm hypotonic saline solution
    b. cool hypotonic saline solution
    c. warm isotonic saline solution
    d. cool isotonic saline solution

24. The most common cause of haemoabdomen is:
    a. abdominal trauma
    b. splenic masses
    c. abdominal viscera rupture
    d. iatrogenic

25. Urine output in postoperative care of acute abdominal disease should be above:
    a. 1–2ml/kg/h
    b. 3–4ml/kg/h
    c. 5–6ml/kg/h
    d. 7–8ml/kg/h

26. The rates of dehiscence between stapled and sutured intestinal anastomoses show that:
    a. staples are better than sutures
    b. the rates are similar for both
    c. sutures are better than staples
    d. staples will help when there has been poor surgical technique

27. Pyloromyotomy is carried out to:
    a. remove the pylorus
    b. examine the pylorus
    c. increase the diameter of the pylorus
    d. decrease the diameter of the pylorus

28. Small stab incisions into the gastric serosa during GDV surgery are used to assess:
    a. arterial bleeding to determine gastric wall viability
    b. the possibility of gastric wall necrosis
    c. the viability of the splenic arteries and veins
    d. adhesions between the pyloric antrum and the right body wall

29. The ileo-caeco-colic junction is the most common site for:
    a. linear foreign bodies
    b. intestinal strangulation

    c. gastric dilation volvulus
    d. intussusception

30. A product that should be avoided as an enema solution as it could result in colonic mucosal infection is:
    a. warm water
    b. lactulose
    c. mineral oil
    d. soap

UROGENITAL SURGERY

31. An example of an acquired disease of the urogenital system is:
    a. ectopic kidney
    b. hydronephrosis
    c. utererocoele
    d. agenesis

32. Recommended fluid therapy infusion rates for all animals undergoing surgery is:
    a. 5ml/kg/h
    b. 10ml/kg/h
    c. 15ml/kg/h
    d. 20ml/kg/h

33. The ideal suture material for use within the bladder is:
    a. catgut
    b. polyglycolic acid
    c. polydioxanone
    d. silk

34. Operating microscopes are invaluable for surgery of the:
    a. vagina
    b. prostate
    c. bladder
    d. ureter

35. The surgical treatment to correct an ectopic ureter is known as:
    a. neoureterostomy
    b. ureteronephrectomy
    c. cystotomy
    d. urethrostomy

36. Urethostomy incisions are sutured with:
    a. horizontal mattress
    b. ford interlocking
    c. simple continuous
    d. simple interrupted

37. The stage of the oestrus cycle when a pyometra is likely to occur is:
    a. anoestrus
    b. oestrus
    c. pro-oestrus
    d. dioestrus

38. After surgery the bladder wall reaches full strength within:
    a. 0–6 days
    b. 7–13 days
    c. 14–21 days
    d. 22–29 days

39. Prostatic omentalisation is indicated for:
    a. prostatic cysts
    b. prostatic neoplasia
    c. urolithiasis
    d. colposuspension

40. Urine output in a healthy dog undergoing surgery should be equal to:
    a. 0.05ml/kg/h
    b. 0.5ml/kg/h
    c. 1.0ml/kg/h
    d. 2.0ml/kg/h

THORACIC SURGERY

41. The premedicant agent that may induce excitement and agitation in non compromised patients is:
    a. acepromazine
    b. diazepam
    c. medetomidine
    d. buprenorphine

42. Following thoracic surgery abrupt re-expansion of the lungs may open previously collapsed vessels resulting in:
    a. hypothermia
    b. hyperthermia
    c. hypotension
    d. hypertension

43. The presence of a chest drain tube in the pleural cavity will induce the production of the following volume of pleural fluid:
    a. 0–1ml/kg/day
    b. 2–10ml/kg/day
    c. 11–15ml/kg/day
    d. 16–20ml/kg/day

44. A standard self-retaining retractor useful in larger patients is a:
    a. Gelpi
    b. West
    c. Weitlaner
    d. Finochietto

45. An intercostal thoracotomy approach severely limits access to the:
    a. contralateral hemithorax
    b. pericardium
    c. mediastinum
    d. bronchus

46. Normal animals can tolerate removal of up to:
    a. 10% normal lung capacity
    b. 25% normal lung capacity
    c. 50% normal lung capacity
    d. 65% normal lung capacity

47. The site for thoracocentesis is between intercostal spaces:
    a. 2nd–4th
    b. 4th–7th
    c. 8th–10th
    d. 11th–13th

48. A double-valve Denver peritoneal-venus catheter is used in:
    a. pleurodesis
    b. intermittent suction
    c. passive pleuroperitoneal shunting
    d. active pleuroperitoneal shunting

49. An imbalance of the Starling forces results in:
    a. pneumothorax
    b. hydrothorax
    c. chylothorax
    d. haemothorax

50. A basket weave suture pattern may be used to repair:
    a. diaphragmatic rupture
    b. multiple intercostals ruptures
    c. flail chest
    d. restrictive pericarditis

THE CARDIOVASCULAR SYSTEM

51. The valve between the right atrium and the ventricle is the:
    a. mitral
    b. pulmonic
    c. aortic
    d. tricuspid

52. An anaesthetic induction agent that maintains cardiac output and is not arrhythmogenic is:
    a. ketamine
    b. propofol
    c. thiopentone
    d. etomidate

53. Pledgets may be useful to:
    a. temporarily occlude vessels
    b. buttress sutures in great vessels
    c. retract phrenic nerves
    d. securing large cannulae

54. The forceps used to dissect around vascular structures are:
    a. Mixter
    b. Satinsky
    c. Cooley
    d. Debakey

55. Pacemaker implantation is indicated in:
    a. pulmonic stenosis
    b. sinus bradycardia
    c. constrictive pericarditis
    d. pericardial cysts

56. A Gianturco is an example of a:
    a. vascular access sheath
    b. percutaneous balloon
    c. pericardiocentesis catheter
    d. vascular occlusion coil

57. Transcatheter closure is a procedure that may be used to treat:
    a. patent ductus arteriosus
    b. pericardial effusion
    c. persistent right aortic arch
    d. pulmonic stenosis

58. One of the most commonly used suture materials in cardiovascular surgery is:
    a. polyglycolic acid
    b. polypropylene
    c. linen
    d. catgut

59. Branham's sign may be seen during surgical repair of patent ductus arteriosus and if severe may result in:
    a. hypercapnia
    b. hypoxia
    c. systole
    d. asystole

60. The most common presentation of pulmonic stenosis is:
    a. valvular
    b. subvalvular
    c. infundibular
    d. supravalvular

ENT SURGERY

61. The type of ear pinna neoplasia which commonly affects white cats is:
    a. histiocytoma
    b. mast cell tumour
    c. fibrosarcoma
    d. squamous cell carcinoma

62. An example of a glandular disorder that can become a causative agent of otitis externa is:
    a. ceruminous hyperplasia
    b. demodecosis
    c. systemic lupus erythematosus
    d. dermatophytosis

63. A lateral wall resection is indicated in patients whom show:
    a. chronic proliferative changes in the ear canal beyond the vertical canal
    b. neoplastic disease of the ear canal and tympanic canal
    c. minimal hyperplasia of the epithelium of the external auditory meatus
    d. Complete ear canal stenosis

64. A myringotomy describes an incision into the:
    a. tympanic membrane
    b. nasopharynx
    c. tympanic bulla
    d. external auditory meatus

65. Temporary damage to facial nerves due to stretching during surgery is termed:
    a. Horner's syndrome
    b. vestibular disorientation
    c. neuropraxia
    d. vestibular dysfunction

66. Primary conformational changes which are seen in BAOS include:
    a. pharyngeal hypertrophy
    b. laryngeal collapse
    c. tracheal hypoplasia
    d. tonsillar hypertrophy

67. Propofol is recommended for anaesthesia for diagnostic procedures as it:
    a. can be given in small incremental doses
    b. impairs laryngeal function
    c. is a potent respiratory depressant
    d. reversed the effect of analgesics

68. Haemorrhage during surgical procedures to the trachea should be controlled:
    a. by lowering blood pressure
    b. with swabs applied with pressure
    c. by means of diathermy
    d. with the use of artery forceps

69. Patients recovering from surgical interference to the larynx should be fed:
    a. liquid food from a low position
    b. canned solid food from a low position
    c. liquid food from a raised position
    d. canned solid food from a raised position

70. The rhinarium describes the:
    a. soft hairless part of the nose
    b. comma-shaped openings allowing air to pass
    c. lateral accessory cartilage
    d. tube of the nostril

71. Nasal aspergillosis is an infection which is:
    a. parasitic
    b. bacterial
    c. viral
    d. fungal

72. The prognosis for untreated nasal conditions is poor, with survival times averaging:
    a. 1 month or less
    b. 6 months or less
    c. 12 months or less
    d. 18 months or less

73. Dehiscence is a problem after surgery to the secondary palate and may result from:
    a. good blood supply
    b. complete mobilisation of tissue
    c. sutures placed at correct tension
    d. lack of available tissue

74. The nasopharynx is described as:
    a. extending from the caudal choate to the larynx
    b. caudal to the oral cavity
    c. cranial to the nasal passages
    d. immediately rostral to the larynx

75. The term dysphonia describes difficulty in:
    a. smelling
    b. vocalising
    c. swallowing
    d. tasting

76. Surgical management of laryngeal paralyses which can be described as extralaryngeal includes:
    a. arytenoid lateralisation
    b. castellated laryngofissure
    c. ventriculocordectomy
    d. partial arytenoidectomy

77. The laryngeal pathology often seen in young Bull Terriers is:
    a. laryngeal stenosis
    b. laryngeal tumours
    c. laryngeal trauma
    d. laryngeal collapse

78. Postoperatively, patients who have had surgery to the larynx should be placed in:
    a. left lateral recumbency
    b. dorsal recumbency
    c. right lateral recumbency
    d. sternal recumbency

79. The aims of tracheal wound healing include all the following except:
    a. encouragement of stenosis
    b. retention of normal flexibility
    c. retention of inherent resistance to collapse
    d. re-establishment of normal mucociliary function

80. A temporary tracheostomy is indicated for all the following except:
    a. bypass of upper airway obstruction
    b. ventilatory management
    c. access to the lower airway
    d. long-term maintenance of a patent airway

ORTHOPAEDICS

81. The method of lavage for contaminated wounds is:
    a. soaking in normal saline
    b. low pressure lavage with normal saline
    c. cover with swabs and lavage with Hartmann's
    d. high pressure lavage with Hartmann's

82. Some fractures are better left unsupported preoperatively to prevent:
    a. the provision of significant analgesia
    b. heavy dressings acting as pendulums
    c. exudates from the wound
    d. adequate immobilisation of the limb

83. A fracture that has a small associated puncture wound is described as an open fracture at:
    a. Class I
    b. Class II
    c. Class III
    d. Class IV

84. Perioperative broad spectrum antibiotic cover should be given intravenously:
    a. 10 minutes prior to surgery
    b. 20 minutes prior to surgery
    c. 30 minutes prior to surgery
    d. 40 minutes prior to surgery

85. Patients who have had a cast applied should be kept hospitalised for a period of:
    a. 12 hours
    b. 24 hours
    c. 36 hours
    d. 48 hours

86. A bladder which is emptied too frequently in an incontinent patient may result in
    a. further infections
    b. irreversible flaccidity of bladder
    c. damage to the muscular network of the bladder wall
    d. removal of stimulus to urinate

87. All of the following are commonly used as donor bones for skin grafts except:
    a. distal metatarsals
    b. iliac crest
    c. proximal humerus
    d. medial tibia

88. The benefit of a power drill over a hand-held one is:
    a. it allows more control
    b. it is easier to sterilise
    c. it allows pins to slip
    d. it is self cleaning

89. Burrs could be used to cut:
    a. casts
    b. deep bone
    c. joint cartilage
    d. inaccessible bone

90. The thread design of the AO/ASIF screw makes it:
    a. more difficult for the screw to pull out
    b. easier to get better purchase in soft bone
    c. more difficult to screw the implant in
    d. easier to create more micro-trauma

PRE- AND POSTOPERATIVE NURSING

91. An example of an idophor skin disinfectant is:
    a. chlorhexidine gluconate
    b. isopropyl alcohol
    c. triclosan
    d. povidone iodine

92. Degreasing of the surgical area can be achieved by the use of:
    a. chlorhexidine gluconate
    b. isopropyl alcohol
    c. triclosan
    d. povidone iodine

93. Paediatric patients are classified as those animals up to:
    a. up to 6 weeks of age
    b. up to 12 weeks of age
    c. up to 18 weeks of age
    d. up to 24 weeks of age

94. A common site for arterial catheterisation during surgery is:
    a. carotid
    b. jugular
    c. lingual
    d. femoral

95. The Seldinger technique is used in:
    a. urinary catheterisation
    b. femoral artery catheterisation
    c. saphenous vein catheterisation
    d. central venous catheterisation

96. In relation to canine blood groups the term DEA denotes:
    a. dog eosinophil antibody
    b. dog eosinophil antigen
    c. dog erythrocyte antibody
    d. dog erythrocyte antigen

97. Maximum blood donation volume in a dog is:
    a. 10–12ml/kg
    b. 13–15ml/kg
    c. 16–18ml/kg
    d. 19–21ml/kg

98. To ensure antibiotic plasma concentration is at its peak level at commencement of surgery antibiotics should be given approximately:
    a. 30 minutes before surgery
    b. 1 hour before surgery
    c. 1 hour 30 minutes before surgery
    d. 2 hours before surgery

99. Blocking of intercostals nerves post-thoracic surgery can be achieved by:
    a. epidural anaesthesia
    b. surface anaesthesia
    c. intra-articular anaesthesia
    d. infiltration anaesthesia

100. The estimation of blood loss by weighing used swabs and subtracting dry weight is measured as:
    a. 1g = 0.1ml blood
    b. 1g = 1ml blood
    c. 1g = 10ml blood
    d. 1g = 100ml blood

THEATRE PRACTICE

101. An example of a clean contaminated surgical procedure is:
    a. cystotomy
    b. ovariohysterectomy
    c. colostomy
    d. enterectomy

102. An example of an effective surgical scrub solution is:
    a. hypochlorite
    b. surgical spirit
    c. chlorhexidine
    d. glutaraldehyde

103. The electrical safety acronym PAT stands for:
a. positive atom test
b. patent airway test
c. patient appliance test
d. portable appliance test

104. A suitable method of sterilisation for a flexible endoscope is:
a. hot air oven
b. ethylene oxide
c. autoclave
d. boiling

105. All of the following Acts control disposal of waste except:
a. Medicines Act 1968
b. Controlled waste regulations 1992
c. Environmental Protection Act 1990
d. Control of Pollution Act 1974

106. An 'ostomy' is the suffix used to denote:
a. a temporary surgical opening
b. surgical removal of organs
c. a surgical creation of an opening
d. examination with various equipment

107. A keratectomy describes:
a. repair of congenital ectropion
b. removal of a diseased eye
c. repair of unwanted cilia
d. removal of diseased corneal tissue

108. A gastropexy describes:
a. anchoring of the stomach to the abdominal wall
b. resection of the small intestine
c. joining two ends of intestine after surgery
d. relieving constriction of the pyloric sphincter.

109. The following tasks are all duties of the surgical assistant except:
a. preparing the instrument trolley
b. cutting sutures
c. preparing the operating site
d. swabbing the surgical site

110. Thumb forceps should be held with the:
a. concave side facing up
b. thumb and ring finger through the rings
c. pencil grip
d. ratchets firmly closed

INSTRUMENTATION AND STERILISATION

111. Once sterilised items can be considered sterile if stored correctly for up to:
a. 4 weeks
b. 6 weeks
c. 8 weeks
d. 10 weeks

112. An instrument with a gold handle has an insert made of:
a. martenstic stainless steel
b. titanium
c. autenistic stainless steel
d. tungsten carbide

113. A disadvantage of internal fixation when compared to external fixation is a:
a. greater range of sites
b. earlier return to normal
c. efficient immobilisation of fractures
d. higher risk of infection

114. The term used to describe a deformity of a bone that results from a poorly healed fracture is:
a. union
b. malunion
c. delayed union
d. non-union

115. An example of a plate that could be described as ASIF is:
a. Sherman
b. Dynamic compression
c. Venables
d. Lanes

116. The preferred suture needle size for facial and blood vessel suturing is:
a. 7/0
b. 5/0
c. 3/0
d. 0

117. Cancellous screws are:
   a. intended for use with the metaphysis
   b. not self tapping
   c. intended for use within the diaphysis
   d. useful for removing debris

118. An example of an absorbable suture material which keeps its tensile strength retention for 60 days is:
   a. Polyglactin 910
   b. Poliglecaprone 25
   c. Polydioxanone
   d. Polypropylene

119. A simple continuous suture pattern would be used with:
   a. diaphragmatic closure
   b. closure of the GI tract
   c. intradermal skin closure
   d. closure of hollow viscera

120. An example haemostasis that could be described as physical is:
   a. pressure bandage
   b. silver nitrate
   c. tourniquet
   d. suction

Answers to multiple choice questions

CHAPTER 1

1 c
2 d
3 b
4 d
5 d
6 b
7 d
8 d
9 c
10 a

CHAPTER 2

11 d
12 a
13 b
14 d
15 a
16 b
17 d
18 d
19 b
20 a

CHAPTER 3

21 d
22 a
23 c
24 b
25 a
26 b
27 c
28 a
29 d
30 d

CHAPTER 4

31 b
32 d
33 c
34 d
35 a
36 d
37 d
38 c
39 a
40 d

CHAPTER 5

41 b
42 c
43 b
44 d
45 a
46 c
47 b
48 d
49 b
50 b

CHAPTER 6

51 d
52 d
53 b
54 a
55 b
56 d
57 a
58 b
59 d
60 a

CHAPTER 7

61 d
62 a
63 c
64 a
65 c
66 d
67 a
68 b
69 b
70 a
71 d
72 b
73 d
74 a
75 b
76 a
77 d
78 d
79 a
80 d

CHAPTER 8	CHAPTER 9	CHAPTER 10	CHAPTER 11
81 d	91 d	101 b	111 b
82 b	92 b	102 c	112 d
83 a	93 b	103 d	113 d
84 c	94 d	104 b	114 b
85 b	95 d	105 a	115 b
86 d	96 d	106 c	116 b
87 a	97 c	107 d	117 a
88 a	98 d	108 a	118 c
89 c	99 d	109 c	119 c
90 a	100 b	110 c	120 c

Index